The Summer's Approach

Creating Heaven
Through Your Plate

A Wholistic Eating & Self-Healing Guide

Shelley Summers

Including a Recipe Section

Creating Heaven ON Your Plate

Warm Snow Publishers
Torreon, New Mexico

© 1996 by Shelley Summers

Author photos by Mary Zaremba

Published by:
Warm Snow Publishers, P.O. Box 75, Torreon, NM 87061 USA
(505) 384-1102

ISBN: 0-9629923-5-6
Library of Congress Cat. Card No.: 95-060836

Printed and bound in the United States of America. Printed on acid-free papers

Cataloging-in-Publication Data

613   **Summers, Shelley Easton, 1949-**
SUM   Creating heaven through your plate : a wholistic eating &
          self-healing guide / by Shelley Summers. - 1st ed. Torreon,
          N.M. : Warm Snow Publishers, ©1996.

          320 p.; 25.5 cm.
          Includes bibliography and index.
          Summary: Presents an approach to natural healing which
       begins with eating the easiest-to-digest foods (along with food
       supplements) to balance the body's environment and ener-
       gize the natural healing processes of the body.
          ISBN 0-9629923-5-6
          95-060836

       1. Self-care, Health 2. Applied kinesiology I. Title
                                            613_dc20

Foreword

It is my great privilege and pleasure to invite you to embark on a personal transformational journey as you "digest" and "assimilate" what Shelley Summers has offered in this book

My own journey was greatly influenced by her loving wisdom many years ago, during the time that she was collecting data for this book. I am one of the over 5000 bodies that conversed with her about how it wanted to get well. She facilitated for me, a clarifying growth process, both physiologic and spiritual, that goes far beyond being well, but rather touches upon the accessing of my evolutionary potential for radiant health. In understanding the concepts put forth in this book, you too will have a better knowing of how to feed your body-mind-spirit self, so that the joy of health is on your plate.

You may wonder, do we really need another book about food and diet? Are we not already obsessed with the minutia of prescribed oral regimens, lists of do's and don'ts, timetables and rules? I suggest the answer is yes and no. Yes, as a culture we're oriented toward oral gratification, especially for emotional nourishment. Therefore, let's face it, we will continue to want to feed ourselves until we find what we're missing, be it vitamin or mineral deficiencies or love. And yes, we need this book! Because it provides pathways for satisfying the hungry beast so that the beautiful spirit may be fed. And no, we do not need another diet book. I suggest that you ban your previous concept of the word diet, possibly as having been a vehicle of deprivation, and allow diet, to simply mean *"n. - mode of living; now only with especial reference to food."* (dictionary definition.)

This book will guide you in simple educational steps to make rational, conscious choices about how and under what circumstances you will feed yourself. It will allow access to a greater state of health for every level of being.

There are some surprises here, pearls of wisdom, even for professional nutritionists. Apparently, what our minds have deduced is best for our bodies is not identical with what our bodies indicate. There is freedom here as well. For all of us that have been taught to count calories, or more recently, fat content, we can look forward to being freed of such patently inadequate, thus unsuccessful food management concepts. Also the question of food sensitivities is addressed in a new perspective. It typically has meant that when sensitive to foods, we're limited in what we can take in, and so deprived. But, becoming "sensitive" to food may also mean becoming attuned to what nourishes us. Could it not be, that the body in it's wisdom, provides the symptoms of nutritional needs and reactions in order to guide us toward greater sustenance and fulfillment?

Shelley's wisdom about how to nourish ourselves comes from several sources. There are the collected observations of working nutritionally with so many people, most of whom DID become more well. That alone is a great testimonial to the effectiveness of the simple dietary outlines given here. But, there is more. Shelley is an initiate into the mysteries of mother earth, including its abundance. She has mastery of the wisdom of plants, especially flowers, having developed and made available hundreds of new flower essences indigenous to the southwestern United States. She shares a knowing that not only underlies the day to day decisions of how and what to eat, but also encompasses how to be nourished by our environment as it is today. I encourage you, as you read this book, to remember that as finding wholesome, unaltered food becomes a challenge because of strained environmental resources, so does our creative power respond, to transform whatever we put into our bodies into what we want. Here is a quote from the author, from one of the "Heaven-to-Earth" newsletters that she has shared over the past few years —

"It looks and feels like there is a 'universal cleansing' going on....and our bodies are being immersed in it. It's like no cleansing I have ever seen . . . if you know anything about homeopathics, it's like a 'constitutional' cleansing. It seems that we can no longer use our bodies and food to 'ground' ourselves to this planet. I found myself eating and not being able to feel anything solid from it. My body's sense of what it needs is shifting. My body has gotten more efficient and needs less and less bulk, but more and more life force. I can feel my intestines taking 'food' from air, from connecting with a plant or animal, from the love of others and the universe. It's like the body was a cup that needed regular filling and now the cup no longer exists....and the need to fill it just evaporated. All of this is creating a new and wondrous sense of PRESENCE in the body. There's an interesting paradox of feeling full and empty at the same time . . . that line of duality has closed itself into a circle."

by Debbie Malka M.D., Ph.D.

CONTENTS

Disease, About Parasites, The Illeocecal Valve and Parasites, Computer Stress, Diabetes, Physical Aspects and Eating Patterns, About Insulin, Changing Diabetes, The Spiritual Aspects of Diabetes, Dyslexia, Eating Disorders, About the Causes, Straight Talk About Food, Eyestrain and Eyesight, About Eyestrain, About Eyesight, About the Gallbladder, Living Without a Gallbladder, About Gallstones, Hair Loss, Heart Problems, Headaches, Herpes, Hormone Imbalances, About Hormones in General, Female Hormones, Becoming a Woman, Premenstrual Syndrome, Irregular Periods, Menopause, Male Hormones, Becoming A Man, About ALL Male Hormones, Thyroid, Hypoglocemia, Insomnia, Mercury Poisoning and Other Heavy Metal Problems, Multiple Sclerosis, Skin Problems, Acne, Eczema and Psoriasis, Smoking, About Other Vices, Surgery Preparation, Temporal Mandibular Joint (TMJ), To Fix the Joint, Ulcers and Other Stomach Problems, About Heartburn, About Stomach Valve Problems, About Ulcers, Urinary Tract Health, Bed Wetting, Bladder/Kidney Infections, Weight, Over the Comfort Zone, Under the Comfort Zone

Chapter 1
Creating Heaven Through Your Plate

Creating Heaven in our lives is our birthright. Physical bodies taught me that they have to feel light and healthy so we can use them as a base for creating Heaven in our lives. I mean, when you feel GOOD, you see life from a different point of view.

Creating Heaven Through Your Plate is an approach that works with your body by feeding it the easiest-to-digest foods along with food supplements. This creates an environment in the body that allows it to redirect its energy, focus and nutrients. Bodies are so intelligent! When you create this balanced environment, they just start healing themselves because they know what to fix and how to fix it. So now you need a guide to help you change your overall approach to health and food. And yet do it in a way that doesn't turn your life upside down.

In my personal search for health back in the 70's, I did what many of you did. For years I read every new nutrition book that hit the marketplace. And like many of you, I found alot of information and alot of confusion!!!

I mean, by the time you've read all these conflicting ideas, (*"You should only eat this"* or *"You should only eat that"*) you don't know what to do! Like many of you, I tried to follow 'this way' and 'that way'; I tried to watch how my body and mind felt as I ate and followed yet another method; and I never found THE way. I mean, I sometimes adopted a particular notion that I felt 'worked' for me, but in general I was still confused. And, worst of all, I didn't necessarily feel any difference in my health. I know that many of you have watched your health deteriorate even when you were doing EVERYTHING you could to stop it.

After ten years of this kind of search, I found muscle-response testing or applied kinesiology. I was ecstatic; here was a technique that allowed you to ask questions of a body DIRECTLY. In my typical style, I studied this 'body-asking' technique and then literally threw out all the old nutritional belief systems. I started asking bodies about foods and what they wanted to eat to build a solid foundation of health. And by following what my own body said, I found an aspect of creating Heaven in my life through food.

This book, then, is the result of asking these questions to over 5,000 bodies and helping these people find their own pathways to Heaven through their food.

A NEW APPROACH

Over the next year I studied every body I could get my hands on and as I used the muscle-testing technique I was opened to my psychic abilities. (It didn't take long for me to realize that all those words of wisdom I'd heard in my head as I grew up were coming from what I now call my 'spirit' or 'spiritual self.') Then, a wonderful blending of knowingness and muscle-testing led me through the maze of nutrition. I asked bodies general diet questions like *"Can you assimilate and digest* _____ *with ease?"* and *"Are you deficient in Vitamin ____?"* then studied the responses. Some very interesting information started to become apparent:

1) Bodies KNOW what they need. They have just become confused from garbage we've fed them through our mouths and through our minds!

2) If you give them a break from the flow of garbage, if you give them a healthy basis to start from, bodies KNOW how to get healthy!

There are definitely certain foods that almost all bodies have difficulties digesting and other foods that seem to be easy to digest. Over time some general patterns emerged about which foods fell into which categories. And some time-sequence patterns also became apparent. They are the foundation of this approach.

3) Bodies like to get healthy in an easy, gradual manner. Quick fixes just don't create a foundation of health that the body can grow on.

As a general rule bodies seem to like to take a little time to heal themselves. When asked about the options of say, doing a gallbladder flush (like fasting with apple juice for three days then drinking down olive oil) and flushing out gallstones or doing six months of herbs and dissolving the stones, most bodies wanted the slow method. When flushes were indicated, the body needing them is usually either very sick or already very healthy.

4) Bodies don't see some foods as good and others as bad! It's just that certain foods we ingest will be harder for the body to deal with; that is, it will take more energy, enzymes, vitamins, minerals and time to deal with, say, a chocolate bar than an apple. Basically, there are easy-to-digest foods, hard-to-digest foods and everything in-between.

5) Along with this lack of judgment, bodies are not into denial as a mode of operation. If you can eat yogurt then why not make it into a treat?

6) Most major health problems are not going to be solved by JUST cleaning up the diet. Not to say diet isn't an important part; it is. But it became obvious working with persons with cancer, MS, EBV, candida, AIDS, lupus, and other problems, that emotional, mental and spiritual problems are the basis of serious ill-health. Getting physical-level health balanced can give people the basis to work with the other levels of their dis-ease; but diet alone will not be the answer.

After working with this approach myself, I found I was eating with a totally new viewpoint. Now, I decide what I am going to eat by asking my body. I mean, why not feed myself the most 'perfect food' I can give it in that moment?

So now I stand in front of the fridge and ask my body what it wants, *"Proteins?" "Starches? Fruits? Veggies?"* As I ask about each category, I watch the feeling in my body; I can feel it light up, feel a craving come on, or feel my attention drawn to my taste buds as they go, *"Yum-yum!"* Or I can feel repulsed by that group of foods, get a nasty taste in my mouth, or hear my body go *"Yuck"* if it doesn't want a particular food or group of foods.

I usually go through all the food categories, then go back to the ones that had a positive reaction. I look at the different foods I have in the house in that category and see if there is something more specific my body wants. Then and only then, do I go to my taste buds and give them any say in what I will decide to eat!

ABOUT TASTE BUDS

You have to stop giving your taste buds any power over your decisions of what to eat. Taste buds get messages from all kinds of emotional reactions and rarely listen to messages that come from the whole body! At least, not until your body gets on a path of health.

Taste bud reactions will tell you to eat chocolate or 'just have another slice' when it's the worst thing to do in that moment. I mean, we all hear these voices when we are stressed! The trick is to recognize that taste bud reactions are suspect. They may not tell you the truth! And who wants to listen to a 'voice' that may NOT ALWAYS be telling you the truth?

When we get stressed, we need to learn to eat light and easy, so that we can focus the use of our internal nutrients into dealing with that stress. Eating 'difficult-to-digest' foods at a time of stress just adds to the stress level! And why would you want to do that to yourself? Only because you got trained to do just that!

This training is just one of those 'I'm-not-okay kid reactions' that we need to release and grow beyond. So, when you feel your taste buds going into reactions, put that reaction aside and feel out your whole body. Is your whole body, every single part, saying "Yes, eat that!" If it is, even if the food is the biggest, best, gooiest chocolate brownie in the world, bless it and enjoy the hell out of it!

HOW THIS APPROACH WORKS

When you follow this approach, you will start by giving yourself a Health Assessment Rating. This assessment will help you determine which Basic Diet Approach you should begin following. Following the Basic Diets means you will eat the easiest-to-digest foods along with easy-to-digest supplements.

When you take foods out of your diet that you cannot digest and assimilate with ease, you remove a major stress from your system. Now the energy, enzymes, vitamins and minerals that have been used to try to deal with stress can be refocused by the body. Nutrients can now be used to heal the body instead of defending it against the toxins you made, by eating something you couldn't digest!

Basically, this approach to eating HONORS the body by giving it a break. This allows the body to create a pathway to health and as this pathway develops, the body starts using the available nutrients to heal itself. One of the things the body heals is the level of digestive enzymes so it can digest all different kinds of food.

After a couple of months, the results of this increase in enzymes means that you can start adding more foods into your diet!!! You can start moving through the follow-up diets. And with the second follow-up diet, Phase 2 'Getting There,' you get to work more specifically with any personal problems.

And the final payoff? Most people, after following this approach for 12-18 months, are able to eat almost everything again and yes, that includes coffee and chocolate. Of course, there are food boundaries to stay within to maintain health, but now it's done with a new relationship between body and food. People are able to make food choices from a place of health. They are learning to create Heaven through their plates!

NO DENIAL!

Denial and eating just don't work together! I have a major sweet tooth and I feed it. But I feed it with foods that are healthy for my body. And I also honor my taste buds and sometimes feed them foods that are rich and decadent! I mean, most of us learned to eat and desire sweets to some degree; and this isn't a problem in itself. Of course, overdoing the eating of sweets is something else again.

In the recipe section of this book you will find all kinds of ideas for sweets (and other dishes.) Now, don't let your mind start screaming, "But sweets are fattening!!" Desserts are only fattening when you either eat too much of them or they contain ingredients that you can't digest properly. Besides, you know, if you deny yourself some goodies, somewhere along the line you'll break down and go for something REALLY hard on your system.

Denial induces self-judgment and you can't do more harm to your body (or your life) than to judge it. Of course, this statement just moved us out of the physical realm of eating and into the emotional depths of the body. But, guess what? There is no way to separate these two! When your body is out of balance your emotions will probably be out of balance, too.

So, one of the best ways to get your emotions under control is to get your body healthy.

ABOUT CRAVINGS

Cravings come from three basic sources: 1) the need for deficient vitamins and minerals, 2) hypoglycemia and other physical imbalances, and 3) emotional reactions. It is important to take care of the physical level of cravings so you can deal with the emotional ones.

Food cravings are a very important message from the body. Your body knows when it needs certain vitamins and minerals and it will send a message throughout your body, asking for these nutrients. Then you crave something but you don't know what it is. So, you eat what you think will satisfy the craving only to find that the craving is back a half hour later (if not sooner.) So you eat something else and find the cycle being repeated.

What's happening to you is simple. Your body needs a nutrient, but your mind and taste buds are not totally in tune with the whole process. They don't know what you can actually digest and assimilate to get these needed nutrients. So you will crave something that your body knows CONTAINS the nutrients it needs. But it doesn't understand, until after you've eaten that something, that you can't digest it OR get the nutrients out of it. So you crave something else, eat it, have the same reaction and set a pattern in motion.

This happens all the time for women before their periods. The body's need for minerals starts to go up 7-10 days before a woman's period. These minerals are needed to change the hormone levels and trigger the end of the cycle. With this increased need for minerals, major cravings can start.

Hypoglycemia (or low blood sugar,) candida, EBV, environmental poisonings, and so on, can create a wide range of cravings for foods, sugars, and caffeine. America hits the vending machines mid-afternoon, looking for something to deal with the regular drops in energy and the cravings that go with them. Eating right can start to change these reactions within a few days.

Once you get your nutrient levels up to proper maintenance level and deal with specific problems, you can pretty well bet any other cravings are emotional reactions. With the physical elements out of the equation, you can learn to deal with emotional cravings from a more balanced place.

WHAT YOU CAN EXPECT FOLLOWING THIS APPROACH

Bodies all vary in the way they heal; what you may think is a major problem, like acne, may be way down on the body's list of what should be healed first. Eventually the body will correct most problems, given enough nutrients and enough time. But there are some overall changes you can watch for as you follow this program:

**Taking indigestible foods out of the diet immediately creates a great release of energy. How your body will use this energy is a personal reaction, but most people start feeling their overall energy levels come up. They start going through their days without the 'normal' dips of energy, especially that mid-afternoon slump when America hits the vending machines.

**After three to four weeks of following the Basic Diet, you may find that you have become sensitive to foods off the diet. Following the diet has NOT MADE you sensitive to these foods! The reality is that you were already sensitive to them, you just haven't been clear enough to feel it before!

This sensitivity has a couple of positive sides. One, you are feeling, possibly for the first time, exactly what a particular food has been doing to your system. I mean, it's one thing for me to tell you what might be difficult for bodies to deal with and another thing for you to feel it! And two, even as you get stronger and healthier, a level of sensitivity and awareness will stay with you. I have had a number of persons say they have reached the point where they can just look at a food and know whether they should eat it or not!

**For most people some level of weight loss occurs. Extra weight frequently stems not from overeating but from eating foods that are not properly digested and from lack of various nutrients! By just taking these indigestible foods out of the diet and by ingesting the proper nutrients, most people easily lose 5-15 pounds. I'll never forget the guy who freaked out when I told him his body said he couldn't digest meat. He didn't think he could live without it. My response was, *"Look. You don't have to go hungry. There isn't a food in this work-up that will make you fat, so eat, eat, eat."* A month later I got a call from him. He said, *"You couldn't have a happier camper! I am eating three times more food than I have ever eaten in my life and I've lost 20 pounds!"*

If you have that special body-type that needs to put ON weight or if you are at your ideal weight, you need to make sure you eat much more food in general on this program.

**Most people also experience some of the following: the clearing of headaches, more emotional balance, clearer skin, regular bowel movements, no heartburn, raised energy levels, improved sleep, and/or stabilized weight.

ADDITIONAL INSIGHTS

Over the years, I have worked with a wide range of people, in terms of their bodies, age, life-styles and interests. I started to see a pattern. There is a fairly obvious ratio between a person's health and what era they grew up in! I repeatedly have seen people born before 1935 start on their diets and get healthy very fast; faster than all the other groups! I could feel a basic, constitutional level of health in their bodies, and my mind was always filled with pictures of what the food supplies were like when they were growing up. I mean, they didn't have refrigerators so their foods were fresh; being a milkman was a common occupation; the butcher was probably someone you talked to; people lived near their food sources; and there were no chemical fertilizers, pesticides, and food additives..

The next age group, born between 1935-1955, is split into two groups. First, there are people who are basically healthy, who are having some problems just because living is intense. They have developed vitamin and mineral deficiencies and their health is starting to show some wear and tear. These people tend to heal quickly, too. I usually get pictures of these people coming from 'strong stock'; of having been blessed with 'strong genes.'

But the second group weren't blessed with such good beginnings; they are usually having many more physical problems (and spiritual problems) and they heal more slowly.

Us baby boomers were just starting to get the first doses of food preservatives, fertilizers, and pesticides in our foods; those businesses boomed after WWII. We still had access to some quality in our food supply, but it was definitely starting to go downhill. I had to teach my mother, when she was 70 years old, how to cook fresh veggies because we grew up with frozen and canned stuff (yuck!) The upper end of this age group actually had an advantage in that they didn't have the chemicals in their foods when they were kids and developing their bodies.

The trends I started seeing in the next age group sent chills down my spine! The people born after 1955 split into two groups, like the above age group. But there are considerably fewer basically healthy people and the level of physical problems they all are manifesting are more developed. I see 20 year olds with gallbladder problems, serious levels of hypoglycemia, circulation problems, and higher levels of vitamin and mineral deficiencies. Most of the persons in this group heal consistently but more slowly than their elders.

And the Kids! There are some healthy kids out there but I've seen problems in children that used to be considered 'old age' problems. I have seen high levels of hypoglycemia in 2 and 3 year olds! And liver imbalances. And gummed up intestines. And truly scary general health. It is NOT NORMAL to have two, three or four flus or colds a year; it means we are a sick population!

Here we are, the richest nation in the world, with an incredibly immense array of foods available to us, and we are truly in a national health crisis!!! Our general food supply is killing us with empty calories, toxic chemicals and massive amounts of indigestible fats. I knew we'd crossed over the line a few years ago when people started calling McDonalds a restaurant and showing ads of sweet grandpas taking their infant grandchildren there for food!!!

Somewhere, from the time of the first 'fast food' place to now, we changed our attitude toward these kinds of foods in our diets. It seems to me that it used to be a 'treat' to go get a shake and fries; but you ate at home to get good food, food that would make you grow and be healthy. I heard about a study released recently that said people were eating at fast food places on the average of 7 times a week!

Bodies just can't handle it!

Chapter 2
About the Basic Diet

A FEW THINGS TO KEEP IN MIND

I can pass on to you all the information I have obtained from talking to bodies, but YOU ARE THE ONE WHO LIVES IN YOUR BODY. Don't let anyone, EVER, tell you that what you feel or sense about your body is wrong. Developing and learning to trust your own knowingness is a major, underlying part of this diet approach.

This whole program is designed as a guide, but you have to trust your own body reactions to foods. If, after two or three weeks (or even two or three days!) on the program, you feel that something you are eating may be causing a problem, take it out of your diet. By all means, TRUST YOURSELF!

The first three Basic Diets are all cleansing diets. Their main purpose is to give your body a rest in a gentle, balanced manner. We don't want to send your body into a major cleansing mode; that can be more stressful than helpful. If you are not experiencing any physical symptoms like gas or low energy, and you are feeling fit, then doing intense fasting can be a wonderful process, but remember, bodies like moderation.

You can do this program and continue on with your normal life activities. I wouldn't suggest starting any intense physical activities but starting a basic walking program can be helpful. (Check out the section on exercise in Chapter 10.)

All the Basic Diets are great 'stress diets.' When life is running at full tilt and your stress levels edge up to 'total overwhelm,' many nutrients are diverted to just deal with the situation at hand. Unless you are ingesting extra nutrients to deal with the stress, it is likely that your digestive enzyme production will suffer (let alone your whole body.) This is a great time to eat easy-to-digest foods.

HAVE FUN with this new way of eating!!! Think about the foods you are eating as easy, nurturing and loving for your body.

GET CREATIVE!!! Think about all the kinds of meals you like, look at what you can eat and then figure out how you can substitute 'this for that' and get the same general idea. Instead of having a bowl of rice with lamb curry, you can have a bowl of quinoa with vegetable curry.

If you have a busy life-style or cooking just isn't your thing, then I suggest the following: Set aside a couple of hours once a week and cook a bunch of stuff. Then you can easily throw a few things together and reheat! (See Table 1 in the Appendix for some ideas.)

ENZYME LEVELS

Enzymes are proteins that 'function as biochemical catalysts.' In other words, enzymes break down food to its molecular structures making them available for use by the body.

Enzymes are made in the body, using large amounts of vitamins and minerals. If you are deficient in any of these nutrients, your body just cannot make the needed enzymes to utilize your foods. There is nothing special you need to do to bring these enzyme levels up; following this program will give your body a stress-free healing period by taking food stresses out of your body and giving it the nutrients it needs. Your body will bring its enzyme levels up all by itself.

ALLERGIES

If you know or suspect that you are allergic to any particular food, obviously, don't eat it. If this food is within the diet you are following, after a couple of weeks you might want to try a small piece of that food and see what it does. Sometimes just a couple of weeks can make a big difference.

Remember that allergies are just your body's overwhelm-reaction to something in the food. The reaction can come from the body's lack of enzymes to deal with that particular food structure. Remember to trust yourself. Also, check out the Allergy section in the Dis-ease and Dis-comfort chapter.

MUCUS REACTIONS

Anytime you eat something your body cannot digest easily, you will get a rather immediate reaction. Once you have eaten something and your body realizes it can't digest that food, it will go into a defense mode creating mucus. Mucus will surround the offending particles to protect the body from them, to ease their movement through the intestines and sinuses and to stop your body from trying to absorb them.

After a couple of weeks on the appropriate diet, you can use this reaction to aid you in determining whether a food you are considering eating is digestible. Take a small bite and wait. Mucus reactions will appear within a few seconds and up to twenty minutes. If you sneeze, get a runny nose, find yourself clearing your throat, or get a coating of white film covering the back of your throat or tongue, you are having a mucus reaction.

These body indications say, *"Don't eat that!" "I can't digest that!"* And I'd suggest you don't eat it. Usually it's just not worth the discomfort.

There is some major confusion out there about mucus reactions in the body. Specific foods, like diary products, do not CAUSE mucus. The mucus reaction that people get from drinking milk is one of the body's defense reactions! When a body's enzyme levels are high, it can not only digest milk but fully use it and enjoy it!

READING LABELS

Get into the habit of reading the labels on products, especially reading the ingredient lists. Ingredients are listed by volume, the largest ingredient being listed first, the smallest ingredient, last. If there is an ingredient listed that is off your diet, avoid the food. But keep all this in perspective! If a food you need to avoid is listed as the last ingredient, it may be that a very small amount is all you get from eating a normal serving. You have to decide whether ingesting that ingredient will be a problem for you or not. Breads are a good example. The first two Basic Diets call for eating only sprouted grain breads for the first four months and they call for only eating maple syrup, malt syrups and rice bran syrup as sweeteners in that same time span. When you look at the ingredients in many of the sprouted breads, you may find honey or molasses listed.

Here is where your discretion comes into play. When sweeteners are added to the bread-making process, they are used to make the yeasts grow. One or two tablespoons of sweetener per loaf of bread are normal additions. And, in this process, most of the sugars are eaten up by the yeasts, so they can give off gases that make the bread rise. So, when you eat a slice or two of bread, the actual amount of honey or other sweetener you are ingesting is very small.

Again, use your discretion in making your choices and TRUST your body knowingness. If you are not sure about a food, either stay away from it or test eating it as if you were allergic to it. (See above section on Mucus Reactions and Chapter 10, Allergies.)

COUNTING CALORIES

Why? I really can't see any reason to get obsessive about how many calories you're eating and how many you will burn doing some activity. I mean, you know if you're eating too much and if you are getting enough exercise or not!

Relax and learn to enjoy eating healthy! But if you are really interested in checking out calorie info, look up the calorie levels for fruits and veggies. Doing one of the Basic Diets, you will be eating 80% fruits and veggies which contain low levels of calories.

DEALING WITH TOXINS

A word about toxins. Our world is getting more polluted by the day and there is no way any of us can avoid contact with some unwanted chemicals. I grow most of my own food, but I can't control what comes out of the sky with the rain. The best way I can see to deal with toxins is to be careful about what you choose to eat AND to get healthy. When your body is healthy, it has the ability to deal with toxic chemicals. But when it's unhealthy, the toxins just become part of the problem.

Buy foods that are fresh and organic when you can. Choose meats from sources that you can verify. Check their quality in growing and handling. Choose fish when you can verify their origin. You want fish from a relatively clean source.

CHOOSING WHICH DIET TO FOLLOW

The next thing you need to do is read the Health Assessment Chapter to determine which Basic Diet you should follow. Once you have a general idea which health category you fit into, you can move on to the specific Basic Diet you should follow.

Those of you with minor health problems will be following Basic Diet #1--The Basic Balancer. Those of you with mid-level health problems will be directed to Basic Diet #2--The Deep Cleanser for a time. Those of you with more serious problems like candida, high levels of hypoglycemia, EBV, and Chronic Fatigue Syndrome will need to follow Basic Diet #3--The Super Cleanser and additional suggestions made in the appropriate chapters on your specific problems. The schedules at the end of the Health Assessment will give you suggestions on how long to follow each program.

So, take a deep breath, remember that you can have fun with your food while you get yourself healthy, and turn the page!

Chapter 3
Your Health Assessment

Bodies are truly miraculous! They can deal with amazing amounts of stress on emotional, mental, spiritual and physical levels and still keep going. Unfortunately, all this stress takes a toll on the levels of nutrients, and then, deficiencies develop.

I've worked with all kinds of bodies and never found one that didn't have at least one or two vitamin and/or mineral deficiencies. As these nutrient levels go down, the body is forced to pull nutrients from 'less important' body functions. As vitamins and minerals continue to be pulled out of less vital areas, little problems start to creep up, simple things like hangnails, frequent gas or heartburn. And as this pattern continues, other things start to show; your skin gets dry, or your energy level drops or you hear yourself saying *"I just can't do what I used to do."* As deficient conditions continue, things just slowly (and sometimes, not so slowly!) go to new levels of dis-comfort and dis-ease.

Look over the groups of symptoms below. The first group lists 'simple-deficiency' dis-comforts and dis-eases and the last group lists problems associated with 'deep level deficiencies.' If you have symptoms in the last group it is likely you will have some of the ones listed in all the groups.

Each group has a suggestion as to which diet plan you should start following. The schedules at the end of the chapter will give you an idea as to how long each diet should be followed.

First Group
Go to Basic Diet #1--The Basic Balancer, Chapter 4, page 22, if you have any of the following:

acne, occasional
afternoon fatigue,
    spaciness, or sleepiness
backaches
bloodshot eyes
bruising easily
canker sores
bleeding gums
cracks at corner of mouth
cold hands/feet

colds/flus, one-two yearly
craving sweets
dandruff, itchy scalp
dull or dry hair
digestion tract is off,
    gaseous or constipated
5-15 extra pounds
hangnails
    fingernail ridges,
    spots or moons

mucus in back of throat
nervous or anxious
PMS--slight swelling
    of breasts or abdomen,
    acne, vulnerability,
    emotional
sensitivity to sunlight
skin 'goose bumps'
vulnerable feeling
self-judging

Second Group

Go to Basic Diet #2--The Deep Cleanser, Chapter 5, page 36, if you have any of the following symptoms. Also read the special sections in the Dis-ease and Dis-comfort chapter.

acne
allergies to foods,
    pollens, and molds
bad breath regularly
bed wetting,
    incontinence,
    bladder infections
blood pressure imbalance
body odors,
    sour skin smell,
    vaginal odors, B.O.
cholesterol imbalance
colds/flus frequently

cramps in muscles,
    night cramps
edema
hair loss
hay fever
headaches, minor and/
    or occasional
hives
hot flashes
insomnia
irritability
kidney pain
kidney infections

lung mucus
mood swings
PMS--cramps,
    retaining fluids, acne,
    cravings, scarring
self-judgment
sexual problems
sleep without being rested
swollen glands
urination, frequent and/
    or up through the night
vision problems,
    bad night vision
yeast infections

Third Group

Go to Basic Diet #3, Chapter 6, page 51, if you have any of the following; and read any of the special sections in Chapter 10, Dis-ease and Dis-comfort:

alcohol desires
anemia
appetite loss
asthma
atherosclerosis
blister-type bumps
    esp. on fingers
blood chemistry imbalance
cataracts
colitis
diarrhea

depression
dizziness
eczema
fainting
infertility
gallstones
goiters
headaches, migraines
hemorrhoids
hepatitis
herpes

hormone imbalances
impotence
joint pains, problems
'lactose' intolerant
psoriasis
skin rashes
sterility
thyroid imbalances
ulcers
varicose veins

Fourth Group

Go to Basic Diet #3, Chapter 6, page 51 and read it along with the special considerations discussed in Chapter 10, Dis-ease and Dis-comfort.

AIDS
arthritis
birth defects
cancer

candida
diabetes
EBV, Epstein-Barr Virus
Chronic Fatigue Syndrome

epilepsy
heart disease
lupus
Multiple Sclerosis

DIET APPROACH SCHEDULES

Though you have to be the ultimate judge of which diet approach you start with and when you move on to the next phase, I can give you a basic idea. The following schedules will give you the normal time span for each diet approach.

FOR ADULTS **MONTHS ON EACH APPROACH:**

	Basic 3	Basic 2	Basic 1	Phase 2	Getting There	Core Diet	Semi Final
Group 1			2	2	2	2	2
Group 2		1	2	2	2	2	2
Group 3	1	2	2	2	2	2	2
Group 4	2 to 3	2 to 3	2 to 3	2 to 3	2	2	2

FOR CHILDREN (12 & under) **MONTHS ON EACH APPROACH:**

	Basic 3	Basic 2	Basic 1	Phase 2	Getting There	Core Diet	Semi Final
Group 1			1	1 to 2	1 to 2	1 to 2	1 to 2
Group 2		1	1 to 2	1 to 2	2	2	2
Group 3		2	2	2	2	2	2
Group 4		2 to 3	2 to 3	2	2	2	

FOR PREGNANT WOMEN ONLY **MONTHS ON EACH APPROACH:**

	Basic 3	Basic 2	Basic 1	Phase 2	Getting There	Core Diet	Semi Final
Group 1			1	1	1	1	1
Group 2		1	1	1	1	1	1
Group 3	1	1	1	1	1	1	1
Group 4	1	1	1	1	1	1	1

Chapter 4
Basic Diet #1, The Basic Balancer

GETTING INTO IT

Take a look at the Basic Balancer diet listed below. The foods on the YES side are the easiest foods for almost all bodies to digest. There are individual food explanations following the work-up. If you are choosing to do the Basic Balancer, make a copy of the diet and put it on the front of the refrigerator.

MAKE A COMMITMENT TO YOURSELF TO DO THIS. GET EXCITED!

I suggest that you plan on following this diet work-up for TWO MONTHS. Then, if you are feeling good and health is manifesting itself, move on to the second level of the program. You can choose to stay on this diet for longer, if you wish.

Remember: Trust your own senses. If there is something on this plan that doesn't seem to agree with you, don't eat that food for another month and then try reintroducing it. See the section on 'How Do I Reintroduce Foods' in Chapter 7.

The foods on the YES side are basically optional; that is, if you don't want to eat fish or yogurt, or anything else on the YES side, you don't HAVE to. It's the stuff on the NO side that you really want to stay away from for now. Just make sure that you stay within the percentages for the different categories to make sure you get enough protein in your diet.

If you are having a child follow this program, be sure to make note of the differences listed throughout the diet and see Chapter 9, 'Special People and Their Situations' for more information.

Please make note: I don't use the food category called 'carbohydrates.' This group of foods is made up of fruits, veggies, beans, legumes and starches, like grains and soy products. I think it is important to divide this group into individual sections because of some of the future digestive rules you will be following later in the diet.

BASIC DIET #1, THE BASIC BALANCER

YES FOODS	NO FOODS
FRUITS: figs, dates, apricots, bananas, avocados, coconut----------------------	All other fruits
VEGGIES: all veggies including potatoes, and corn/cornmeal----------------------	the cabbage family: broccoli, cauliflower, cabbages, brussels sprouts, kale, collard greens, kohlrabi

YES FOODS	NO FOODS

YES FOODS

DAIRY PRODUCTS: eggs, yogurt, kefir and kefir cheese, and sour cream---------------------------- All other dairy products

MEATS: fish and chicken---------------------------------- All other meats and shellfish

NUTS and SEEDS:-- All nuts and seeds

GRAINS: 100% sprouted grains and quinoa and their flours--------------------------------------- amaranth, barley, buckwheat, couscous, kamut, millet, oats, rice, rye, spelt, teff, wheat, their flours and pastas

SWEETENERS: 100% maple syrup---------------------- All other sweeteners

OILS: butter only-- All other oils

SOY PRODUCTS: miso and tamari--------------------- All other soy products

SPROUTED BEANS & LEGUMES ONLY------------ All regular beans and legumes

HERBS & SPICES: all cooking herbs & spices, medic- inal herbs, all teas plus black & green ones-- NO goldenseal

SPECIAL ITEMS: Carob powder-------------------------- Coffee, chocolate, alcohol, brewer's and nutritional yeasts, vinegar and all condi- ments (catsup, mustard, horseradish, pick- les, mayo, anything with vinegar, see Table 2 in Appendix.)

PERCENTAGES OF FOODS:
    FOR ADULTS:
        60% veggies
        20% fruits
        20% everything else (dairy, fish, chicken, maple syrup, and butter.)
        20% of your veggies can be raw, if you want them. Raw juices are not included in this percentage.
    FOR PREGNANT WOMEN:
        50% veggies
        20% fruits
        30% everything else (dairy products, fish, chicken, maple syrup, and butter.)
        20% of your veggies can be raw, if you want them. Raw juices are not included in this percentage.

FOR CHILDREN UNDER 12:
   20% fruits and veggies
   80% everything else (dairy products, fish, chicken, maple syrup and butter.)
   20% of your veggies can be raw, if you want them. Raw juices are not included in this percentage.

SUPPLEMENTS:
   See Chapter 8, On Supplements.

NUTRITIONAL RULES:
   1) Eat something as soon as you get up in the morning and then, eat a little something every two hours after that.
   2) No shellfish.
   3) <u>For Everyone</u>: Fruits can be eaten with anything except other fruits. Leave a half hour between different fruits. <u>For Children under 3</u>: Keep fruit and veggies separate.
   4) Beans and legumes must be sprouted.

BASIC BALANCER EXPLANATIONS

FRUITS
Figs, Dates, Apricots, Bananas, Coconut and Avocados,
ONLY fresh, cooked, dried or juiced

One of the consistent body symptoms I have seen over the years is hypoglycemia. Bodies that experience sugar imbalances have troubles with fruit sugars. These sugars just digest too quickly and raise the blood sugar level, causing a hypoglycemic reaction.

Fruits listed in the Basic Balancer seem to digest slowly, and for almost all people, do not cause sugar reactions, even though some of them, like the dates, are very sweet to the taste. These are the first fruits that baby's bodies like. These fruits can be eaten in any form; dried, fresh, cooked or juiced.

For now, all other fruits are out because they tend to cause hypoglycemic/sugar level reactions. And, by the way, apples and pears are the last fruits to come back into the diet. They seem to have high and quick sugar levels; eating them is like eating spoonfuls of sugar.

VEGGIES
All vegetables including potatoes, corn and cornmeal, EXCEPT: cabbages,
broccoli, cauliflower, brussels sprouts, kale, collard greens, or kohlrabi

Of all the foods we eat, vegetables have more variety in tastes and textures than anything else. They can be crisp, crunchy and cold or mushy, smooth and hot. Herbs and spices actually fall into this digestive category and lend themselves very well to their cousins.

Almost everyone thinks of potatoes and corn as starches; but they are digested by the same enzymes that digest other veggies. They are starchy veggies, but that's not the same as starches like grains, that are digested by pancreatic enzymes.

The whole cabbage family needs to be out of the diet for now. They can all be difficult to digest, causing gas and bloating.

I seriously suggest that you find someone who grows and sells organic veggies and reintroduce yourself to this wondrous family of foods. Check out the new wave of Community Supported Agriculture farms in your area (see Table 7 in the Appendix.) I grow all my veggies and dehydrate or freeze enough to make soups and stews all winter long; the life-force that transfers itself into my body when I eat these veggies is worth all the work.

Remember, veggies are not fattening. You can eat yourself silly with them and have little or no problem, except maybe feeling comfortably stuffed. See Table 2 in the Appendix for a list of vegetables.

DAIRY PRODUCTS
Eggs, Yogurt, Kefir and Kefir Cheese, and Sour Cream ONLY

ABOUT EGGS
I stick eggs into the dairy products category because they are a protein that needs hydrochloric acid to digest, just like other dairy foods, and they are in the dairy case at the grocery stores. That is where the similarities stop.

Eggs have got a very bad rap by science, big business, the media and the medical profession. It's true that many allergy tests show people are 'allergic' to the albumin that makes up egg whites. Fortunately, this allergic reaction is quickly cleared when the body is given proper levels of vitamins and minerals. Also, the level of cholesterol in eggs has been sighted as a problem. I have not found this to be a problem at all! When I was just starting to do this work, I met an elderly couple who consulted me specifically about high cholesterol problems. They had been on a doctor's high cholesterol diet for 2 years but their cholesterol levels had not gone down. I put them each on a diet that included a dozen eggs a week and butter! Within two months their cholesterol levels started going down and after 6 months leveled off at normal blood cholesterol readings! Bringing their bodies into balance was the key.

Eggs are one of the easiest proteins to digest. And when taking proper levels of vitamins and minerals, rarely do people have problems with eggs. If you have been told you are allergic to eggs, don't eat them for a couple of weeks. When you feel your system has stabilized itself, try eating a bite or two of a well-cooked egg yolk and white, all by itself. Watch for mucus reactions, stomach or intestinal reactions, headaches or any other subtle or obvious body or emotional reactions. If you do not note any reaction, you can then choose to eat them or not.

ABOUT DAIRY PRODUCTS
The milk molecule is a very complex structure and it takes large amounts of both hydrochloric acid (HCL) and lactose enzymes to properly break it down so that it is usable by the body. Most people are lacking high levels of HCL and lactose enzymes and therefore, have allergic reactions to dairy products.

In the process of making soured and cultured dairy products such as yogurt, kefir, cottage cheese, cream cheese, sour cream, buttermilk and cheeses, the milk molecule is broken. Yogurt is called 'predigested' because the milk molecule is so thoroughly broken down that little HCL and lactose enzymes are needed in the body to complete the process. Kefir and kefir cheese are also acidophilus cultures, like yogurt. Their molecular structure is also broken down to the point that small amounts of HCL and lactose enzymes will complete the digestive process.

Kefir is available in health food stores as a drink with the consistency of eggnog. It usually has fruit and sweeteners added to it and it is delicious, but these additions may cause you some problems. Ask your health food store to order plain kefir; then you can use it like buttermilk or yogurt in making salad dressings, or add your own fruits and sweeteners for a drink. Date Kefir is the BEST!!!

Kefir cheese is similar to cream cheese with more tang. Kefir cheese is just kefir with the excess water removed. It can be spread on essene breads hot from the toaster oven or broiler or used to make a cheesecake with yogurt!

Sour cream was one of those surprises I found when I first started talking to bodies. It repeatedly came up as easy to digest. Once I started thinking about it, through, it made sense; it's mostly the fat of the milk, which like butter, seems to be easy to digest. And the souring process breaks the milk molecule down.

All of these products can be used as a substitute for milk by diluting them down with water and sweetening them with maple syrup. A little maple syrup whipped into some sour cream makes a great whipping cream; kefir cheese, yogurt, sour cream and eggs will make cheesecakes; spread kefir cheese on a toasted slice of essene bread; ENJOY!

MEATS
Fish and chicken ONLY

Meats and fish are foods that, like dairy products, take hydrochloric acid in the stomach to break down their molecular structures. High levels of HCL are needed to digest most meats, but fish and chicken are two of the easiest 'meat' proteins to break down. They only use small amounts of HCL.

All the other meats, including turkey, need higher amounts of HCL to properly digest and most people just don't have enough HCL to do the job; so for now, turkey, lamb, pork, beef and all other meats are out.

Shellfish are a no-no. There are two main problems with them. They live near shore, for one; if 'near shore' means near a populated area, then the likelihood is toxin levels are high. The second problem with shellfish comes from the protein structure that makes them up. This particular structure is very hard for most bodies to break down, hence many people's allergic reaction to shellfish.

NUTS AND SEEDS
Avoid all of them

Take a break from these wonderful taste treats. Nuts and seeds are great sources of proteins, oils and nutrients but they are very difficult to digest; that is, they take large amounts of HCL and bile (the soap-like substance from the liver and gallbladder that breaks down fats.)

Even when nuts and seeds are added back into the diet, I suggest people go light on eating them. I like to use them as complements to other foods, like having a few peanuts with my veggie and quinoa curry or having a few walnuts in my carob or chocolate brownies.

GRAINS
Sprouted grains only and Quinoa

Grains have been the basis of civilizations for as far back as people can remember. Grains or starches are digested by a number of enzymes, the major one coming from the pancreas. They are quickly transformed into sugars and give us energy and nutrients.

That is, they do if we can digest them properly. Most people can't! I'm not totally clear on how we arrived at this desperate point of ill-health, though I've got a few suspicions.

ABOUT THE PANCREAS AND GRAINS

First, it seems the pancreas needs huge amounts of vitamin B's, for one thing. Now, stress eats up vitamin B's like crazy, so it's not surprising that most people are deficient in them. This deficiency, in itself, would put the pancreas under stress and disable it's functioning.

The second suspicion is pancreatic stress is from sugar. Did you know that at the turn of the century the average intake of sugar was two pounds a year; now that average is running close to 140 pounds!!! I know that I go through 100 pounds of honey a year, most of which goes into my coffee and tea; the point is, sugar amounts add up fast. There is just no way that human bodies can adjust to that level of change without experiencing it as stress.

The third suspicion is spiritual in nature. I think that people and the planet we live on are going through a major growth spurt of our conscious awareness. We are becoming a very small world; and as we become a more connected world, we become aware that the pain and suffering of one living thing becomes the pain and suffering for all of us. This connectedness creates change and it brings us more and more in line with our spiritual selves.

Traditionally, the energy field or chakra in the body that connects body and spirit together is centered right over the pancreas. There's no way around it, going through spiritual growth puts the pancreas in stress. Whether you agree with my spiritual understandings or not, the physical reality seems to be consistent in humans: we are not digesting sugars and starches well.

ABOUT HYPOGLYCEMIA

Now, not being able to digest starches is a major problem even though it is easily corrected, given the proper diet, nutrient intake and time. There is another side effect of this pancreatic stress that is just as important to deal with specifically. When the pancreas is stressed it seems to lose its ability to control one of its other major functions, that is, the release of appropriate amounts of insulin into the bloodstream. Insulin is a hormone that is made by the pancreas and is released on demand. Insulin acts like a waiter, it 'serves' sugar out of the bloodstream and into the cells.

From my work I would guess that 85% of the population is running some level of hypoglycemia or low blood sugar because of pancreatic stress. Typical symptoms for hypoglycemia are: mid-afternoon dips in energy or overall fatigue, spaciness or the lack of ability to concentrate, craving foods and sugars, mood swings, irritability and snappiness, headaches, depression and dizziness.

If you have one or more of these symptoms, it's likely that you are hypoglycemic. For information on this situation, see the chapter Dis-ease and Discomfort and its section on hypoglycemia.

Taking starches out of the diet relieves the stress the pancreas is under and immediately problems like those listed above start to clear. Patience is needed here because even though symptoms may clear quickly, it may take a year or more to really heal the pancreas. BUT, following the right diet should start changing the symptoms somewhere within a few days and up to two weeks, so that you don't have to deal with the symptoms as your pancreas heals.

ABOUT SPROUTED GRAINS

For most people once a grain has been sprouted, their bodies recognize it as a vegetable and no longer as a starch that requires pancreatic enzymes. Therefore, eating sprouted grains and sprouted grain products doesn't stress the pancreas. If you have been suspecting a wheat allergy, it is very likely that you will have no problems eating sprouted wheat.

And there are some wonderful all sprouted grain breads, muffins, cereals, and flours out there in the marketplace. You can make french toast with sprouted breads and pie crusts from sprouted cereals and carob brownies with panocha (sprouted wheat flour.) Check out Table 3 for a list of sprouted grain products, Table 1 for ideas on how to use them and the Recipe chapter for more information.

ABOUT QUINOA

Quinoa is a wonder food! It's a small 'grain' that looks like millet (or bird seed) but comes from an herb plant similar to lamb's quarters. It acts like a grain but it digests as a fruit!! You can cook it just like rice, in about 20 minutes; you can use the flour to make brownies and muffins and pancakes; you can use quinoa flakes to make cereals and cooked quinoa makes great Tabouli-type salads, all this and it digests with the same enzymes that digest fruits!

Using quinoa does not trigger the pancreas to produce or release pancreatic enzymes. So here's a food that will fill the space created by not using regular starches. Since most pastas are made with wheat (and that includes semolina and durum) they are out of the diet for now; but check out the quinoa info on Table 5 of the appendix. There's a company that makes quinoa and corn noodles!

Every once in awhile, I will find quinoa is too alkaline for certain body-types. If you try quinoa and it does NOT set well, try cooking it in water with grated lemon rind. This practice brings the acidity level up and helps balance the ph, making quinoa easily digestible for everyone.

SWEETENERS
100% Maple Syrup ONLY

Are you shocked? Most people are! But bodies love maple syrup (and taste buds don't normally complain, either!) It seems that maple syrup is very slow to digest so it doesn't cause a sugar rush in the bloodstream. Hypoglycemics can usually take spoonfuls of maple syrup without reactions and when candida levels are low, this sugar doesn't seem to feed the yeasts.

Many of the recipes in this book use maple syrup, so don't deny those cravings for something sweet. Just give it the right sweetener and other ingredients!

There is a problem with all the other natural sweeteners at this point in your diet. They are just too quickly absorbed into the bloodstream. While you are sorting out whether you are hypoglycemic or not, using maple syrup will help keep the blood sugar level nice and even.

OILS
100% real butter only

Well, if the maple syrup didn't have you going, this one probably will! I was shocked, too. When I first started doing diet work-ups for clients, butter would repeatedly be the only oil that someone could use. And after I saw people getting well, saw cholesterol levels dropping, and heard healing stories from clients, I had to let my surprise go.

When you stop and think about it, the concentrated oils that we use, whether they come from vegetables, nuts and seeds, or animals, are not natural. It makes sense to me that our bodies would recognize and deal with butter as a molecular structure it has dealt with before in milk.

There are numerous studies that show hydrogenated oils to be indigestible and very hard on the system. All the oils that are firm or solid like margarines have been hydrogenated; I suggest you do NOT eat them, ever. Check out what Adelle Davis had to say about this even twenty years ago in *Let's Eat Right to Keep Fit*. In general, we have to start thinking about fats in a totally different way. Our bodies need a certain amount of oils in the diet to supply, digest and utilize fat-soluble vitamins, linoleic acid, and the two vitamin B's cholin and inositol. Fats need to be healthy and usable. So enjoy using a little butter (1-2 sticks a week)! Sweet (unsalted) and lightly salted butter are recommended.

SOY PRODUCTS
Miso and Tamari only

All soy products come from soybeans. Beans are digested as starches so they take pancreatic enzymes to digest. Since most people initially have difficulty making enough of these enzymes, soy products present some problems. So, for now, take tofu, soy cheese, tempeh, soy powders and soy milk out of the diet.

Miso and tamari (natural soy sauce) are fermented to the point where most bodies do not recognize them as starches any longer. They seem to take little or no further digesting. There is no problem using either product when they contain rice or wheat or some other grain, because that grain has also been fermented. People with yeast problems like candida need to stay away from fermented foods, and so, should not eat either miso or tamari.

BEANS AND LEGUMES
All sprouted beans and legumes

Beans and legumes (lentils and peas) are notorious gas producers. Any time a food causes gas, it means it is rotting and putrefying in the intestines. The reason beans do this is simple: human bodies do not have the enzymes needed to digest them.

When beans are growing, they are full of vegetable sugars, but when these beans are dried, the sugars are converted into a starch. Our bodies do not have the enzymes needed to break down that starch and it seems that we don't have the ability to develop these enzymes, either. For centuries South American peoples have eaten beans and their bodies STILL get gas.

There is a simple way to take care of this problem and make beans and legumes not only digestible but delicious and fun. Sprout them! When you sprout beans and legumes, you reverse the vegetable sugars-to-starches process. As the sprouts grow, the starches are converted back into vegetable sugars. Once this process is complete, the body digests them as a vegetable.

You can cook the beans and use them just like you normally would. I make chili, refried beans, kidney bean salad, black bean soup, and baked beans all with sprouted beans.

Beans and legumes are easy to sprout. (See 'How to Sprout Beans and Legumes' in the Recipe section.) As they sprout, the vitamin and mineral levels skyrocket. And I have to warn you: sprouted beans are addictive! I think that our bodies recognize the high levels of nutrients available in the sprouted beans and literally crave them.

With a mischievous glint in my eye, I have taken my kidney bean salad to parties, then sat back and watched. After people try the salad, the addictive Need sets in and you see them going back for seconds;, then thirds; and then fourths, as they cover their faces, trying to hide their embarrassment. They can't believe they are eating all these beans! I mean, normally you'd have to closet yourself up for a week after four helpings of beans!

A few days later I start getting calls. *"What did you do to those beans? I didn't get any gas from them!"*

I have a quick and dirty trick concerning beans. I start with 4-5 cups of dried beans, so I end up with 10-12 cups of sprouted beans. I cook them all and put them in different size containers, then freeze them. Cooked beans are great coming out of the freezer (they come out just as good as they went in which isn't so for all foods.) I just don't want to have to think about sprouting beans all the time, so when I want to use them, I just take frozen ones out of the freezer and add them to whatever I'm doing. I like to keep a couple different kinds in the freezer and have fun with them!

HERBS AND SPICES
All cooking herbs, all spices, all medicinal herbs, and
all teas including black and green teas, except NO goldenseal

This whole category is enormous. All these dried plants are treated as veggies by the body and most people don't have any problems with them. When I have seen troubles in this area, it usually has had to do with blood chemistry problems.

The kind of symptoms you may experience if your blood chemistry is out of balance are: quick reactions to smells, like perfumes or freon, quick reactions to sugars, herbs, or certain foods, a sense that you are not always completely in your body, rapid up and down swings of energy, and/or mental or emotional confusion.

If you suspect you have a blood chemistry imbalance, don't use any herbs or spices for a month or so. Then start slowly introducing them back into your diet, one at a time. Check out the chapters on hypoglycemia and EBV.

I haven't seen many people having problems with small amounts of caffeine, so occasionally using black and green teas may work in your body. I recommend staying away from them if you have any concerns about your reactions to them. Then after a couple of weeks on the Basic Balancer, try a cup of black tea and see how your body reacts.

A word about salt. Salt is one of those nutrients that is essential to life and our bodies crave it. But like all out-of-balance cravings, the desire for too much salt indicates an imbalance in the body usually linked to mineral deficiencies.

So, how much salt is too much? The general rule seems to be a range of salt on a weekly basis, somewhere between 1/4 tsp. to 1/2 tsp. weekly! I suggest that you claim your own salt shaker, fill it once a week and use it sparingly until it's gone.

And I can hear some of your howls! I'll never forget the friend who was riding in my back seat when she asked me how much salt her body wanted. When I relayed the information, she was immediately in the front seat, screaming, "What?"

The body needs a balance of minerals, including sodium. But bodies prefer having these nutrients delivered in natural forms from food. Cut back on the salt for awhile, a few weeks, then try some salty food you used to eat. As your body comes to balance, your taste buds will balance out too.

A word about goldenseal. This root herb became very popular in the 60's and 70's because it acts like a natural antibiotic. The problem with it, besides its terrible taste, is that it also acts as natural insulin in the body, so it lowers the blood sugar levels! Because of the high levels of hypoglycemia in this country, I suggest avoiding the use of goldenseal. Instead of goldenseal, I recommend the use of propolis, a product that bees gather from plants, which also acts as a natural antibiotic. It also is antiviral, antifungal, antimicrobial and antibacterial. Propolis is resinous, which makes it hard for the body to digest; so I recommend taking it in extract or tincture form. See the section on Herbs in the Supplement Chapter for more information.

SPECIALTY FOODS
Carob powder is a YES, NO Coffee, Chocolate, Alcohol
NO Brewer's and Nutritional Yeast, NO Vinegar or Condiments

ABOUT CAROB
Carob beans come from the pod of an evergreen tree that grows in the Mediterranean. It's touted as a chocolate substitute, though you won't find many chocolate lovers who agree with that.

Carob digests as a protein and it is a very easy-to-digest one. Check out the suggestions in Table 1 about this fun food and the recipes for Carob-Quinoa brownies.

Skip the carob chips for now; the oils in them are intense.

ABOUT COFFEE
Coffee is out for now.

Coffee is a wonderful beverage but it has it's difficulties. It is out of the Basic Diets, but take heart, it will come back into the diet if you want it.

Coffee has a number of problems. First, there are some very strong, natural chemicals in it that can upset the blood chemistry and slow down the healing process. This is why coffee is out of the Basic Diets. Second, the way that we make coffee, by pouring hot water directly on the grounds, creates some serious body reactions. When hot water comes in contact with coffee grounds, it leaches out all the oils and the acids. These two substances create digestive problems; the oils are indigestible and the acids conflict with the natural stomach acids. The acids and oils also interact with the caffeine, creating most of the negative side effects people experience from coffee and associate with caffeine.

There is a better way to brew coffee and you can read about it in Beverage section of the Recipes. But for now, stay away from coffee. If you want (or need) caffeine, use black or green teas.

ABOUT CHOCOLATE

Chocolate is out for now.

Like coffee, chocolate has some harsh natural chemicals that can slow down the healing process. And the natural oils, the cocoa butter, demands high quality and high levels of bile to break down, making it a food you want to avoid while you do the Basic Diets. And, again, like coffee, chocolate can come back into the diet, though it will need to be dealt with carefully.

ABOUT ALCOHOL

Alcohol is out for now.

This restriction usually doesn't raise an eyebrow. We've all come to a cultural agreement that alcohol is 'a problem.' Remember that bodies don't carry that kind of judgment and eventually most bodies can deal with alcohol, with a little extra nutrient help. But some bodies and psyches have very physical problems with alcohol. Read the section on Alcohol in Chapter 10, Dis-Ease and Dis-Comfort.

ABOUT SUPPLEMENTAL YEASTS

Brewer's yeast, which is the yeast by-product of making beer, and nutritional yeast, a yeast grown on molasses, are great sources of vitamin B's and other nutrients, but they are digested as proteins. They take large amounts of HCL to digest and therefore, cause problems for most people. Few people use these supplements because they don't like the taste. But mixed with the right foods, these yeasts can be wonderful (I can't imagine my popcorn butter not having brewers yeast in it!)

For now, let them alone.

ABOUT VINEGAR

The problem with vinegar is its acidity level. When your system gets out of balance, the Ph (acid/alkaline) balance suffers and becomes 'delicate.' Vinegar can throw this delicate situation into a tail spin so it is important to avoid it for now. Even the small amounts of vinegar in the condiments (catsup, prepared mustard, horseradish and pickles) can be a problem.

Ph imbalances will manifest symptoms similar to hypoglycemia with one obvious difference. If you have ever felt that you are half in and half out of your body, you are experiencing a Ph imbalance.

Ph imbalances are one of the first things that bodies will correct on the proper diet since imbalances in the acid/alkaline levels affect all other functions in the body.

FOOD PERCENTAGES

Work out your food percentages 'by volume'; that is, if you eat 10 cups of food a day, following the Adult ratios below, you would be eating 6 cups of veggies (that's alot!) and 2 cups of those veggies could be raw, 2 cups of fruit, and 2 cups of eggs, yogurt, kefir, sour cream, fish, chicken, maple syrup, and butter.) 'Volume' for salad-type veggies is measured in packed cups.

FOR ADULTS
60% veggies, 20% fruits, 20% everything else and 20% raw veggies

To keep the Basic Balancer a cleansing and healing experience, we have to keep the level of fruits and vegetables high in the diet. Eating too many starches, proteins, sweeteners or oils (foods that require high amounts of enzymes to digest) doesn't give the body a rest. Eating 80% fruits and veggies and 20% everything else puts the body in a cleansing mode without robbing it of vitality.

If you feel that you want more of a cleanse, eat 90% fruits and veggies and 10% everything else, with no raw foods for the first month, except for juices. For the second month do 80% fruits and veggies and 20% everything else. By the end of this program, the ratio of fruits and veggies to everything else will settle into a regular body pattern. Most adult bodies settle into a maintenance program of 70% fruits and veggies, 30% everything else.

FOR PREGNANT WOMEN
70% fruits and veggies, 30% everything else and 20% raw veggies (except for juices)

The Basic Balancer has a higher percentage of 'everything else' because your baby will need good levels of protein and fats available to it throughout the pregnancy. Enjoy!

FOR CHILDREN UNDER 12
20% fruits and veggies, 80% everything else,
(dairy products, fish, chicken, maple syrup, and butter,)
20% of you veggies can be raw (not including raw juices.)

As you can see, children need a higher level of proteins, fats, starches, sweeteners and oils than adults. Their bodies are in constant 'growing mode' and they need heavy-duty building blocks to create a healthy adult body. We adults are only doing general maintenance plans, even when we are healing. Read Chapter 9 on children for more information about how to handle your kids' healing.

NUTRITIONAL RULES
1) Eat every two hours, 2) No shellfish, 3) You can eat fruits with anything
except other fruits. Separate different fruits by 1/2 hour. (See note for children under 3.)
4) Beans and legumes must be sprouted.

When I started talking to bodies, I made long lists of all the different nutritional rules I found in the 'popular theory' books. There were only four 'rules' that I found bodies consistently wanted to follow; occasionally I saw a body that fit one of the remaining rules.

1) The first rule you need to follow is eating when you first get up in the morning and then eating something every two hours after that, until you go to bed.

About two hours after you eat something, the simple sugars are pulled out of the intestines and into the bloodstream. So, the sugar levels will naturally start to drop and there lays the problem. When the body is healthy, this drop in the blood sugar level is compensated for and the blood sugar levels are kept even; but, because of the high percentages of hypoglycemia, most people's bodies cannot regulate themselves and hypoglycemic reactions start.

When you eat a little something every two hours, you keep sugars coming from the intestines and this helps keep the blood sugar levels nice and even. As people heal, the times between eating can get elongated; but for now, eat something every two hours.

Like I said, this 'eating every two hours' doesn't have to be a meal. If you've got a sweet tooth, a spoonful of maple syrup or a maple syrup candy may do it. A few dates or dried apricots, a slice of sprouted bread, a glass of juice or a real meal will all do just fine.

After a few days of watching the clock and remembering to eat every two hours (set yourself an alarm until it becomes a habit,) you will find that your body will start telling you when the time has passed! It will start screaming at you that "it is time to eat something!"

Don't worry about 'getting fat from eating so much.' Remember that many peoples' weight has to do with eating things that can't be digested properly. And following this diet, you will be eating 80% fruits and veggies. You REALLY have to work at putting on weight from eating too many fruits and veggies! Especially since the high calorie foods you can eat, like sour cream and butter and maple syrup, can only be 20% part of your overall diet!

2) Avoid shellfish. They are almost always a problem for the digestive system. See the previous section on Meats for more info.

3) You can eat fruits with anything except other fruits. Separate different fruits by 1/2 hour.

Mixed fruits confuse the pancreas. The only time I have consciously experienced a hypoglycemic reaction was years ago when I was doing my first cookbook. I was working on the beverage section and had three blenders going, with three different fruit smoothies. After going to each blender several times and tasting each of them, I found myself standing in the middle of the kitchen trying to remember why I was there and what I was doing.

An internal voice said, *"You just ate three different fruits and are as hypoglycemic as hell, Silly!"* Oops! I grabbed a bite of protein and went outside and lay on the grass until my sugar level balanced itself out again.

I was amazed that most people have those kinds of hypoglycemic reactions throughout their days. I wondered how people function!!!

4) Beans and legumes must be sprouted. As explained above, unsprouted beans and legumes are indigestible. See the recipe section on beans and legumes for easy directions on how to sprout them.

FOLLOW THROUGH

So, now it's time to skip ahead to Chapter 7, How Do I ....?, which will answer some of the questions that might arise, like How Do I Do This Alone? or With Family?, How Do I Eat Out?, How Do I Reintroduce Foods, or How Do I know What an Emotional Food Reaction Is?

Read Chapter 8, On Supplements, so you can decide what vitamins and minerals you need to add to your new eating patterns. And read Chapter 9, Special People and Their Situations, if you are pregnant or planning to have a child follow the eating program.

Check out the product lists in the Appendix for more information on all sprouted breads, quinoa pastas, maple syrup candies, and more. Then after two months on the Basic Balancer, when you feel obviously better, move on to the Phase Two Diet, Chapter 11.

Now, get to it and enjoy yourself!

Chapter 5
Basic Diet #2, The Deep Cleanser

This diet approach is almost identical to the Basic Balancer diet; but there are a few very important exceptions. The Deep Cleanser diet is just what its name implies; it is an approach that will give you a deep level of cleansing without pushing most bodies into a healing crisis.

I suggest you do this approach for one month if your Health Assessment put you in the Second Group and two to three months if you are in the Third or Fourth Group.

The major differences between this approach and the next level up, the Basic Balancer, are the restrictions on corn, cornmeal, sour cream, and chicken, the difference in the food percentages and higher levels of supplements. I know this doesn't seem like much of a difference, but it is!

These restricted foods represent a distinctive increase in the need for certain enzymes that people in the Second, Third and Fourth Groups are having difficulty producing. And the diet includes just enough proteins and carbohydrates in the food percentages to keep the body from going parasitic on itself and breaking down muscle, organ or bone tissue to keep the blood chemistry balanced.

This approach can also be used by anyone wanting to do a deep cleansing without going on a total juice or water fast.

Please make note: I don't use the food category called 'carbohydrates.' This group of foods is made up of fruits, veggies, beans, legumes and starches, like grains and soy products. I think it is important to divide this group into individual sections because of some of the future digestive rules you will be following later in the diet.

THE BASIC DIET #2, THE DEEP CLEANSER DIET

YES FOODS	NO FOODS
FRUITS: figs, dates, apricots, bananas, avocados ---	all other fruits
VEGGIES: all veggies including potatoes-------------	cabbage family, corn and cornmeal
DAIRY PRODUCTS: eggs, yogurt, kefir and kefir cheese--	all other dairy products
MEATS: fish only----------------------------------	all other meats and shellfish
NUTS & SEEDS:------------------------------------	all nuts and seeds
GRAINS: 100% sprouted grains & quinoa & their flours---	regular grains, flours, pastas
SWEETENERS: 100% maple syrup-------------------	all other sweeteners

YES FOODS	NO FOODS

YES FOODS

OILS: butter only--

SOY PRODUCTS: miso and tamari------------------

SPROUTED BEANS & LEGUMES ONLY---------

HERBS & SPICES: all cooking herbs & spices,
       medicinal herbs, all herbal teas--------------

SPECIAL ITEMS: Carob powder----------------------

NO FOODS

all other oils

all other soy products

all regular beans and legumes

NO goldenseal, black or green teas

coffee, chocolate, alcohol, brewer's
and nutritional yeasts, vinegar and
all condiments

PERCENTAGES OF FOODS:
    FOR ADULTS:
        70% veggies
        20% fruits
        10% everything else (dairy, fish, maple syrup, and butter)
        No raw veggies (except for juices)
    FOR PREGNANT WOMEN:
        60% veggies
        20% fruits
        20% everything else
        No raw veggies (except for juices.)
    FOR CHILDREN UNDER 12:
        20% fruits and veggies
        80% everything else
        No raw veggies (except for juices.)

SUPPLEMENTS:
    See the Chapter 8, On Supplements.

NUTRITIONAL RULES:
    1) Eat something as soon as you get up in the morning and then eat a little something every two hours after that.
    2) No shellfish.
    3) For Everyone: Fruits can be eaten with anything except other fruits. Leave a half hour between different fruits. For Children under 3, keep fruit and veggies separate.
    4) Beans and legumes must be sprouted.

DEEP CLEANSER EXPLANATIONS
Most of the following explanations are the same as in the Basic Balancer Diet
with a few additions and changes, which are marked with ***

FRUITS
Figs, Dates, Apricots, Bananas and Avocados
ONLY fresh, cooked, dried or juiced

One of the consistent body symptoms I have seen over the years is hypoglycemia. Bodies that experience sugar imbalances have troubles with fruit sugars. These sugars just digest too quickly and raise the blood sugar level, causing a hypoglycemic reaction.

The fruits listed in the Basic Balancer seem to digest slowly, and for most people, do not cause sugar reactions, even though some of them, like the dates, are very sweet to the taste. These are the first fruits that baby's bodies like. These fruits can be eaten in any form; dried, fresh, cooked or juiced.

For now, all other fruits are out because they tend to cause hypoglycemic/sugar level reactions. And, by the way, apples and pears are the last fruits to come back into the diet. They seem to have high and quick sugar levels; eating them is like eating spoonfuls of sugar.

VEGGIES
All vegetables including potatoes, EXCEPT: cabbages, broccoli, cauliflower,
brussels sprouts, kale, collard greens, or kohlrabi, and NO corn and cornmeal

Of all the foods we eat, vegetables have more variety in tastes and textures than anything. They can be crisp, crunchy and cold or mushy, smooth and hot. Herbs and spices actually fall into this digestive category and lend themselves very well to their cousins.

Most people think of potatoes and corn as starches; but they are digested by the same enzymes that digest other veggies. They are starchy veggies, but that's not the same as starches like grains, that are digested by pancreatic enzymes.

But when some bodies reach a certain point of ill-health, their pancreas' will react to the starchy molecules as if they were a starch. This will stress the system, so for now, avoid corn and cornmeal.

The whole cabbage family needs to be out of the diet for now. They can all be difficult to digest, causing gas and bloating.

I seriously suggest that you find someone who grows and sells organic veggies and reintroduce yourself to this wondrous family of foods. Check out the new wave of Community Supported Agriculture farms in your area (see Table 7 in the Appendix.) I grow all my veggies and dehydrate or freeze enough to make soups and stews all winter long; the life-force that transfers itself into my body when I eat these veggies is worth all the work.

Remember, veggies are not fattening. You can eat yourself silly with them and have little or no problem, except maybe feeling comfortably stuffed. See Table 2 in the Appendix for a list of vegetables.

DAIRY PRODUCTS
EGGS, YOGURT, KEFIR AND KEFIR CHEESE ONLY

ABOUT EGGS

I stick eggs into the dairy products category because they are a protein that needs hydrochloric acid to digest, just like other dairy foods, and they are in the dairy case at the grocery stores. That is where the similarities stop.

Eggs have got a very bad rap by science, big business, the media and the medical profession. It's true that many allergy tests show people are 'allergic' to the albumin that makes up egg whites. Fortunately, this allergic reaction is quickly cleared when the body is given proper levels of vitamins and minerals. Also, the level of cholesterol in eggs has been sighted as a problem. I have not found this to be a problem at all! When I was just starting to do this work, I met an elderly couple who consulted me specifically about high cholesterol problems. They had been on a doctor's high cholesterol diet for two years but their cholesterol levels had not gone down. I put them each on a diet that included a dozen eggs a week and butter! Within two months their cholesterol levels started going down and after 6 months leveled off at normal blood cholesterol readings! Bringing their bodies into balance was the key.

Eggs are one of the easiest proteins to digest. And when taking proper levels of vitamins and minerals, rarely do people have problems with eggs. If you have been told you are allergic to eggs, don't eat them for a couple of weeks. When you feel your system has stabilized itself, try eating a bite or two of a well-cooked egg yolk and white, all by itself. Watch for mucus reactions, stomach or intestinal reactions, headaches or any other subtle or obvious body or emotional reactions. If you do not note any reaction, you can then choose to eat them or not.

ABOUT DAIRY PRODUCTS

The milk molecule is a very complex structure and it takes large amounts of both hydrochloric acid (HCL) and lactose enzymes to properly break it down so that it is usable by the body. Most people are lacking high levels of HCL and lactose enzymes and therefore, have allergic reactions to dairy products. In the process of making soured and cultured dairy products such as yogurt, kefir, cottage cheese, cream cheese, sour cream, buttermilk and cheeses, the milk molecule is broken. Yogurt is called 'predigested' because the milk molecule is so thoroughly broken down that little HCL and lactose enzymes are needed in the body to complete the process.

Kefir and kefir cheese are also acidophilus cultures, like yogurt. Their molecular structure is also broken down to the point that small amounts of HCL and lactose enzymes will complete the digestive process. Kefir is available in health food stores as a drink with the consistency of eggnog. It usually has fruit and sweeteners added to it and it is delicious, but these additions may cause you some problems. Ask your health food store to order plain kefir; then you can use it like buttermilk or yogurt in making salad dressings, or add your own fruits and sweeteners for a drink. Date Kefir is the BEST!!!

Kefir cheese is similar to cream cheese with more tang. Kefir cheese is just kefir with the excess water removed. It can be spread on essene breads hot from the toaster oven or broiler or used to make a cheesecake with yogurt! All of these products can be used as a substitute for milk by diluting them down with water and sweetening them with maple syrup.

A little maple syrup whipped into some yogurt makes a great whipping cream; kefir cheese, yogurt and eggs will make cheesecakes; spread kefir cheese on a toasted slice of essene bread; ENJOY!

MEATS
Fish ONLY

Meats and fish are foods that, like dairy products, take hydrochloric acid in the stomach to break down their molecular structures. High levels of HCL are needed to digest most meats, but fish is the easiest 'meat' protein to break down. It only uses small amounts of HCL.

All the other meats need higher amounts of HCL to properly digest and most people just don't have enough HCL to do the job; so for now, chicken, turkey, lamb, pork, beef and all other meats are out.

Shellfish are a no-no. There are two main problems with them. They live near shore, for one thing; if 'near shore' means near a populated area, then the likelihood is that the toxin levels are high. The second problem with shellfish comes from the protein structure that makes them up. This particular structure is very hard for most bodies to break down, hence many people's allergic reaction to shellfish.

NUTS AND SEEDS
Avoid all of them

Take a break from these wonderful taste treats. Nuts and seeds are great sources of proteins, oils and nutrients but they are very difficult to digest; that is, they take large amounts of HCL and bile (the soap-like substance from the liver and gallbladder that breaks down fats.)

Even when nuts and seeds are added back into the diet, I suggest people go light on eating them. I like to use them as complements to other foods, like having a few peanuts with my veggie and quinoa curry or having a few walnuts in my carob or chocolate brownies.

GRAINS
Sprouted grains only and Quinoa

Grains have been the basis of civilizations for as far back as people can remember. Grains or starches are digested by a number of enzymes, the major one coming from the pancreas. They are quickly transformed into sugars and give us energy and nutrients. That is, they do if we can digest them properly. Most people can't! I'm not totally clear on how we arrived at this desperate point of ill-health, though I've got a few suspicions.

ABOUT THE PANCREAS AND GRAINS

First, it seems the pancreas needs huge amounts of vitamin B's, for one thing. Now, stress eats up vitamin B's like crazy, so it's not surprising that most people are deficient in them. This deficiency, in itself, would put the pancreas under stress and disable it's functioning.

The second suspicion is pancreatic stress is from sugar. Did you know that at the turn of the century the average intake of sugar was two pounds a year; now that average is running close to 140 pounds!!! I know that I go through 100 pounds of honey a year, most of which goes into my coffee and tea; the point is, sugar amounts add up fast. There is just no way that human bodies can adjust to that level of change without experiencing it as stress.

The third suspicion is spiritual in nature. I think that people and the planet we live on are going through a major growth spurt of our conscious awareness. We are becoming a very small world; and as we become a more connected world, we become aware that the pain and suffering of one living thing becomes the pain and suffering for all of us. This connectedness creates change and it brings us more and more in line with our spiritual selves.

Traditionally, the energy field or chakra in the body that connects body and spirit together is centered right over the pancreas. There's no way around it, going through spiritual growth puts the pancreas in stress. Whether you agree with my spiritual understandings or not, the physical reality seems to be consistent in humans: we are not digesting sugars and starches well.

ABOUT HYPOGLYCEMIA

Now, not being able to digest starches is a major problem even though it is easily corrected, given the proper diet, nutrient intake and time. There is another side effect of this pancreatic stress that is just as important to deal with specifically. When the pancreas is stressed it seems to lose its ability to control one of its other major functions, that is, the release of appropriate amounts of insulin into the bloodstream. Insulin is a hormone that is made by the pancreas and is released on demand. Insulin acts like a waiter, it 'serves' sugar out of the bloodstream and into the cells.

From my work I would guess that 85% of the population is running some level of hypoglycemia or low blood sugar because of pancreatic stress. Typical symptoms for hypoglycemia are: mid-afternoon dips in energy or overall fatigue, spaciness or the lack of ability to concentrate, craving foods and sugars, mood swings, irritability and snappiness, headaches, depression and dizziness.

If you have one or more of these symptoms, it's likely that you are hypoglycemic. For information on this situation, see the chapter Dis-ease and Discomfort and its section on hypoglycemia.

Taking starches out of the diet relieves the stress the pancreas is under and immediately problems like those listed above start to clear. Patience is needed here because even though symptoms may clear quickly, it may take a year or more to really heal the pancreas. BUT, following the right diet should start changing the symptoms somewhere within a few days and up to two weeks, so that you don't have to deal with the symptoms as your pancreas heals.

ABOUT SPROUTED GRAINS

For most people once a grain has been sprouted, their bodies recognize it as a vegetable and no longer as a starch that requires pancreatic enzymes. Therefore, eating sprouted grains and sprouted grain products doesn't stress the pancreas. If you have been suspecting a wheat allergy, it is very likely that you will have no problems eating sprouted wheat. And there are some wonderful all sprouted grain breads, muffins, cereals, and flours out there in the marketplace. You can make french toast with sprouted breads and pie crusts from sprouted cereals and carob brownies with panocha (sprouted wheat flour.) Check out Table 3 for a list of sprouted grain products, Table 1 for ideas on how to use them and the Recipe chapter for more information.

ABOUT QUINOA

Quinoa is a wonder food! It's a small 'grain' that looks like millet (or bird seed) but comes from an herb plant similar to lamb's quarters. It acts like a grain but it digests as a fruit!! You can cook it just like rice, in about 20 minutes; you can use the flour to make brownies and muffins and pancakes; you can use quinoa flakes to make cereals and cooked quinoa makes great Tabouli-type salads, all this and it digests with the same enzymes that digest fruits!

Using quinoa does not trigger the pancreas to produce or release pancreatic enzymes. So here's a food that will fill the space created by not using regular starches.

Since most pastas are made with wheat (and that includes semolina and durum) they are out of the diet for now; but check out the quinoa info on Table 5 of the appendix. There's a company that makes quinoa and corn noodles!

Every once in awhile, I will find quinoa is too alkaline for certain body-types. If you try quinoa and it does NOT set well, try cooking it in water with grated lemon rind. This practice brings the acidity level up and helps balance the ph, making quinoa easily digestible for everyone.

SWEETENERS
100% Maple Syrup ONLY

Are you shocked? Most people are! But bodies love maple syrup (and taste buds don't normally complain, either!.) It seems that maple syrup is very slow to digest so it doesn't cause a sugar rush in the bloodstream. Hypoglycemics can usually take spoonfuls of maple syrup without reactions and when candida levels are low, this sugar doesn't seem to feed the yeasts.

Many of the recipes in this book use maple syrup, so don't deny those cravings for something sweet. Just give it the right sweetener and other ingredients!

There is a problem with all the other natural sweeteners at this point in your diet. They are just too quickly absorbed into the bloodstream. While you are sorting out whether you are hypoglycemic or not, using maple syrup will help keep the blood sugar level nice and even.

OILS
100% real butter only

Well, if the maple syrup didn't have you going, this one probably will!

I'll tell you, I was shocked, too. When I first started doing diet work-ups, butter would repeatedly be the only oil that someone could use. And after I saw people getting well, saw cholesterol levels dropping, and heard healing stories from clients, I had to let my surprise go.

When you stop and think about it, the concentrated oils that we use, whether they come from vegetables, nuts and seeds, or animals, are not natural. It makes sense to me that our bodies would recognize and deal with butter as a molecular structure it has dealt with before, in milk.

There are numerous studies that show hydrogenated oils to be indigestible and very hard on the system. All oils that are firm or solid like margarines have been hydrogenated; I suggest you do NOT eat them, ever. Check out what Adelle Davis had to say about this even twenty years ago in *Let's Eat Right to Keep Fit.* In general, we have to start thinking about fats in a totally different way. Our bodies need a certain amount of oils in the diet to supply, digest and utilize fat-soluble vitamins, linoleic acid, and the two vitamin B's cholin and inositol. The fats just need to be healthy and usable. So enjoy using a little butter (1-2 sticks a week)! Sweet (unsalted) and lightly salted butter are recommended.

SOY PRODUCTS
Miso and Tamari only

All soy products come from soybeans. Beans are digested as starches so they take pancreatic enzymes to digest. Since most people initially have difficulty making enough of these enzymes, soy products present some problems. So, for now, take tofu, soy cheese, tempeh, soy powders and soy milk out of the diet.

Miso and tamari (natural soy sauce) are fermented to the point where most bodies do not recognize them as starches any longer. They seem to take little or no further digesting. There is no problem using either product when they contain rice or wheat or some other grain, because that grain has also been fermented. People with yeast problems like candida need to stay away from fermented foods, and so, should not eat either miso or tamari.

BEANS AND LEGUMES
All sprouted beans and legumes

Beans and legumes (lentils and peas) are notorious gas producers. Anytime a food causes gas, it means it is rotting and putrefying in the intestines. The reason beans do this is simple: human bodies do not have the enzymes needed to digest them.

When beans are growing, they are full of vegetable sugars, but when these beans are dried, the sugars are converted into a starch. Our bodies do not have the enzymes needed to break down that starch and it seems that we don't have the ability to develop these enzymes, either. For centuries South American peoples have eaten beans and their bodies STILL get gas.

There is a simple way to take care of this problem and make beans and legumes not only digestible but delicious and fun. Sprout them! When you sprout beans and legumes, you reverse the vegetable sugars-to-starches process. As the sprouts grow, the starches are converted back into vegetable sugars. Once this process is complete, the body digests them as a vegetable.

You can cook the beans and use them just like you normally would. I make chili, refried beans, kidney bean salad, black bean soup, and baked beans all with sprouted beans.

Beans and legumes are easy to sprout. (See 'How to Sprout Beans and Legumes' in the Recipe section.) As they sprout, the vitamin and mineral levels skyrocket. And I have to warn you: sprouted beans are addictive! I think that our bodies recognize the high levels of nutrients available in the sprouted beans and literally crave them.

With a mischievous glint in my eye, I have taken my kidney bean salad to parties, then sat back and watched. After people try the salad, the addictive Need sets in and you see them going back for seconds;, then thirds; and then fourths, as they cover their faces, trying to hide their embarrassment. They can't believe they are eating all these beans! I mean, normally you'd have to closet yourself up for a week after four helpings of beans!

A few days later I start getting calls. *"What did you do to those beans? I didn't get any gas from them!"*

I have a quick and dirty trick concerning beans. I start with 4-5 cups of dried beans, so I end up with 10-12 cups of sprouted beans. I cook them all and put them in different size containers, then freeze them. Cooked beans are great coming out of the freezer (they come out just as good as they went in which isn't so for all foods.)

I just don't want to have to think about sprouting beans all the time, so when I want to use them, I just take frozen ones out of the freezer and add them to whatever I'm doing. I like to keep a couple different kinds in the freezer and have fun with them!

HERBS AND SPICES
All cooking herbs, all spices, all medicinal herbs and all teas
including black and green teas except NO goldenseal

This whole category is enormous. All these dried plants are treated as veggies by the body and most people don't have any problems with them. When I have seen troubles in this area, it usually has had to do with blood chemistry problems.

The kind of symptoms you may experience if your blood chemistry is out of balance are: quick reactions to smells, like perfumes or Freon, quick reactions to sugars, herbs, or certain foods, a sense that you are not always completely in your body, rapid up and down swings of energy, and/or mental or emotional confusion.

If you suspect you have a blood chemistry imbalance, don't use any herbs or spices for a month or so. Then start slowly introducing them back into your diet, one at a time. Check out the chapters on hypoglycemia and EBV.

I haven't seen many people having problems with small amounts of caffeine, so occasionally using black and green teas may work in your body. I recommend staying away from them if you have any concerns about your reactions to them. Then after a couple of weeks on the Basic Balancer, try a cup of black tea and see how your body reacts.

A word about salt. Salt is one of those nutrients that is essential to life and our bodies crave it. But like all out-of-balance cravings, the desire for too much salt indicates an imbalance in the body usually linked to mineral deficiencies. So, how much salt is too much? The general rule seems to be a range of salt on a weekly basis, somewhere between 1/4 tsp. to 1/2 tsp. weekly! I suggest that you claim your own salt shaker, fill it once a week and use it sparingly until it's gone.

And I can hear some of your howls! I'll never forget the friend who was riding in my back seat when she asked me how much salt her body wanted. When I relayed the information, she was immediately in the front seat, screaming, *"What?"* The body needs a balance of minerals, including sodium. But bodies prefer having these nutrients delivered in natural forms, from food. Cut back on the salt for awhile, a few weeks, then try some salty food you use to eat. As your body comes to balance, your taste buds will balance out too.

A word about goldenseal. This root herb became very popular in the 60's and 70's because it acts like a natural antibiotic. The problem with it, besides its terrible taste, is that it also acts as natural insulin in the body, so it lowers the blood sugar levels! Because of the high levels of hypoglycemia in this country, I suggest avoiding the use of goldenseal.

Instead of goldenseal, I recommend the use of propolis, a product that bees gather from plants, which also acts as a natural antibiotic. It also is antiviral, antifungal, antimicrobial and antibacterial. Propolis is resinous, which makes it hard for the body to digest; so I recommend taking it in extract or tincture form. See the section on Herbs in the Supplement Chapter 8 for more information.

SPECIALTY FOODS
Carob powder is a YES, NO Coffee, Chocolate, Alcohol,
NO Brewer's and Nutritional Yeast, NO Vinegar or Condiments

ABOUT CAROB
Carob beans come from the pod of an evergreen tree that grows in the Mediterranean. It's touted as a chocolate substitute, though you won't find many chocolate lovers that agree with that.

Carob digests as a protein and it is a very easy-to-digest one. Check out the suggestions in Table 1 about this fun food and the recipes for Carob-Quinoa brownies.

Skip the carob chips for now; the oils in them are intense.

ABOUT COFFEE
Coffee is out for now.

Coffee is a wonderful beverage but it has it's difficulties. It is out of the Basic Diets, but take heart, it will come back into the diet if you want it. Coffee has a number of problems. First, there are some very strong, natural chemicals in it that can upset the blood chemistry and slow down the healing process. This is why coffee is out of the Basic Diets. Second, the way that we make coffee, by pouring hot water directly on the grounds, creates some serious body reactions.

When hot water comes in contact with coffee grounds, it leaches out all the oils and the acids. These two substances create digestive problems; the oils are indigestible and the acids conflict with the natural stomach acids. The acids and oils also interact with the caffeine, creating most of the negative side effects people experience from coffee and associate with caffeine.

There is a better way to brew coffee and you can read about it in Beverage section of the Recipes. But for now, stay away from coffee. If you want (or need) caffeine, use black or green teas.

ABOUT CHOCOLATE
Chocolate is out for now.

Like coffee, chocolate has some harsh natural chemicals that can slow down the healing process. And the natural oils, the cocoa butter, demands high quality and high levels of bile to break down, making it a food you want to avoid while you do the Basic Diets. And, again, like coffee, chocolate can come back into the diet, though it will need to be dealt with carefully.

ABOUT ALCOHOL

Alcohol is out for now.

This restriction usually doesn't raise an eyebrow. We've all come to a cultural agreement that alcohol is 'a problem.' Remember that bodies don't carry that kind of judgment and eventually most bodies can deal with alcohol, with a little extra nutrient help. But some bodies and psyches have very physical problems with alcohol. Read the section on Alcohol in Chapter 10, Dis-Ease and Dis-Comfort.

ABOUT SUPPLEMENTAL YEASTS

Brewer's yeast, which is the yeast by-product of making beer, and nutritional yeast, a yeast grown on molasses, are great sources of vitamin B's and other nutrients, but they are digested as proteins. They take large amounts of HCL to digest and therefore, cause problems for most people. Few people use these supplements because they don't like the taste. But mixed with the right foods, these yeasts can be wonderful (I can't imagine my popcorn butter not having brewers yeast in it!) For now, let them alone.

ABOUT VINEGAR

The problem with vinegar is its acidity level. When your system gets out of balance, the Ph (acid/ alkaline) balance suffers and becomes 'delicate.' Vinegar can throw this delicate situation into a tail spin so it is important to avoid it for now. Even the small amounts of vinegar in the condiments (catsup, prepared mustard, horseradish, pickles, see Table 2 in the Appendix for a full list) can be a problem. Ph imbalances will manifest symptoms similar to hypoglycemia with one obvious difference. If you have ever felt that you are half in and half out of your body, you are experiencing a Ph imbalance. Ph imbalances are one of the first things that bodies will correct on the proper diet since imbalances in the acid/alkaline levels affect all other functions in the body.

FOOD PERCENTAGES

Work out your food percentages 'by volume'; that is, if you eat 10 cups of food a day, following the Adult ratios below, you would be eating 6 cups of veggies (that's alot!) and 2 cups of those veggies could be raw, 2 cups of fruit, and 2 cups of eggs, yogurt, kefir, sour cream, fish, chicken, maple syrup, and butter.) 'Volume' for salad-type veggies is measured in packed cups.

FOR ADULTS
70% veggies, 20% fruits, 10% everything else and NO raw veggies

To keep the Deep Cleanser a cleansing and healing experience, we have to keep the level of fruits and vegetables high in the diet. Eating too many starches, proteins, sweeteners or oils (foods that require high amounts of enzymes to digest) doesn't give the body a rest. Eating 90% fruits and veggies and 10% everything else puts the body in a cleansing mode without robbing it of vitality.

By the end of this program, the ratio of fruits and veggies to everything else will settle into a regular body pattern. Most adult bodies settle into a maintenance program of 70% fruits and veggies, 30% everything else.

FOR PREGNANT WOMEN
60% veggies, 20% fruits, 20% everything else and No raw veggies (except for juices)

These percentages reflects the higher level of cleansing needed in this Deep Cleanser Diet. But remember, it is only for a month. After that time, you should move up to the Basic Balancer, which includes more proteins.

FOR CHILDREN UNDER 12
20% fruits and veggies, 80% everything else, and No raw veggies (except for juices.)

As you can see, even though the Deep Cleanser is what its name implies, kids still need high levels of foods other than fruits and veggies.

ABOUT RAW FOODS
Raw veggies are very difficult to digest, unless, of course, they are juiced. The cell walls of vegetables are made of cellulose and there is NOTHING in the human body that will break down cellulose except chewing. Externally, juicing or cooking breaks cellulose down. Adelle Davis has a great explanation about the body's ability to get Vitamin A out of a carrot. The raw levels start at 5% and the cooked levels are around 35%! So, for now don't eat any raw veggies. They will start coming back in with the next level diet. I know that there are many people out there who have gone on Raw Food diets that have had wonderful and miraculous healings. I think these raw food plans work because people are taken off all the other foods that are killing them!

I had the opportunity years ago to work with a group of people who had been seriously ill and who had healed themselves with raw foods. But they were seeing me because they were starting to have new illnesses develop. They had all reached points of vitamin, mineral and protein deficiencies that their raw food diets could not heal. They were shocked, to say the least, when I told them it was time to eat foods that were cooked, that they needed some animal proteins and that they were vitamin and mineral deficient!

"But we eat so well," they cried. I had to remind them that cows have four stomachs and chew their cuds (that is, they regurgitate grass and chew and chew and chew it) to break down the cell walls because their bodies don't have enzymes that break cellulose down either!***

NUTRITIONAL RULES
1) Eat every two hours, 2) No shellfish, 3) You can eat fruits with anything except other fruits. Separate different fruits by 1/2 hour, and 4) Beans and legumes must be sprouted.

When I started talking to bodies, I made long lists of all the different nutritional rules I found in the 'popular theory' books. There were only four 'rules' that I found bodies consistently wanted to follow; occasionally I would find a body that fit one of the remaining rules.

1) The first rule you need to follow is eating when you first get up in the morning and then eating something every two hours after that, until you go to bed.

About two hours after you eat something, the simple sugars are pulled out of the intestines and into the bloodstream. So, the sugar levels will naturally start to drop and there lays the problem. When the body is healthy, this drop in the blood sugar level is compensated for and the blood sugar levels are kept even; but, because of the high percentages of hypoglycemia, most people's bodies cannot regulate themselves and hypoglycemic reactions start.

When you eat a little something every two hours, you keep sugars coming from the intestines and this helps keep the blood sugar levels nice and even. As people heal, the times between eating can get elongated; but for now, eat something every two hours. Like I said, this 'eating every two hours' doesn't have to be a meal. If you've got a sweet tooth, a spoonful of maple syrup or a maple syrup candy may do it. A few dates or dried apricots, a slice of sprouted bread, a glass of juice or a real meal will all do just fine.

After a few days of watching the clock and remembering to eat every two hours (set yourself an alarm until it becomes a habit,) you will find that your body will start telling you when the time has passed! It will start screaming at you that *"it is time to eat something!"*

Don't worry about 'getting fat from eating so much.' Remember that many peoples' weight has to do with eating things that can't be digested properly. And following this diet, you will be eating 80% fruits and veggies. You REALLY have to work at putting on weight from eating too many fruits and veggies! Especially since the high calorie foods you can eat, like sour cream and butter and maple syrup, can only be 20% part of your overall diet!

2) Avoid shellfish. They are almost always a problem for the digestive system. See the previous section on Meats for more info.

3) You can eat fruits with anything except other fruits. Separate different fruits by 1/2 hour.

Mixed fruits confuse the pancreas. The only time I have consciously experienced a hypoglycemic reaction was years ago when I was doing my first cookbook. I was working on the beverage section and had three blenders going, with three different fruit smoothies. After going to each blender several times and tasting each of them, I found myself standing in the middle of the kitchen trying to remember why I was there and what I was doing.

An internal voice said, *"You just ate three different fruits and are as hypoglycemic as hell, Silly!"* Oops! I grabbed a bite of protein and went outside and lay on the grass until my sugar level balanced itself out again.

I was amazed that most people have those kinds of hypoglycemic reactions throughout their days. I wondered how people function!!!

4) Beans and legumes must be sprouted. As explained above, unsprouted beans and legumes are indigestible. See the recipe section on beans and legumes for easy directions on how to sprout them.

FOLLOW THROUGH

So, now it's time to skip ahead to Chapter 7, How Do I ....?, which will answer some of the questions that might arise, like How Do I Do This Alone? or With Family?, How Do I Eat Out?, How Do I Reintroduce Foods, or How Do I know What an Emotional Rood Reaction Is?

Read Chapter 8, On Supplements, so you can decide what vitamins and minerals you need to add to your new eating patterns. And read Chapter 9, Special People and Their Situations, if you are pregnant or planning to have a child follow the eating program.

Check out the product lists in the Appendix for more information on all sprouted breads, quinoa pastas, maple syrup candies, and more. Then after a month or two on the Deep Cleanser, when you feel obviously better, move on the Basic Balancer, Chapter 4, and follow that plan.

Now, get to it and enjoy yourself!

Chapter 6
Basic Diet #3, The Super Cleanser

This diet approach is for the Health Assessment Groups three and four, people who are having more serious levels of health problems. Kids and pregnant women should never follow this diet.

FACING FACTS

Face it, if your Health Assessment put you in the third or fourth group, your body is having some troubles! It took you a long time to arrive at this place; so it's going to take you some time to correct it. Relax. You can do it! What's a year or so of concentrated work on your health in comparison to how long it took you to get here?

There's another fact of life that you also need to face; deep level physical problems always have a spiritual, emotional or mental core. Until you look at whatever THAT problem is, nothing you do on a physical level will CURE you.

Oh, yeah, you can do this diet plan and get better. But if you don't deal with the core of the problem, all you really do is push the problem deeper into the body. Eventually, it will resurface as some other serious dis-ease.

So, do the physical level things you can do: eat right, exercise, get massages, and take advantage of all the wonderful healing techniques that are available. Start thinking about what the core issue of this dis-ease might be. Stop being afraid of whatever it is. It's eating you up now. What could be worse?

GETTING INTO IT

Take a look at the Super Cleanser Diet listed below. You will see that instead of listing a YES side and No side as I did on the Basic Balancer and Deep Cleanser, I have only given you a list of the foods you can eat. This list includes only the easiest foods for most bodies to digest.

Remember to trust your own senses. If there is something on this plan that doesn't seem to agree with you, don't eat it! With problems like candida, you may already be experiencing sensitivities and reactions to food. Make what adjustments you need, using the diet as a guideline.

Make a copy of the diet, making what changes you need and put it on the front of the refrigerator.

MAKE A COMMITMENT TO YOURSELF TO DO THIS FOR YOURSELF! AND GET EXCITED! You can get healthy and enjoy yourself at the same time.

Please make note: I don't use the food category called 'carbohydrates.' This group of foods is made up of fruits, veggies, beans, legumes and starches, like grains and soy products. I think it is important to divide this group into individual sections because of some of the future digestive rules you will be following later in the diet.

BASIC DIET #3, THE SUPER CLEANSER

YES FOODS ONLY

FRUITS:
dates, apricots,
avocados only

VEGGIES:
arrowroot
artichokes
asparagus
beets
carrots
celeriac
celery
chives
cranberries
cucumbers
endive
fennel
garlic

greens:
arugula
beet greens

greens cont'd.
chicory
corn salad
dandelion
escarole
radicchio
watercress

Jerusalem artichoke
jicama
lettuce
mustard greens
okra
olives, black

peas:
green
snap
sugar

peppers:
chili or jalapeno
green/red/yellow

poppy seeds
pumpkins
radishes
sorrel
spinach

squash, summer:
crookneck
patty pan
zucchini

squash, winter:
acorn
banana
butternut
delicata
hubbard
spaghetti

Swiss chard
tapioca
wild rice

DAIRY PRODUCTS: eggs and yogurt only

MEATS: fish only

GRAINS: quinoa, quinoa flour and 100% sprouted sourdough bread only

SWEETENERS: maple syrup and stevia only

OILS: butter only

HERBS and SPICES: only use cooking herbs and spices

SPECIAL ITEMS: Carob powder

PERCENTAGES OF FOODS:
> 70%-80% veggies
> 10%-20% fruits
> 10% everything else (eggs, yogurt, fish, maple syrup, stevia and butter.)
> 0% raw veggies except in juice form

SUPPLEMENTS:
> See Chapter 8, On Supplements.

NUTRITIONAL RULES:
> 1) Eat something as soon as you get up in the morning and then eat a little something every two hours after that.
> 2) No shellfish.
> 3) Fruits must be eaten alone. Leave a half hour between different fruits.

BASIC DIET #3, EXPLANATIONS

FRUITS
Dates, Apricots, and Avocados ONLY fresh, cooked, dried or juiced

One of the consistent body symptoms I have seen over the years is hypoglycemia. Bodies that experience sugar imbalances have troubles with fruit sugars. These sugars just digest too quickly and raise the blood sugar level, causing a hypoglycemic reaction.

The fruits listed in the Super Cleanser are the slowest to digest of all the easy-to-digest fruits. For most people, they do not cause sugar reactions, even though some of them, like the dates, are very sweet to the taste. These are the first fruits that baby's bodies like. These fruits can be eaten in any form; dried, fresh, cooked or juiced.

For now, all other fruits are out because they tend to cause hypoglycemic/sugar level reactions. And, by the way, apples and pears are the last fruits to come back into the diet. They seem to have high and quick sugar levels; eating them is like eating spoonfuls of sugar.

Ph imbalances, yeast problems and diabetes, as well as other problems, can all have difficulty with concentrated sugars. These three fruits usually aren't hard on the system, if taken in small amounts. Anyone with yeast problems should only include dates into their diets when they start following the program. One nice thing about dates is that their sugars don't seem to feed yeast in the bloodstream. Try a few bites and see how you feel. Be careful to not over do them!

Avocados aren't really high in sugars and they are easy to digest, so they are usually fine everyone's bodies. But stay away from them if you seem to have difficulty to fatty foods and butter.

VEGGIES

All veggies except: beans in any form, bok choy, broccoli, brussels sprouts,
cabbages, capers, cauliflower, collard greens, corn, eggplant, horseradish, kale, kohlrabi,
leeks, mushrooms, onions, parsnips, potatoes, rutabagas, salisfy, scallions, shallots,
tomatillo, tomatoes, turnips and turnip greens and yams.

Of all the foods we eat, vegetables have more variety in tastes and textures than anything. They can be crisp, crunchy and cold or mushy, smooth and hot. Herbs and spices actually fall into this digestive category and lend themselves very well to their cousins.

Most people think of potatoes and corn as starches; but they are digested by the same enzymes that digest other veggies. But they are still 'starchy' veggies, and it is likely that at this point in your health, your body may still reaction to the 'starchiness.' So stay away from them for now.

You may have noticed that all the other starchy root vegetables and beans are also out of the diet for now. The whole cabbage family needs to be out of the diet; they can all be difficult to digest, causing gas and bloating. Note the whole nightshade family is out as well as a few miscellaneous veggies like capers and mushrooms.

I seriously suggest that you find someone who grows and sells organic veggies and reintroduce yourself to this wondrous family of foods. Check out the new wave of Community Supported Agriculture farms in your area (see Table 7 in the Appendix.) I grow all my veggies and dehydrate or freeze enough to make soups and stews all winter long; the life-force that transfers itself into my body when I eat these veggies is worth all the work.

Remember, veggies are not fattening. You can eat yourself silly with them and have little or no problem, except maybe feeling comfortably stuffed.

Since all the 'No veggies' are known problem areas, stay away from them for awhile, even if you feel that one of them doesn't cause YOU a problem. Wait a few weeks and let your body get settled into the diet program.

Then reintroduce the food and see what happens. If there are no symptoms after a couple of days, eat some more of it and watch again. Then try this, again, for a third time. If you still don't notice any obvious side effects, include the food into your diet; but if you do notice something 'off,' then let that food stay on the NO side for awhile longer. See Table 2 in the Appendix for a list of vegetables.

DAIRY PRODUCTS
Eggs and Yogurt ONLY

ABOUT EGGS

I stick eggs into the dairy products category because they are a protein that needs hydrochloric acid to digest, just like other dairy foods, and they are in the dairy case at the grocery stores. That is where the similarities stop.

Eggs have got a very bad rap by science, big business, the media and the medical profession. It's true that many allergy tests show people are 'allergic' to the albumin that makes up egg whites.

Fortunately, this allergic reaction is quickly cleared when the body is given proper levels of vitamins and minerals. Also, the level of cholesterol in eggs has been sighted as a problem. I have not found this to be a problem at all! When I was just starting to do this work, I met an elderly couple who consulted me specifically about high cholesterol problems.

They had been on a doctor's high cholesterol diet for two years but their cholesterol levels had not gone down. I put them each on a diet that included a dozen eggs a week and butter! Within two months their cholesterol levels started going down and after six months leveled off at normal blood cholesterol readings! Bringing their bodies into balance was the key.

Eggs are one of the easiest proteins to digest. And when taking proper levels of vitamins and minerals, rarely do people have problems with eggs. If you have been told you are allergic to eggs, don't eat them for a couple of weeks. When you feel your system has stabilized itself, try eating a bite or two of a well-cooked egg yolk and white, all by itself. Watch for mucus reactions, stomach or intestinal reactions, headaches or any other subtle or obvious body or emotional reactions. If you do not note any reaction, you can then choose to eat them or not.

ABOUT DAIRY PRODUCTS

The milk molecule is a very complex structure and it takes large amounts of both hydrochloric acid (HCL) and lactose enzymes to properly break it down so that it is usable by the body. Most people are lacking high levels of HCL and lactose enzymes and therefore, have allergic reactions to dairy products.

In the process of making soured and cultured dairy products such as yogurt, kefir, cottage cheese, cream cheese, sour cream, buttermilk and cheeses, the milk molecule is broken down. Yogurt is called 'predigested' because the milk molecule is so thoroughly broken down that little HCL and lactose enzymes are needed in the body to complete the process.

Yogurt can be used as a substitute for milk by diluting it down with water and sweetening it with maple syrup. There is no reason why you can't take yogurt, make yogurt cheese and use them to make yourself a dynamite cheesecake. Check the recipe section for ideas and ENJOY!

If you have yeast problems, all the dairy products need to be excluded from the diet. But if you've got candida, you probably already know that!

MEATS
Fish ONLY

Meats and fish are foods that, like dairy products, take hydrochloric acid in the stomach to break down their molecular structures. High levels of HCL are needed to digest most meats, but fish and chicken are very easy proteins to break down. They only use small amounts of HCL.

All the other meats need higher amounts of HCL to properly digest than you have at the moment, so for now, all meats are out.

Shellfish are a no-no. There are two main problems with them. They live near shore, for one thing; if 'near shore' means near a populated area, then the likelihood is that the toxin levels are high. The second problem with shellfish comes from the protein structure that makes them up.

This particular structure is very hard for most bodies to break down, hence many people's allergic reaction to shellfish.

When you are having this level of problems, it is very important to have digestible proteins. We don't want you to start such a deep level cleanse (with fruits and veggies only) that you get sick. The addition of simple proteins helps keep the pace of the cleanse at a positive level. The addition of fish in the diet also gives the body proteins to rebuild muscle and organ tissues.

I'm not saying you HAVE to eat fish; do eggs or dairy instead. But get some high-quality, easy-to-digest proteins into your body.

NUTS AND SEEDS
Avoid all of them

Take a break from these wonderful taste treats. Nuts and seeds are great sources of proteins, oils and nutrients but they are very difficult to digest; that is, they take large amounts of HCL and bile (the soap-like substance from the liver and gallbladder that breaks down fats.)

Even when nuts and seeds are added back into the diet, I suggest people go light on eating them. I like to use them as complements to other foods, like having a few peanuts with my veggie and quinoa curry or having a few walnuts in my carob or chocolate brownies.

GRAINS
Quinoa, quinoa flour and 100% sprouted SOURDOUGH bread ONLY

Grains have been the basis of civilizations for as far back as people can remember. Grains or starches are digested by a number of enzymes, the major one coming from the pancreas. They are quickly transformed into sugars and give us energy and nutrients. That is, they do if we can digest them properly. Most people can't! I'm not totally clear on how we arrived at this desperate point of ill-health, though I've got a few suspicions.

ABOUT THE PANCREAS AND GRAINS

First, it seems the pancreas needs huge amounts of vitamin B's, for one thing. Now, stress eats up vitamin B's like crazy, so it's not surprising that most people are deficient in them. This deficiency, in itself, would put the pancreas under stress and disable it's functioning.

The second suspicion is pancreatic stress is from sugar. Did you know that at the turn of the century the average intake of sugar was two pounds a year; now that average is running close to 140 pounds!!! I know that I go through 100 pounds of honey a year, most of which goes into my coffee and tea; the point is, sugar amounts add up fast. There is just no way that human bodies can adjust to that level of change without experiencing it as stress.

The third suspicion is spiritual in nature. I think that people and the planet we live on are going through a major growth spurt of our conscious awareness. We are becoming a very small world; and as we become a more connected world, we become aware that the pain and suffering of one living thing becomes the pain and suffering for all of us. This connectedness creates change and it brings us more and more in line with our spiritual selves. Traditionally, the energy field or chakra in the body that connects body and spirit together is centered right over the pancreas. There's no way around it, going through spiritual growth puts the pancreas in stress.

Whether you agree with my spiritual understandings or not, the physical reality seems to be consistent in humans: we are not digesting sugars and starches well.

ABOUT HYPOGLYCEMIA

Now, not being able to digest starches is a major problem even though it is easily corrected, given the proper diet, nutrient intake and time. There is another side effect of this pancreatic stress that is just as important to deal with specifically. When the pancreas is stressed it seems to lose its ability to control one of its other major functions, that is, the release of appropriate amounts of insulin into the bloodstream. Insulin is a hormone that is made by the pancreas and is released on demand. Insulin acts like a waiter, it 'serves' sugar out of the bloodstream and into the cells.

From my work I would guess that 85% of the population is running some level of hypoglycemia or low blood sugar because of pancreatic stress. Typical symptoms for hypoglycemia are: mid-afternoon dips in energy or overall fatigue, spaciness or the lack of ability to concentrate, craving foods and sugars, mood swings, irritability and snappiness, headaches, depression and dizziness.

If you have one or more of these symptoms, it's likely that you are hypoglycemic. For information on this situation, see the chapter Dis-ease and Discomfort and its section on hypoglycemia.

Taking starches out of the diet relieves the stress the pancreas is under and immediately problems like those listed above start to clear. Patience is needed here because even though symptoms may clear quickly, it may take a year or more to really heal the pancreas. BUT, following the right diet should start changing the symptoms somewhere within a few days and up to two weeks, so that you don't have to deal with the symptoms as your pancreas heals.

ABOUT SPROUTED GRAINS

For most people once a grain has been sprouted, their bodies recognize it as a vegetable and no longer as a starch that requires pancreatic enzymes. But, when bodies reach a certain point of ill-health, they will react to the starchy molecules of sprouted grains as if they were regular grains. Therefore, eating sprouted grains and sprouted grain products will stress your pancreas now.

There is, however, usually one sprouted product that will not cause starch reactions at this point in your healing process, and, that is 100% sprouted sourdough products. Usually people with yeast problems will not have problems with sourdough yeasts, for some reason. So definitely, give it a try.

See Table 3 in the Appendix for information on this kind of product. You can make french toast with sprouted sourdough bread, use it for toast, a pie crust, or make a 'stuffing' or coating for fish.

ABOUT QUINOA

Quinoa is a wonder food! It's a small 'grain' that looks like millet (or bird seed) but comes from an herb plant similar to lamb's quarters. It acts like a grain but it digests as a fruit!! You can cook it just like rice, in about 20 minutes; you can use the flour to make brownies and muffins and pancakes; you can use quinoa flakes to make cereals; and cooked quinoa makes great Tabouli-type salads, all this and it digests with the same enzymes that digest fruits! Using quinoa does not trigger the pancreas to produce or release pancreatic enzymes. So here's a food that will fill the space created by not using regular starches.

For now you will need to avoid all pastas. Unfortunately, the quinoa pastas have corn in them. And I've never run across any pastas that fall within this diet's range.

If you DON'T have EBV, candida or any metal poisoning, stay away from sprouted grain products for one month and, then try to introduce them into your diet. If you DO have one of these problems, stay away from sprouted grains for at least two months.

Every once in awhile, I will find quinoa is too alkaline for certain body-types. If you try quinoa and it does NOT set well, try cooking it in water with grated lemon rind. This practice brings the acidity level up and helps balance the ph, making quinoa easily digestible for everyone.

SWEETENERS
100% Maple Syrup and Stevia

Are you shocked? Most people are! But bodies love maple syrup (and taste buds don't normally complain, either!.) It seems that maple syrup is very slow to digest so it doesn't cause a sugar rush in the bloodstream. Hypoglycemics can usually take spoonfuls of maple syrup without reactions and when candida levels are low, this sugar doesn't seem to feed the yeasts. Check it out for yourself. Many the recipes in this book use maple syrup, so don't deny those cravings for something sweet. Just give it the right sweetener and other ingredients!

There is a problem with all the other natural sweeteners at this point in your diet. They are just too quickly absorbed into the bloodstream. While you are sorting out whether you are hypoglycemic or not, using maple syrup will help keep the blood sugar level nice and even.

ABOUT STEVIA

Stevia is an herb that grows in Peru and is so sweet to the taste that a small flake (the size of a parsley flake) on the tip of the tongue will make you think you just took a spoonful of sugar!

There has been some FDA problems with stevia that are in flux and change as I write this. The FDA banned importing stevia unless it was already in a tea blend or in extract form. Even in extract form, it could not be brought into the country as a sugar substitute. But things are changing. Now I hear people can find loose leaf stevia in some herb and health food stores. And you can still buy stevia extract and stevia in white powder form. See Table 3 in the Appendix for sources. Check out Donna Gates' *The Body-Ecology Diet* and Nicole Walker's *Sugarfree Cooking* for more information and recipes.

Stevia extract has a slight molasses taste and it is extremely sweet. A drop or two in a cup of tea is equal to a spoonful of other sweeteners yet it will not cause sugar reactions in the bloodstream.

OILS
100% real butter only

Well, if the maple syrup didn't have you going, this one probably will! I was shocked, too. When I first started doing diet work-ups, butter would repeatedly be the only oil that someone could use.

And after I saw people getting well, saw cholesterol levels dropping, and heard healing stories from clients, I had to let my surprise go.

When you stop and think about it, the concentrated oils that we use, whether they come from vegetables, nuts and seeds, or animals, are not natural. It makes sense to me that our bodies would recognize and deal with butter as a molecular structure it has dealt with before, in milk.

There are numerous studies that show hydrogenated oils to be indigestible and very hard on the system. All the oils that are firm or solid like margarines have been hydrogenated; I suggest that you do NOT eat them, ever. Check out what Adelle Davis had to say about this even twenty years ago in *Let's Eat Right to Keep Fit*.

In general, we have to start thinking about fats in a totally different way. Our bodies need a certain amount of oils in the diet to supply, digest and utilize fat-soluble vitamins, linoleic acid, and the two vitamin B's cholin and inositol. The fats just need to be healthy and usable. So enjoy using a little butter (1-2 sticks a week)! Sweet (unsalted) and lightly salted are recommended.

SOY PRODUCTS
All soy products are out

All soy products come from soybeans. Beans are digested as starches so they take pancreatic enzymes to break down; since most people initially have difficulty making enough of these enzymes, soy products present some problems. So, for now, take tofu, soy cheese, tempeh, soy powders and soy milk out of the diet. People with more serious health problems need to also stay away from fermented foods, and so, miso or tamari are also out of the diet for now.

BEANS AND LEGUMES
All sprouted beans and legumes are out

Beans and legumes (lentils and peas) are notorious gas producers. Any time a food causes gas, it means it is rotting and putrefying in the intestines. The reason beans do this is simple, human bodies do not have the enzymes needed to digest them. When beans are growing, they are full of vegetable sugars, but when these beans are dried, the sugars are converted into a starch. Our bodies do not have the enzymes needed to break down that starch and it seems that we don't have the ability to develop these enzymes, either. For centuries South American peoples have eaten beans and their bodies STILL get gas.

When the body is operating with serious problems, the overall digestive level usually cannot handle even sprouted beans and legumes. Sometimes the problem with them is the increased possibility of molds and funguses.

Like the sprouted grains, stay away from sprouted beans and legumes for a month or so and then try introducing them into the diet. Watch for body and mucus reactions. And try different kinds of beans. Sometimes a person will have terrible problems with, say, sprouted kidney beans and not with sprouted garbanzos. Go the section on 'Beans and Legumes' in the Super Cleanser diet to learn more about sprouted beans and legumes, when you are ready to reintroduce them. Also see the recipe section on how to sprout them and cook with them.

HERBS AND SPICES
All herbs and spices should be out for one month

This whole category is enormous. All these dried plants are treated as veggies by the body and most people don't have any problems with them. When I have seen troubles in this area, it usually has had to do with blood chemistry problems. I suspect that you may have a blood chemistry imbalance along with other problems that you are manifesting, so for now, don't use any herbs or spices for a month or more. Then start slowly introducing them back into your diet, one at a time. The kind of symptoms you may experience if your blood chemistry is out of balance are: quick reactions to smells, like perfumes or Freon, quick reactions to sugars, herbs, or certain foods, a sense that you are not always completely in your body, rapid up and down swings of energy, and/or mental or emotional confusion.

A word about salt. Salt is one of those nutrients that is essential to life and our bodies crave it. But like all out-of-balance cravings, the desire for too much salt indicates an imbalance in the body usually linked to mineral deficiencies. So, how much salt is too much? The general rule seems to be a range of salt on a weekly basis, somewhere between 1/4 tsp. to 1/2 tsp. I suggest that you claim your own salt shaker, fill it once a week and use it sparingly until it's gone.

And I can hear some of your howls! I'll never forget the friend who was riding in my back seat when she asked me how much salt her body wanted. When I relayed the information, she was immediately in the front seat, screaming *"What?"*

The body needs a balance of minerals, including sodium. But bodies prefer having these nutrients delivered in natural forms, from food. Cut back on the salt for awhile, a few weeks, then try some salty food you use to eat. As your body comes to balance, your taste buds will balance out too.

If you feel you need an antibiotic, I recommend use of propolis, a product that bees gather from plants. It acts as a natural antibiotics as well as being antiviral, antifungal, antimicrobial and antibacterial. Propolis is resinous, which makes it hard for the body to digest; so I recommend taking it in extract or tincture form. See the section on Herbs in the Supplement Chapter for more information.

When you start reintroducing herbs and spices, be sure to read the Herbs and Spice section in the Basic Balancer or Super Cleanser Diet Explanations.

SPECIALTY FOODS
Carob powder is a YES, NO Coffee, Chocolate, Alcohol,
NO Brewer's and Nutritional Yeast, NO Vinegar or Condiments

ABOUT CAROB

Carob beans come from the pod of an evergreen tree that grows in the Mediterranean. It's touted as a chocolate substitute, though you won't find many chocolate lovers that agree with that.

Carob digests as a protein and it is a very easy-to-digest one. Check out the suggestions in Table 1 about this fun food and the recipes for Carob-Quinoa brownies.

Skip the carob chips for now, the oils in them are intense.

ABOUT COFFEE

Coffee is out for now. Coffee is a wonderful beverage but it has it's difficulties. It is out of the Basic Diets, but take heart, it will come back into the diet if you want it. Coffee has a number of problems. First, there are some very strong, natural chemicals in it that can upset the blood chemistry and slow down the healing process. This is why coffee is out of the Basic Diets. Second, the way that we make coffee, by pouring hot water directly on the grounds, creates some serious body reactions.

When hot water comes in contact with coffee grounds, it leaches out all the oils and the acids. These two substances create digestive problems; the oils are indigestible and the acids conflict with the natural stomach acids. The acids and oils also interact with the caffeine, creating most of the negative side effects people experience from coffee and associate with caffeine.

There is a better way to brew coffee and you can read about it in Beverage section of the Recipes. But for now, stay away from coffee.

ABOUT CHOCOLATE

Chocolate is out for now. Like coffee, chocolate has some harsh natural chemicals that can slow down the healing process. And the natural oils, the cocoa butter, demands high quality and high levels of bile to break down, making it a food you want to avoid while you do the Basic Diets. And, again, like coffee, chocolate can come back into the diet, though it will need to be dealt with carefully.

ABOUT ALCOHOL

Alcohol is out for now. This restriction usually doesn't raise an eyebrow. We've all come to a cultural agreement that alcohol is 'a problem.' Remember that bodies don't carry that kind of judgment and eventually most bodies can deal with alcohol, with a little extra nutrient help. But some bodies and psyches have very physical problems with alcohol. Read the section on Alcohol in Chapter 10, Dis-Ease and Dis-Comfort.

ABOUT SUPPLEMENTAL YEASTS

Brewer's yeast, which is the yeast by-product of making beer, and nutritional yeast, a yeast grown on molasses are great sources of vitamin B's and of other nutrients, but they are digested as proteins. They take large amounts of HCL to digest and therefore, cause problems for most people.

Few people use these supplements because they don't like the taste. But mixed with the right foods, these yeasts can be wonderful (I can't imagine my popcorn butter not having brewers yeast in it!) For now, let them alone.

ABOUT VINEGAR

The problem with vinegar is its acidity level. When your system gets out of balance, the Ph (acid/alkaline) balance suffers and becomes 'delicate.' Vinegar can throw this delicate situation into a tail spin so it is important to avoid it for now. Even the small amounts of vinegar in the condiments (catsup, prepared mustard, horseradish and pickles) can be a problem. Ph imbalances manifest symptoms similar to hypoglycemia with one obvious difference. If you have ever felt you are half in and half out of your body, you are experiencing a Ph imbalance. Ph imbalances are one of the first things bodies will correct on the proper diet since imbalances in acid/alkaline levels affect all other functions in the body. See Table 2, Appendix for a list of these foods.

FOOD PERCENTAGES

Work out your food percentages 'by volume'; that is, if you eat 10 cups of food a day, following the Adult ratios below, you would be eating 6 cups of veggies (that's alot!) and 2 cups of those veggies could be raw, 2 cups of fruit, and 2 cups of eggs, yogurt, kefir, sour cream, fish, chicken, maple syrup, and butter.)

FOR ADULTS ONLY
70%-80 veggies, 10% fruits, 10%-20% everything else, NO raw veggies except juices

To keep the Super Cleanser a cleansing and healing experience, we have to keep the level of fruits and vegetables high in the diet. If you feel that you want more of a cleanse, eat 90% fruits and veggies and 10% everything else, with no raw foods for the first month, except for juices. By the end of this program, the ratio of fruits and veggies to everything else will settle into a regular body pattern. Most adult bodies settle into a maintenance program of 70% fruits and veggies, 30% everything else.

NUTRITIONAL RULES
1) Eat as soon as you get up in the morning and every two hours after that time, 2) No shellfish,
3) Eat fruits all by themselves, except for avocados. Separate different fruits
by 1/2 hour, and 4) All beans and legumes are out for now.

When I started talking to bodies, I made long lists of all the different nutritional rules I found in the 'popular theory' books. There were only four 'rules' that I found bodies consistently wanted to follow; occasionally I would find a body that fit one of the remaining rules.

1) The first rule you need to follow is eating when you first get up in the morning and then eating something every two hours after, until you go to bed. About two hours after you eat something, the simple sugars are pulled out of the intestines and into the bloodstream. So, sugar levels will naturally start to drop and there lays the problem. When the body is healthy, this drop in the blood sugar level is compensated for and the blood sugar levels are kept even; but, because of the high percentages of hypoglycemia, most people's bodies cannot regulate themselves and hypoglycemic reactions start.

When you eat a little something every two hours, you keep sugars coming from the intestines and this helps keep the blood sugar levels nice and even. As people heal, the times between eating can get elongated; but for now, eat something every two hours. This 'eating every two hours' doesn't have to be a meal. If you've got a sweet tooth, a spoonful of maple syrup or a maple syrup candy may do it. A few dates or dried apricots, a slice of sprouted bread, a glass of juice or a real meal will all do just fine.

After a few days of watching the clock and remembering to eat every two hours (set yourself an alarm until it becomes a habit,) you will find your body will start telling you when the time has passed! It will start screaming at you that "it is time to eat something!" Don't worry about 'getting fat from eating so much.' Remember many peoples' weight has to do with eating things that can't be digested properly. And following this diet, you will be eating 80% fruits and veggies. You REALLY have to work at putting on weight from eating too many fruits and veggies! Especially since the high calorie foods you can eat, like sour cream, butter and maple syrup, can only be 20% part of your overall diet!

2) Avoid shellfish. They are almost always a problem for the digestive system. And the possibility of high toxin levels is there because of where the grow.

3) Fruits need to be eaten by themselves for awhile. They tend to speed the digestive system and you don't need that situation developing at this time in your healing process. Also separate different fruits by 1/2 hour. Mixed fruits confuse the pancreas. The only time I have consciously experienced a hypoglycemic reaction was years ago when I was doing my first cookbook. I was working on the beverage section and had three blenders going, with three different fruit smoothies. After going to each blender several times and tasting each, I found myself standing in the middle of the kitchen trying to remember why I was there and what I was doing. An internal voice said, *"You just ate three different fruits and are as hypoglycemic as hell, Silly!"* Oops! I grabbed a bite of protein and went outside and lay on the grass until my sugar level balanced itself out again. I was amazed that most people have those kinds of hypoglycemic reactions throughout their days. I wondered how people function!!!

4) All beans and legumes are out of the diet for now. See the explanation section above for more information.

THE NEXT STAGE

I suggest you follow this diet plan for one to three months, depending on how out-of-balance you feel you are. Trust your own knowingness. When you start to feel better, congratulate yourself; then continue on with that plan for another couple of weeks or more. When you really feel your body has 'turned the corner,' that it really is moving in the right direction, then upgrade yourself to the Deep Cleanser Diet. Gradually add those YES foods into your diet, following the instructions in the 'How Do I Reintroduce Foods' section. Remember, the problems your body is having will take some time to heal themselves. And you must deal with the emotional aspects of your specific problems as well. So, be patient with yourself, don't take any of life too seriously, and let yourself heal on all levels.

FOLLOW THROUGH

So, now it's time to skip ahead to Chapter 7, How Do I .....?, which will answer some of the questions that might arise, like How Do I Do This Alone? or With Family?, How Do I Eat Out?, How Do I Reintroduce Foods? or How Do I Know What an Emotional Food Reaction Is? Read Chapter 8, On Supplements, so you can decide what vitamins and minerals you need to add to your new eating patterns. And read Chapter 9, Special People and Their Situations, if you are pregnant or planning to have a child follow the eating program.

Check out the product lists in the Appendix for more information on all sprouted breads, quinoa pastas, maple syrup candies and more.

Go to Chapter 10 and read about your specific area of Dis-Ease and Dis-Comfort, so that you can incorporate suggestions from there into your new eating plan.

Now, get to it and enjoy yourself!

Chapter 7
How Do I ......?

HOW DO I KNOW HOW MUCH WATER TO DRINK?

Our bodies are mostly water; water that is in constant motion and flow into us, through us and back out of us. Without some regular intake of water, we'd all eventually die. But just how much is enough? There are some 'theories' out there that say, *"You should"* (I always get nervous when I hear that word 'should') *"You should drink eight glasses of pure water every day."*

Guess what? I have asked lots of bodies about this belief and some of them have actually said they needed that much water. But, many more of them have said that they needed a whole lot less! Four to six cups is more common.

Some bodies say they want pure water to meet their daily needs for water and others say that they consider the water they get in foods, like juices and soups, to be part of the total intake needed. One of the things you have to be aware of concerning water consumption is the reality that some vitamins and minerals are water-soluble; that is, they break down in water, are carried into the body in water, and get flushed out of the body in water. Adelle Davis cites a number of studies in *Let's Eat Right to Keep Fit* that show the harm that can be done to the body by drinking too much water!

So, how do you decide how much water you need? Drink when you are thirsty! There is a very intricate system in your body that triggers the response-need for water. Let it work for you. All you need to do is obey it when it directs you to drink something. Then, have a glass of water. If that satisfies the thirst, great. If it doesn't satisfy you, try something else, like a glass of juice or a cup of tea. If that doesn't do it, try taking a tablet of kelp or a piece of seaweed. It may be your body needs some minerals to balance and hold the liquid.

I know my body doesn't need eight glasses of water on a daily basis. On dry, arid days in New Mexico, I can drink water (and pee it right back out) all day long and still be thirsty. On the other hand, I can open a beer, sip on it for hours and have my thirst quenched! (Obviously, I don't mind warm beer in the least.) Now, I'm not saying that you should run out and do the same thing. What I am saying is, find out what works in YOUR body! Try different things and see what comes naturally for you. And if you find that sometime in the future, the pattern changes, watch it, see if it indicates a problem or not and go on from there.

Needs for water can change just with the seasons changing or with the lunar cycles waxing and waning. They can change with age and activity. They can change when you move from one area to another. There is another consideration you have to take into account. If you are cleansing and releasing toxins into the bloodstream, you NEED to drink enough water to keep toxins flowing out of your body or you may experience constipation! Remember, if you are having to force yourself to drink water because you THINK it's good for you, get out of your head and back into your body. Trust yourself. You are the one who lives in there!

HOW DO I DO THIS ALONE?

Human nature has a humorous side to it. People are in constant RE-action to their fellow humans' intentions. One of these reaction scenarios you may find when you follow this program is other peoples' desire to get you to eat something off the diet. It's like they feel superior if you 'fall off the wagon.' Don't worry about it one way or the other. If you give in to temptation and eat something off the diet, at least enjoy it while you do it. So it makes you feel crappy, so what? Let that become an impetus to stay with the program and feel good. Just try to limit your indulgences to once a week!

Even now, if I eat something I know will be a body stress, I fill it with gold light (as in, blessing it) and then proceed to thoroughly enjoy it!

If you live alone, you already know life has fewer distractions in it and following a program like this can be relatively easy. But, being human, it is likely that you need a support system. So ask a good friend to do the program with you; then you can share ideas for meals, actually go to someone's house to eat who understands what you need to ingest without giving you flak, and you can share the changes happening in your bodies and lives.

HOW DO I DO THIS WITH A FAMILY?

When you are the brave one in the family, the one who does the new things first, it can be a lonely place. And trying to stay with the program while you are fixing meals for the rest of the family can be REALLY difficult. Here are a few tricks:

**Cook a bunch of food for yourself once a week so that you don't have to think about your own meal planning so much.

**Before you start cooking family meals, eat something that is within your program. You will be less likely to fall to temptation if your body is already feeling satisfied. One of the worst things you can do to yourself in these situations is try to cook on an empty stomach!

**Make sure that you have decadent treats for yourself. "Ooh" and "Ah" over them as you enjoy them. Let the rest of the family know that you are treating yourself, not denying yourself!

**Make as many of the family meals fall within your diet range as possible. They can all happily live with chicken and veggies and quinoa instead of steak, rice and veggies for awhile.

Remember, being the brave one means you are the one creating the pathway to health for the whole family. You don't have to try to talk them (or anyone else, for that matter) into believing you are doing the 'right' thing. Get yourself healthy and let THAT show them. I have never advertised for clients. My clients have always been my advertising! After a couple of months on the program, people start walking up to them and saying things like, *You look great! What are you doing?"*

HOW DO I FOLLOW THE PROGRAM AND EAT OUT?

There's no way around it, some things on the menu are definitely going to be out for awhile. But that doesn't mean you can't have a good time!

One of things you can do is scout out restaurants that will tend to have a wider variety of dishes. Chinese places are good examples. You can choose from a large number of veggie and chicken dishes, as well as fish. Just don't eat the rice, noodles or cookies and you'll be fine. Oh, and watch the sauces.

Ask for substitutions. A chicken and rice dinner can become a chicken and baked potato dinner with a simple request. Or ask for more veggies or a bowl of soup in place of the rice.

Check out the vegetarian restaurants in town. Some of these places can just be dynamite! And check out the breakfast places for omelettes and potatoes. Some Southwestern and Mexican food restaurants will have chicken enchiladas in corn tortillas, just ask for them without the cheese.

One kind of food that is usually out for awhile is Italian. It's rare to find things on the menu that don't have some kind of pasta in them, but check out the places you love. Maybe they can come up with something spectacular for you.

Usually the hidden things you need to watch out for are the lousy oils and margarines restaurants use, the salad dressings, the sauces, chemicals that are added to foods like MSG and citric acid, and waitpersons who won't be up front with you about what's in some food or other.

If you really want to check out what the menu has to offer, ask for a bite of the foods you are interested in! Then do a 'mucus reaction' test on them!

Forget about eating desserts out, for now. It's very unlikely that you will find a commercial dessert made with the ingredients you can have. Just make sure that you follow an evening out with a dessert party at home! (Check out some of the decadent recipes in the back of the book!)

HOW DO I FOLLOW THE PROGRAM AND TRAVEL?

Obviously, following the eating-out suggestions above is a place to start. Remember, travelling is a high level stress! Even if you love where you're going and love what you're doing, there are so many stresses on your system, it's hard to count them! You're not sleeping in your own bed and it's likely you don't have your own pillow with you. (I always travel with mine.) Your whole day's normal rhythm is off and it's possible you're not even in the same time zone anymore! Your eating schedule is probably different, let alone your activity schedule.

One of the hardest things on your body at this point is to eat different foods. The closer you can stick to the diet plan you are on at the moment, the better. Doing the Basic Balancer or the Deep Cleanser while you travel would be great since they're good stress reducing diets. You will find that you will have MORE energy for enjoying the rest of the experience by treating your body well.

If you are going to a place where you will have more control over your food than checking out menus, do some preparation for yourself. Take foods along with you that you might have a hard time finding in a regular market, like sprouted grain breads or quinoa. Carry some dried fruits or fresh ones for the first day or two you're travelling. If you're driving some place, take a cooler along; yogurt, sour cream and butter will travel well for a few days, at least. And you can always bag up some carob brownies; who cares if they get smashed? Even the crumbs will be great!

The important thing is to think ahead and plan to be good to yourself! Take extra vitamin and minerals to aid the clearing of the stress without taking nutrients away from your healing process.

There are some precautions you can take while you travel so you don't pick up parasites. Check out the information on parasites in Chapter 10 in the section on Colitis and Other Intestinal Distress.

HOW DO I REINTRODUCE FOODS INTO MY DIET?

"Gradually" is the answer to the above question. Once your body experienced difficulty digesting a particular food, it established a 'negative rapport' with that food. Once that pattern was established, your body immediately embarked on a certain course of action whenever that food was ingested. It probably had mucus reactions, allergic reactions or other stress and toxin reactions.

Taking this particular food out of the diet for a time doesn't guarantee that your body just forgets the reaction patterns it established. If your body was only experiencing minor problems with that food, then it may still remember how to properly react and digest it by putting out the right amount of enzymes. So it may just accept the reintroduced food like an old friend.

On the other hand, your body may have totally 'forgotten' the proper way of digesting that particular food. Your body may need to be reintroduced to the food in a gentle and gradual manner so that it can establish a new blueprint or pattern.

Follow these simple instructions when you reintroduce any foods into your diet:

1) Hold the food without eating it. Just imagine yourself ingesting it and enjoying it. Imagine your body recognizing the food and remembering how to digest and utilize it WITHOUT any stress reactions.

2) If you have mental or emotional reactions to the food as you are holding it, don't eat it!! You may find yourself saying, "I CAN'T eat this." or "This can't be good for me!" or you may feel nauseated, weak or headachy. These reactions only indicate you are not ready to reintroduce that food yet.

3) If you do not register any reaction to the food, then take a small bite of it. Again, watch your body for reactions. Did you get a mucus build up? Or sneeze? Or feel nauseated? Review the section on mucus reactions on page 16.

4) If you had only pleasant reactions to the food, then eat a little more all by itself. This helps your body reestablish a new blueprint for digesting and utilizing the food.

5) The next time you eat this food, do it in combination with other foods that you know you have no problems with. Be sure to follow all the nutritional rules on that particular diet. Again, watch and see if any reactions manifest.

If there are no reactions, you may assume that your body has successfully reintroduced that food and you may continue to include it in your diet. If you have any reactions at any point along this reintroducing process, you may be having an emotional reaction to the food as well as a physical reaction. Be sure and read the next section on emotional reactions of foods.

HOW DO I KNOW WHAT AN EMOTIONAL REACTION TO FOOD IS?

Emotional reactions to food are fairly wide spread. And *"What exactly is an emotional food reaction?"* you ask. I can answer that best by explaining how they happen.

Years ago I had a client, a ten-year old, who had major emotional reactions to food. His body said he could digest and assimilate a number of things he had serious reactions to when he did eat them. I got that he was having emotional reactions to the foods; then, I got the full story from his parents.

This kid had been taken away from his natural mother because of neglect. She was having serious drug and alcohol problems and was not feeding this two-year old. He was surviving by raiding his neighbors garbage cans!! That's why social services was called in the first place!

One of his major emotional reactions as a ten-year-old was to strawberries; as I listened to his adopted mom's story, I started getting pictures of him eating rotting and molding berries from the trash. That's sickening enough to make anyone develop emotional reactions to foods!!!

One of my ex-husbands had an obvious food reaction. He hated coconut with a passion. One day I was talking to his mother about making something special for a dinner we were planning for him and she suggested a coconut cream pie.

I said, *"But he hates coconut."* And through her laughter, she said, *"Oh, he still has THAT?"* She went on to explain that when he was seven, he had eaten a bunch of coconut just before he came down with the stomach flu. He had thrown all the coconut back up and had been sick for three days. But in his seven-year-old brain, he had decided that *"Coconut makes me sick!"* and he had been living that reality out for years!!! Mom said that she had repeatedly tried to convince him that he had only had the flu. She thought he would eventually just 'grow out of it.'

Obviously, it doesn't take much to cement a reaction into the body! I mean, I have always had the visual of a small girl sitting at the kitchen table eating something; in walks her Dad and he's upset about something. He tells her Mom and she also gets upset. Maybe voices are raised. Maybe tears are shed. But the next few bites of food the little girl ingests are the ones that can implant the emotional reactions in her body; from that point on, every time she eats that particular food, she may feel upset and never know why.

Emotional reactions within the body can happen on other levels besides food. Here's another great example of emotional reactions. I was out clothes shopping with a girlfriend one day (a rarity for me) and we were having a hilarious time. All of a sudden she went into a tail spin of depression; and, it was present in a flash. I asked her what was wrong, but she didn't know, though she had recognized the sudden change. I psychically looked at the reaction and realized it had to do with a smell. Moments before a woman had walked by with very strong lilac perfume on and the reaction was linked to that.

So I explained it to my friend and watched her face fall as she realized what had triggered her depression. She said that her grandmother had beaten her regularly and she always wore lilac perfume!!! The association had been made in her body and thereafter every time she smelled lilac perfume it brought up all the fears and reactions of being beaten. Once she worked on disassociating the smell from the past, she no longer had the reaction.

Here's a few key things to watch for to identify emotional food reactions:

1) Note that strong feelings about a particular food may indicate an emotional reaction pattern. If you passionately dislike something it's a good bet you have attached a negative emotional association to the food. Of course, frequently, food 'dislikes' can also be a clear message from the body that you are physically allergic to a particular food. My body is 'allergic' to vinegar because it is so acidic

but I found I just avoided eating things with vinegar in them. I just didn't care for the taste. That's not the same as having an emotional reaction to it.

2) If there seems to be NO logical reason for your body to have a reaction to a particular food, then it may be an emotional reaction.

3) If you notice that whenever you eat, say, banana squash, you always feel heavy or depressed later but you don't have any problem with acorn or hubbard squash or delicatas, then you can start looking for an emotional reaction.

Say you are eating all of the different fruits with no negative reactions, but don't feel so good when you eat peaches. That is definitely a reaction that is not linked to digestion or assimilation; all the fruits need basically the same amount of enzymes to break them down with ease so it's not a digestion problem. And there are similar sugar-content fruits in the group so it's not a hypoglycemic/diabetic problem.

Similar foods tend to have similar reactions. Red meats as a group are harder to digest than poultry meats. If you only react to one food in a group, then, it's likely you are having an emotional reaction.

4) If contact with a particular food 'pulls' you out of the present and into some floaty sense of the past, it's likely there's a reaction. When I have talked with someone about an emotional reaction and identified the food, they will frequently have images pop in their heads about it. All of a sudden they remember what the emotional reaction was in response to. I can't remember how many times I have heard someone say, *"I know exactly where this comes from!"* And then proceed to tell me their story. As the pictures roll by, people will also have other memories 'click' into place and they'll say, *"Oh, now that old pattern makes sense."* Some odd personal behavior finally takes on reason and makes sense!

Besides these four general areas, anything can happen. People are very creative in their interpersonal communications, so you may create any number of physical responses to emotionally reactive food. For example, some foods may always give you nightmares and that may be an emotional reaction.

Whatever you experience, if you have a repetitive reaction to a food, DON'T EAT IT!!! Follow the guidelines in the next section and learn how to disassociate the emotion from the food. Once the food is free of this connection, you will most likely be able to eat it again. The little survivor who ate out of trash cans I mentioned earlier reprogrammed his association with strawberries and now eats them without breaking out in a rash.

HOW DO I DEAL WITH AN EMOTIONAL REACTION TO FOOD?

Reprogramming the brain is relatively simple. It just takes a little concentrated effort and understanding. Once you have identified an emotionally reactive food, or you suspect a particular food, you can run through the simple guidelines below. I suggest only dealing with one food at a time. The whole process will take from 5 to 15 days, so you can finish with one reaction and then start dealing with another. Have some of the 'offending' food available. It doesn't need to be much, just a handful. Usually foods are not 'case sensitive'; that is, if you are dealing with a emotional reaction to oats, you can hold whole oats or rolled oats or oat flour and have the same basic reactions. If you do have a 'case sensitive' reaction then deal with it in it's specific form.

1) To start the process, set aside a few minutes every day to devote to this pattern change.

2) At that time create a quiet space where you won't be disturbed. (In a busy household, sometimes the bathroom is a good place to hide away for a few minutes.)

3) Take a couple of deep breaths and relax. Step away from everything else in your life and put your focus on your body.

4) Pick up the chosen food and hold it in your hands. You will be holding it for the next four to five minutes. Just let yourself become aware of any body sensations or reactions. You might feel a knot developing in your stomach. Or you might get cold. Your shoulders might get tight. You might feel spacy, dizzy or sick to your stomach. You might hear yourself thinking negative thoughts. And you might see flashes of memory. Just watch and observe the sensations.

5) Do this routine every day until no new reactions appear, or you are only getting reruns. Three to five days is the average time people take on this part of the process.

6) Once you feel you have all the information (reactions) you are going to get, then visualize separating the reactions from the food. A food shouldn't make you want to get up and run away or tighten your shoulders into knots or any of the other reactions you have noted. Let the reactions remain in the past situation where they belong! Visualize pushing them into the past.

7) Repeat the process of holding the food daily. Watch for the reactions. If any of them are still there, work on separating them from the food. Visualize the food free and clear of any reactions. See it for what it is, a wondrous creation in the universe. Repeat this process for at least 3 days.

8) Once you feel the reactions are totally separated from the food, then eat a little of it. Again, watch for reactions. If you don't see any reactions, eat a little more. If you do see reactions go back to #6 and separate the food from the emotions again. Wait a day or two and eat some more of the food.

9) You can go back and repeat the whole process or parts of it as needed. If the food is still giving you trouble, don't eat it for a month or two and then repeat the whole procedure. Just because you think it's time to deal with an issue, doesn't mean that your body or the universe are in agreement!

HOW DO I EAT AS A VEGETARIAN AND STAY HEALTHY?

To be a complete vegetarian and stay healthy, you have to keep your vitamin and mineral levels out of deficiency ranges. And to do that, you have to read and understand about them and how they work in the body, as well as really being in touch with your body's messages. See the appendix for book suggestions.

You can't assume that you will get all the nutrients you need without some concentrated effort on your part. Being a complete vegetarian means taking alot more responsibility for your body's needs than people who include eggs, dairy, fish and meats in their diets. But, it is quite possible.

I was a vegetarian for five years because my body and Spirit wanted me to get lighter. I have no moral problems with eating meat; hearing carrots scream as they are pulled from the ground by some unconscious gardener took care of any moral reasons. But meats are heavy in the system and I needed to get used to a lighter, internal physical feeling.

During this period, I was a fire fighter for the US Forest Service and never lacked for energy. I spent five days out in a 'spike camp' once. That's where they fly you in a helicopter and leave you until the job is done. I ate everyone else's apples, cookies and peanut butter sandwiches because steaks and bologna sandwiches were the only other choices! And I still had more energy than most of the crew.

Then I ran into a problem with being a vegetarian after living in Santa Fe for nine months. I was doing massive amounts of spiritual growth and going along just fine until I had to move from one house to another. Suddenly, I just couldn't pick up my packing boxes; all my strength had drained away.

That night I went out to eat at a Japanese restaurant. As I looked over the menu, an internal voice said, *"Number 4. Eat it. You need it."* I about dropped out of the chair. Number 4 was Chicken Teriyaki!

I asked my guidance directly, *"What was that?"* and the response came back the same, *"Number 4. Eat it. You need it."* One of the things I've always done is follow my guidance, so I ordered and ate the chicken. And much to my surprise, my body loved it. I mean, I thought I would never eat meat again! There had been times that just smelling it had made me nauseated! But here I was eating chicken!

The next day I sat down and asked Spirit what was going on with this meat-eating thing and I heard, *"You are just getting too spacy from the spiritual work you have done. It's time to eat meat again as a way to stay more connected with your body. We want you to eat meat two to three times a week."*

I had to laugh! Growth had come full circle; first I was told to avoid meat to get more spiritual and then I was told to eat meat so I could continue to do my spiritual work!

Over the years I have seen this pattern vary; sometimes my body wants meat every day for four to five days and then it may not want any for weeks at a time.

I suggest that you follow your heart and body on the subject of eating meat and keep your mental processes out of the picture. Remember, what you need to eat in nutrients is linked back in time to what your ancestors ate. And remember, bodies like moderation.

Following this diet plan can be easier for you as a vegetarian than it is for other people because you are already in the habit of using veggies in a variety of ways. To make sure that you get enough protein, make sure that you eat enough quinoa and sprouted beans and legumes, at least until the other proteins, like nuts and seeds, and grains come back into the diet. If you are including dairy products and eggs in your diet, stay within the proper percentages and you will probably get more than enough protein.

If you get the urge to try some fish or chicken, trust yourself and your connection to your body. And if you never touch meat again, that's fine too!

Chapter 8
On Supplements

A FEW BASICS

Talking about additional supplements in the diet can be difficult because there are so many misconceptions out there in the world. So, for now, try to forget everything you have learned about vitamins and minerals.

The need for additional supplements is obvious, even when you are eating 'right' you may be experiencing physical symptoms that indicate you have developed some vitamin and mineral deficiencies. To speed the process of healing up, you need to include some supplemental additions to your foods. It is important to remember that it may take six months to a year to bring vitamin and mineral deficiencies out of the hole, and that's with the concentrated effort of eating stress-free!

The kind of supplements I recommend are mostly foods in concentrated form, like alfalfa tablets or liquid or powdered herbs. Bodies were designed to recognize and deal with foods, so giving them concentrated forms of these substances allows them to treat the supplements just like any other food; the body will break it down, use what it needs, store what it can and easily flush the rest!

It is also VERY important to give the body a full range of nutrients. Just because you take a vitamin B supplement doesn't automatically mean that will take care of a B deficiency. Vitamins and minerals interact in the body; they aid each other in keeping the organism working properly. You want to make sure that you take a supplement or number of supplements that cover the whole range of vitamins and minerals.

Because of this need for a balance of nutrients, it can be difficult to take individual vitamin and mineral tablets. I'm sure that most of you know the frustration (let alone the expense) of trying to figure out what you're deficient in and how to take care of the deficiency. You always wonder, *"Am I taking enough?"* or *"Am I taking too much?"* or *"Am I taking the right combination?"*

Over the years the companies who make these regular vitamin and mineral tablets have improved the pills digestibility, but that doesn't mean that they are easy to digest and utilize. If you are having problems digesting regular food, what makes you think you will be able to digest a bunch of pills?

In 1986, a suit was brought against a manufacturer by a woman who found hundreds of calcium tablets in the bottom of septic system, tablets that she had ingested to NOT develop a calcium deficiency. But the tablets were indigestible so she didn't get any benefit from them at all. She won the suit and all the manufacturers changed their formulas to make them digestible. Laws were enacted that required companies prove digestibility, at least on calcium supplements.

I'm not saying that vitamin, mineral and other supplements should never be taken. They can be of great use, but only when you can digest and utilize them. Unfortunately for those of you who have been taking lots of pills, I generally see the same levels of deficiencies in you as I see in those who aren't taking supplements. If you have been taking an oil-based Vitamin E but are not digesting oils well, it's likely you are flushing some very expensive substances down the toilet! I suggest for now that you try something a little easier on the body.

Store any supplements either in the fridge or in a cool, dark place. When you are more in touch with your body needs, you can pull them back out and use them.

ABOUT DIGESTIVE AIDS

I don't recommend taking supplements of HCL, pancreatic enzymes, or lactose enzymes if you are using them as substitutes. Taking them means that you are once again telling your body there is a problem it can't handle. It's much better to stay away from the offending foods and heal your body.

But there are times when taking digestive aids can be beneficial. If your body, or some organ or system within it, has 'forgotten' how to make a digestive enzyme, it may need help creating a new, healthy blueprint.

I suggest that digestive aids not be added into the diet until it becomes obvious the body is NOT creating digestive enzymes on its own. As you move from one phase of this program to the next, you should be able to reintroduce new foods with little or no problem. But if you repeatedly try to incorporate a new food and respond negatively (with heartburn, gas, or constipation) then you might want to try an enzyme aid. Of course, you might be having an emotional reaction, too, so check that out also.

To properly use digestive enzymes, ingest both the difficult food and its needed enzyme aid. Use HCL for protein digestion, pancreatic enzymes for starches, lecithin for oil digestion, and complex or combination enzymes for fruits and veggies. If the digestion of the food is obviously better, then repeatedly use the aid for about a month while eating that food. Then stop eating the food for a month and let your body rest.

After a month's rest, try eating the food again WITHOUT the digestive aid. If it has created a new blueprint and learned or remembered how to make the needed enzyme, you won't have any trouble digesting the food. If your body is still having troubles digesting the food, use the enzyme aid for another month, rest for a month and try the food again.

AS A GENERAL RULE

In the Appendix, Table 4 lists the possible vitamin and mineral deficiencies that create specific problems. Because of the interaction of nutrients in the body, sometimes a specific nutrient will not be the direct cause of a problem.

For example, a lack of calcium can cause leg cramps, especially at night, but you may have plenty of calcium in the blood and not enough Vitamin B's to utilize it, thus the cramps. Taking extra calcium, in this case, would not end the night cramps.

Always think of bringing the vitamin and mineral levels into balance as well as bringing deficiencies into line. Over the years, as I worked on more and more bodies, a pattern emerged concerning deficiencies and levels of health.

Check out the chart on the following page. As a general rule:

HEALTH ASSESSMENT	POSSIBLE DEFICIENCIES
Group One	Vitamins: B, C, Minerals: Iodine, Zinc
Group Two	Vitamins: A, B, C, D, E Minerals: Iodine, Magnesium, Phosphorus, Zinc, Trace Minerals
Group Three	Vitamins: A, B, C, D, E, and Trace vitamins Minerals: Copper, Iodine, Magnesium, Manganese, Phosphorus, Zinc, Trace Minerals
Group Four	Vitamins: All, Minerals: Any or All

ABOUT VITAMINS

There are a number of excellent products out there that will give your body a wide range of vitamins and will trigger your body to utilize the vitamins and minerals available in the blood. Here are products I have asked bodies about for years:

Alfalfa
    Alfalfa juice powder
    Alfalfa juice capsules
    Alfalfa tablets
Barley Grasses
Bee Pollen
    capsules
    loose
    tablets
Blue-Green Algaes
    Cell-Tech Blue Green
    Spirulina
    Sun Chlorella
Chlorophyll
    powder or liquid

Liquid Vitamins
    Flora-dix
        Children's Formula
        Herbs and Iron
        Multi-Vitamin Formula
    Green Gold
    Liquid Life
Nettles
    capsules
    tea
Wheat Grass
    Wheat Grass Juice powder
    Wheat Grass Juice capsules
    Wheat Grass tablets

And there are some new companies with new products like Six Tastes, Synergy, Greens +, Futurebiotics, Green Gold, Liquid Life and Body Booster coming on the market all the time. Keep your eyes open and check out products that you are drawn to. I like the feel of many of these mixed sprouted grass products.

The two most commonly used vitamin supplements are Alfalfa products and the Flora-dix formulas (though there are many new liquid vitamin products on the market. I just haven't had time to check all of them out on numerous bodies.) After them, the list of supplements called for descends in this order: Bee Pollen, Barley Grasses, Blue-Green Algae, Wheat Grass or Chlorophyll, Nettles, and Spirulina. All of these products are wonderful but it has become obvious in talking to bodies that certain supplements work better than others at certain stages of healing.

For instance, Blue-Green Algaes, the mixed grass products and Bee Pollen definitely have high spiritual connections in the body as well as physical healing abilities. If you take them before you are vibrationally ready for them, they can push your healing so quickly that you end up in a healing crisis! One of the points of this whole approach is to help you feel better as quickly as possible. Pushing yourself into feeling sick just isn't positive.

Some of these supplements are relatively inexpensive, some seem to be very expensive. But take a look at the cost of individual vitamin and mineral supplements and figure you would have to buy bottles of all of them. THAT gets truly outrageous!

The following individual explanations will give you more information about the specific supplements. And the charts at the end of each section list the suggested amounts of nutrients to take for the different Health Assessments and Basic Diet Programs. Also read the sections in Chapter 10--DIS-EASE and DIS-COMFORT for your specific problems. There is additional information on vitamins, minerals and herbs you may want to take to speed up your healing.

Remember that you are the one who lives in your body; you are the only one who really knows if a supplement feels right or not. Trust yourself. Try Alfalfa or liquid vitamins for a couple of weeks and see how they feel. If they are not working for you, then try the supplements on down the list, one at time, and see how they feel. It is very common as people reach the end of the program that their bodies want a variety of nutrients. They also find that they switch from one to another as they need different vitamins and minerals. I keep most of these supplements around and take different ones at different times.

But for now, while you are going through this program, it's best to try to stay simple. Use one multivitamin and one multi-mineral supplement until you feel you are clearly in touch with your body. Then, as you get more in touch with your body's needs, you can feel out if you need more than one supplement to meet your needs.

ABOUT MINERALS

The number of products available that will give you a full range of minerals (in food form) is limited. But the few things that work well are really great!

The most commonly used mineral supplements are Kelp and Dulse, with Alfalfa, Mezotrace, Body Booster and Spirulina coming next in line. Check out the specifics on taking them in the next few pages. Following is a list of commonly used mineral supplements:

Body Booster	Kelp	Spirulina	Dulse
liquid	tablets	capsules	capsules
Mezotrace	capsules	tablets	tablets
tablets	liquid	loose	liquid
	loose		loose

ABOUT TAKING SUPPLEMENTS

1) *"Make it easy on yourself!"* All of these vitamin and mineral supplements are recognized by the body as food, so it really doesn't seem to matter if you take them with food or if you take them all by themselves! If it's easier to remember to take your supplements with meals, then do that; if it's easier to remember to take them some other time, then do that.

Occasionally I will see someone who NEEDS to take supplements with foods; I think the upset stomach, nausea, and whooziness that these people have experienced is a stomach and body reaction to the intensity of nutrients available from a concentrated food supplement. Taking the nutrients with food usually dilutes the intensity enough to stop the upsets. So, if you are having any of these symptoms, be sure and take your supplements WITH food.

2) I suggest you divide supplements you take in half and take part of them in the morning and part of them in the evening. Bodies are very efficient machines; they run on a rhythm and at a certain pace. You just can't dump a whole lot of nutrients into the system and expect your body to be able to use all the overload. It will use what it can, store what it can and flush the rest. Unfortunately, Vitamin B's are water-soluble and they are one of the things your body will flush instead of store. So if you spread out your supplement intake, you give your body two or three boosts of nutrients in a day instead of one massive shot. Levels of deficiencies come into balance much faster this way.

3) Link your taking of supplements with something else you do every day, like eating or brushing your teeth. I don't have much routine in my life so I tend to be terrible about taking something on a regular a.m. and p.m. basis. I can usually remember in the morning, but the night dose fades with the sunset! So, I learned that when I take my supplements in the morning, I immediately put my night-time dose on my pillow or under the sheets! Then I can't crawl into bed and forget taking them!

Another cute trick: if you tend to forget taking your supplements all together, stick the end of your toothbrush in, say, your Alfalfa tablet bottle and the later dose on your pillow! Or even keep them in the car (weather permitting) on your car seat! Whatever works!!!

4) Some sensitive people can experience such a lift in energy after taking certain supplements that they can't go to sleep for hours afterwards. If you experience an obvious 'lift' when taking vitamins and minerals, then be sure to take the evening dose with meals, unless, of course, you WANT to be up all night!

ABOUT EACH SUPPLEMENT

The dosages listed on the following charts are meant to be a guide. Trust your body and follow the information there. The dosages are also meant for the average adult. If you are larger or smaller than 'average,' adjust your dosages accordingly. Remember, taking more than you actually can utilize it just a waste of money and body energy.

FOR CHILDREN'S DOSAGES — Between the ages of 3 and 12, children need to have high quality nutrients available in the bloodstream on a constant basis. Use of the liquid vitamins is usually more acceptable to the kids than tablets and capsules. For this age range, 3 to 12, cut the adult dosages in half. As the kids heal, start asking them how much they think they need. If it sounds reasonable, follow their advice! Teenagers need to follow the Adult Dosages and increase their mineral intake.

ALFALFA

This herb is a godsend! Check out the Herbs and Vitamins/ Minerals list in the Appendix, Table 5. As you can see Alfalfa is listed as containing high amounts of all the vitamins and almost all the minerals. What alfalfa doesn't have within it are a few nutrients that are needed only in minute amounts or are easy to get in food.

Alfalfa is an inexpensive supplement to purchase and gives you the most for your money. Since it is also high in most of the minerals, if you use alfalfa, you can cut the use of a mineral supplement in half!

The only 'problem' I have seen with taking alfalfa is the form it is in. Some people have digestive trouble with the binders that are used to form the alfalfa into a tablet. If you choose to use Alfalfa tablets and experience some digestive upset or if you know you are sensitive to taking tablets, then try taking the herb capsules or even blending alfalfa powder in water like a tea.

Most of the companies who market vitamin and mineral supplements include an alfalfa product or two. I haven't seen most bodies having a preference about the brand, though I like to buy ones that feel fresh and potent and are small and easy to swallow! There are only a few manufacturers of supplement products in this country and they make most of the pills, capsules and powders we take. Formulas and ingredient sources may vary but not by much!

The wholesale herb business is BIG and getting bigger by the day and the supply of herbs doesn't have much controls. Usually the smaller herb companies are the ones who are keeping good quality controls in place. In the international herb business it is well known that there are no pesticide, insecticide and chemical fertilizer controls on the growing of herbs! So try to find sources (or maybe even create them) where you buy your herbs from someone you call by name!

Table 1, Recommended tablets or capsules of alfalfa, twice daily

	Super Cleanser	Deep Cleanser	Basic Balancer	Phase 2	Phase 3	Phase 4 Core	Semi Final	Gradu- ation
1st Group			6	6	5	4	3	3
2nd Group		8	8	6	6	5	5	4
3rd Group	10	10	8	8	8	6	6	5
4th Group	10	10	10	8	8	7	6	5

BEE POLLEN

Bee pollen is really flower and plant pollen, that is, plant sperm. Bees happen to be the ingenious creatures that gather it from flowers. Bees use pollen as their protein source, it's about 20% of their diets. Bee Pollen is right up at the top of the list of Wonders of the World. Just the life force is incredible. And within pollen are ALL the nutrients we need to survive and be healthy; it is the only food that can make this claim!!! Check out the chemical analysis in the Appendix, Table 6. This stuff is really incredible.

Bees are vulnerable to chemical sprays. The overuse of pesticides years ago created a crisis and bee populations declined rapidly. Farmers quickly learned that they had to wait and spray plants AFTER the plant flowers had been pollinated and the bees were OUT of the fields. After all, if that male plant sperm isn't spread around, plants can't produce or reproduce! So, the quality of both pollen and honey is high and the levels of chemicals will always be low.

A quarter teaspoon of pollen is equal to a multivitamin and mineral tablet; though usually bodies want extra minerals to create a complete balance. And because bee pollen has all the known enzymes, coenzymes, fatty acids, fats, oils, proteins, carbohydrates, amino acids, and micronutrients we need to be healthy, it helps the body remember and create new blueprints and patterns of health.

Bees gather the pollen, carry it in their leg sacks and deliver it to the hive. There, they ball it up and 'hand' it to a bee just inside the 'door,' who takes it to its storage space. Bee keepers will put a pollen trap on the hive; it's a very small 'door' that stops the bees from being able to carry the balled pollen into the hive, so they drop it at the doorstep. The pollen is caught in a 'trap' below the door.

You can buy bee pollen 'balls' or granules by the pound in most health food stores. It is also available in pressed tablets and in capsules. There are some differences between pollens that are bee-collected and pollens that are hand-collected; some people feel that the differences are major and they say people should only eat hand-collected pollen. But I haven't found bodies really had a preference one way or the other. Check it out for yourself.

Different plant pollens taste different. I bought some pollen a few years ago that had a strong flavor of cedar to it; it was delicious but I tired of the taste quickly. Here in New Mexico, I like to buy 'spring' pollen because desert plants that bloom from midsummer to fall have very strong and bitter pollens. I'll never forget this one batch of pollen that had brown pollen balls mixed throughout. I picked one, tasted it and thought I'd died and gone to heaven! They tasted like brown-sugar candies!

You may see 'Spanish Pollen' in your stores. This pollen does come from Spain and more specifically from Spanish alfalfa fields. It always has a consistent taste, where local pollens may vary in taste from season to season and year to year.

If you choose to add bee pollen to your supplement routine, take care in introducing it. I had a client years ago who put her hubby in the hospital by giving him pollen! Her body loved it and she just assumed that if bee pollen was good for her, it would be good for him. So, she sprinkled a tablespoon of pollen on his breakfast cereal and said, *"Here, honey. You'll love this!"* Well, his body had a violent reaction to the pollen, he went into anaphylactic shock and they were on their way to the hospital!!! It is relatively rare for someone to have such an intense reaction, but it obviously happens.

If you choose to add pollen to your diet, take a few granules and see if you have any allergic reaction. Symptoms include a tightness in the throat, sneezing, mucus, an upset stomach, or nausea. If you have reaction, choose a different supplement. Just because you are sensitive to pollens in the air doesn't automatically mean you will have reactions to ingesting bee pollen. Some people with allergies find ingesting pollen 'cures' their allergies and others find it irritates them. To heal allergies you have to change the body's inability to cope with foreign particles. Bring the body into nutritional balance and you will 'cure' allergies.

If you have no negative reactions to the bee pollen, repeat the process of ingesting small amounts for several days in a row. Check and double check for any reactions. Then go ahead and increase the amounts ingested by 1/4-1/2 tsp. increments over the next week.

I suggest you really enjoy eating pollen! Think about the work it took to get that incredible life-force into your life! Taste all the different colored pollen 'balls' and remember you are tasting flowers!

Table 2, Recommended daily amounts of bee pollen, twice daily

		Super Cleanser	Deep Cleanser	Basic Balancer	Phase 2	Phase 3	Phase 4 Core	Semi Final	Graduation
tablets or capsules	1st Group			5	5	4	4	3	3
teaspoons				1 1/2	1 1/2	1	1	3/4 - 1	1/2 - 1
	2nd Group		6	5	5	5	4	4	3
			2	1 1/2	1 1/2	1 1/2	1	1	1/2 - 1
	3rd Group	6	6	5	5	5	5	4	4
		2	2	1 1/2	1 1/2	1 1/2	1 1/2	1	1
	4th Group	6	6	6	5	5	5	4	4
		2	2	2	1 1/2	1 1/2	1 1/2	1	1

BLUE-GREEN ALGAES

Blue-green algaes are the basis of all aquatic life on this planet. If they can sustain all those life-forms, including huge whales, you have to figure algaes could sustain humans as well. The major kinds of freshwater blue-green algaes are Blue-Green and Chlorella, and Spirulina is the ocean-grown blue-green algae. See Table 3 of the Appendix for brands of algaes.

Look for a brand that is freeze-dried. If the algae is heat-dried, it can become indigestible.

All algaes are high in vitamins, minerals and proteins, though freshwater ones seem to be easier for most people to digest. Also, there is a high vibrational level associated with all algaes and they can just be too stimulating an energy to deal with when first starting the diet program. I suggest you wait a few months before introducing them into your supplement routine. Then, watch for toxin overload.

Table 3, Recommended amounts of algae, twice daily

	Super Cleanser	Deep Cleanser	Basic Balancer	Phase 2	Phase 3	Phase 4 Core	Semi Final	Gradu-ation	
1st Group			5	5	4	4	3	3	tablets or capsules
			1 1/2	1 1/2	1	1	3/4 - 1	1/2 - 1	teaspoons
2nd Group		6	5	5	5	4	4	3	
		2	1 1/2	1 1/2	1 1/2	1	1	1/2 - 1	
3rd Group	6	6	5	5	5	5	4	4	
	2	2	1 1/2	1 1/2	1 1/2	1 1/2	1	1	
4th Group	6	6	6	5	5	5	4	4	
	2	2	2	1 1/2	1 1/2	1 1/2	1	1	

Table 4, Recommended amounts of spirulina, twice daily

	Super Cleanser	Deep Cleanser	Basic Balancer	Phase 2	Phase 3	Phase 4 Core	Semi Final	Gradu-ation	
1st Group			8	8	6	6	5	4	tablets or capsules
			1 1/2	1 1/2	1	1	3/4	1/2 - 1	teaspoons
2nd Group		10	10	8	8	6	6	5	
		2	2	1 1/2	1 1/2	1	1	3/4 - 1	
3rd Group	10	10	10	8	8	8	6	6	
	2 1/2	2	2	1 1/2	1 1/2	1 1/2	1	1	
4th Group	10	10	10	10	8	8	6	4	
	2 1/2	2 1/2	2	2	1 1/2	1 1/2	1 1/2	1 1/2	

CHLOROPHYLL

Chlorophyll is your basic, natural plant juice. It's been around for eons, since people started squeezing liquids from plants. Most of the chlorophyll on the market comes from alfalfa, which makes it a great multivitamin source. You may find that it is cheaper to buy chlorophyll than it is for other plant juices.

If you choose to take Chlorophyll in liquid, powder made into liquid, tablets or capsules, it is a good idea to take a small dose of another vitamin supplement. Chlorophyll, depending upon what plants it was made from, may need extra vitamin B supplements added into the diet to get the right balance of all the nutrients, else the chlorophyll source is alfalfa.

Table 5, Recommended daily amounts of chlorophyll, twice daily

		Super Cleanser	Deep Cleanser	Basic Balancer	Phase 2	Phase 3	Phase 4 Core	Semi Final	Gradu- ation
tablets or capsules	1st Group			5	5	4	4	3	3
liquid teaspoons				1 1/2	1 1/2	1	1	3/4 - 1	1/2 - 1
	2nd Group	6		5	5	5	4	4	3
		2		1 1/2	1 1/2	1 1/2	1	1	1/2 - 1
	3rd Group	6	6	5	5	5	5	4	4
		2	2	1 1/2	1 1/2	1 1/2	1 1/2	1	1
	4th Group	6	6	6	5	5	5	4	4
		2	2	2	1 1/2	1 1/2	1 1/2	1	1

DULSE, KELP AND SEAWEEDS

Check out the vitamin and mineral information in Table 5. Kelp is listed in almost every category! All the seaweeds are great sources of minerals and they contain all these nutrients in a food form!

The seaweeds (Kelp and dulse are the easiest to find) are much the same in what they can provide you, except for one thing.

If you have edema or swelling anywhere, it is possible you are dealing with a sodium/potassium imbalance. Dulse has a better balance of these two interactive minerals than the other seaweeds, so I suggest that you find a dulse source. Dulse is also a better mineral source for people dealing with high blood pressure. Other than these two particular situation, any of the seaweeds will do just fine. See the following page for recommended amounts.

Table 6, Recommended amounts of dulse, kelp, or seaweed, twice daily

	Super Cleanser	Deep Cleanser	Basic Balancer	Phase 2	Phase 3	Phase 4 Core	Semi Final	Gradu- ation	
1st Group			5	5	4	4	3	2 to 3	tablets or capsules
			10	10	8	8	6	4 to 6	drops
2nd Group		6	6	5	5	4	4	3	
		12	12	10	10	8	8	6	
3rd Group	6	6	6	5	5	4	4	4	
	12	12	12	10	10	8	8	8	
4th Group	6	6	6	6	6	5	5	4	
	12	12	12	12	12	10	10	8	

LIQUID MINERALS

Again, there are new products on the market all the time, and now you can purchase liquid mineral sources. You can purchase liquid kelp and dulse, which surprisingly enough, do not taste salty, but are almost sweet. You can also buy a number of other types of liquid minerals. The one I am most familiar with is Body Booster (See Table 3 for sources and follow their dosage directions.) The amounts you may need to take of these non-seaweed liquid minerals is considerably higher than the liquid seaweeds. But, don't let that be a deterrent.

LIQUID VITAMINS

There are great liquid vitamin products on the market that are combinations of herbal extracts high in vitamins and some minerals. The best thing about these liquid herbs is they take no digestion and go directly into the bloodstream. People taking this form of vitamin supplement have told me they frequently feel an immediate uplifting in their energy and well-being after taking their morning and evening doses.

I realize the cost of these products can seem high, but remember they are giving you a well-rounded source of vitamins in a highly usable form. If you like how the liquid vitamins feel and work in your body, ask your health food outlet or distributor about buying a case at a discount.

The first liquid multivitamin I became familiar with was the Flora-dix formulas. Most bodies use the Multi-Vitamin formula well, but if you have been diagnosed with an iron deficiency anytime in your life or suspect you might have an iron deficiency, take the Herbs and Iron formula. Some of the formulas have yeast, orange juice and/or honey in them and these things are off the first three of the Basic Diets; but don't be concerned. The small amounts of these ingredients in the formulas and in your overall diet shouldn't present a problem unless you are yeast sensitive. If you are, try the yeast-free formula or another supplement all together. Flora-dix is also available in tablet forms, which makes it easy to travel and continue your use. The Children's formula is just great. You can add it to an infant's bottle with ease and kids of all ages usually love the taste.

Within the last few years I have also worked with several other liquid multivitamins like Liquid Life and Green Gold. Whichever source you find, make sure it has a complete vitamin base or mix it partially with a green-based powder.

Table 7, Recommended amounts of liquid vitamins in teaspoons, twice daily

	Super Cleanser	Deep Cleanser	Basic Balancer	Phase 2	Phase 3	Phase 4 Core	Semi Final	Gradu-ation
1st Group			1 1/2	1 1/2	1	1	3/4	1/2
2nd Group		1 1/2	1 1/2	1 1/2	1	1	3/4	1/2
3rd Group	2 - 2 1/2	2	2	1 1/2	1 1/2	1	1	1
4th Group	2 - 2 1/2	2	2	1 1/2	1 1/2	1 1/2	1	1

* chart note: 2 tablets Flora-dix equals 1 tsp.

MEZOTRACE

This mineral supplement is unique. My first encounter with it was at a health food trade show years ago. I was walking down the aisle and my hands were drawn to this big greenish rock like iron to a magnet.

The rock turned out to be Mezotrace. It is mined from one of only two known deposits in the world! This substance woke up a cellular memory in my body that I hadn't realized was asleep. I took Mezotrace for five months and could feel it waking up this deep memory of a different body concept. After the five months passed, I felt like the memory was wide awake and I no longer needed the physical reminder.

I have seen this 'awakening' in everyone who has taken this mineral supplement, so I suggest you treat it as one of those high vibrational substances that you only take after numerous months on the diet program. When you do take it, watch for cleansing reactions that could send you into a healing crisis. Increase the dosages slowly and keep taking other mineral sources for dietary needs.

Table 8, Recommended amounts of mezotrace in tablets, twice daily

	Super Cleanser	Deep Cleanser	Basic Balancer	Phase 2	Phase 3	Phase 4 Core	Semi Final	Gradu-ation
1st Group			3	3	2	2	2	O - 1
2nd Group		3	3	3	3	2	2	O - 1
3rd Group	4	4	4	3	3	2	2	O - 1
4th Group	4	4	4	3	3	3	2	O - 1

NETTLES

Nettles is one of those lowly herbs that has a bad 'reputation' because of its stinging ability, but is wonderful beyond belief! Not only is it high in all the vitamins (though it is not listed in the Herb/Vitamin chart,) it helps balance the blood chemistry, acts as a relaxant, and will fertilize your house and garden plants!

Table 9, Recommended amounts of nettles in capsules, twice daily

	Super Cleanser	Deep Cleanser	Basic Balancer	Phase 2	Phase 3	Phase 4 Core	Semi Final	Gradu-ation
1st Group			5	5	4	4	4	3
2nd Group		5	5	5	5	4	4	3
3rd Group	6	6	5	5	5	5	4	4
4th Group	6	6	6	5	5	5	4	4

SPROUTED GREEN GRASSES

Anytime a seed is sprouted, the vitamin and mineral levels skyrocket. The seed is actually creating the nutrients it needs to grow into a healthy plant. When these sprouted plants are juiced and dried, we get the benefit of all those wonderful nutrients.

For years there were only a few companies making sprouted barley or wheat grass products, but because of the healing success in the body, numerous companies are now making single-grass or mixed-grass powders, capsules and tablets. All the companies I have had connection with are conscientious and conscious about maintaining the quality of their products. So, find a product that feels good to you.

Sprouted barley seems to be the preference of most bodies. The first two barley grass formulas I worked with were the Barley Green and Green Magma formulas. Barley Green is usually purchased through a distributor system and Green Magma is sold through regular retail outlets like health food stores.

The main ingredient in both products is dried juice from young barley leaves. Both products, unfortunately, have small amounts of cooked, dried and powdered brown rice in them. The rice itself might cause some digestive problems but nutrients in the dried juice seem to counterbalance the negative affects for most people. The Barley Green formula also contains dried and powdered kelp which also helps with the digestion of the brown rice and gives additional minerals.

If you choose to avoid the rice until it comes back into your regular diet, then choose another brand of barley grass capsules, tablets or powder. See Appendix, Table 3 for information on other barley grass products and companies. And for more information on barley grasses, see Table 6 for a chemical analysis.

Sprouted wheat grass was first popular in the fresh-juice form, which is still the best way to take it. But that's not convenient, unless you can pick it at the local juice bar. Tablets and capsules are easier and still retain high levels of nutrients. Remember that kamut and spelt are varieties of wheat.

The mixed-grass powders and tablets are great products and they represent a new direction in food supplements. In general, I am still finding that bodies like to start out with a single-grass supplement. Then as they heal, as they move out of healing-crisis range, they like to shift to a mixed-grass formula.

If you are drawn to do a mixed-grass formula from the start, go every slow in introducing it, building up to the suggested dosage over a two to three week period. Make sure that you aren't pushing too many toxins too quickly. If you are, you may feel weak, tired, headachy, or overloaded. Back off to a single-grass vitamin supplement for a couple of weeks, letting your body recover yet still keeping your vitamin levels high.

If you are drawn to mixed-grass formulas after doing the diet for two-four months and if you feel spiritually ready to move to another level, then slowly switch to a mixed-grass formula. Again, watch for toxic or spiritual overload. Remember, the body is the last aspect of self to catch up to change. It will catch up, you just need to give it some time. See the charts on the following page for recommended amounts.

Table 10, Recommended amounts of single sprouted grasses in capsules, twice daily

	Super Cleanser	Deep Cleanser	Basic Balancer	Phase 2	Phase 3	Phase 4 Core	Semi Final	Gradu- ation
1st Group			5	5	4	4	4	3
2nd Group		5	5	5	5	4	4	3
3rd Group	6	6	5	5	5	5	4	4
4th Group	6	6	6	5	5	5	4	4

Table 11, Recommended amounts of mixed sprouted grasses in capsules, twice daily

	Super Cleanser	Deep Cleanser	Basic Balancer	Phase 2	Phase 3	Phase 4 Core	Semi Final	Gradu- ation
1st Group			3	3	3	3	2	2
2nd Group		3	3	3	3	3	2	2
3rd Group	3 to 4	3 to 4	3 to 4	3	3	3	3	3
4th Group	3 to 4	3 to 4	3 to 4	3	3	3	3	3

HERB SUGGESTIONS

There is one use of herbs that I want to discuss in a general sense and that is the use of herbs as preventatives. There are numerous herbs that will help with specific problems both as healers and preventatives. But you have to be careful with all of the herbs because of the multi-functions they perform. The only natural substance I am aware of that will act as a healer and a preventative WITH-OUT possibly interfering with other body functions is propolis.

Propolis is actually a resin that plants ooze in the early spring and summer as they bud out. You have to be up early, early in the morning to even see it. It looks like clear dewdrops until you touch it; then you will find out that it's sticky.

Bees gather propolis, mix it with some enzymes and pollen and cover the whole inside of their hives with it. They are susceptible to certain microbes and fungi and propolis is antimicrobial and antifungal, as well as antibacterial, antiviral and an antibiotic!

I suggest using propolis in tincture or extract form because it is a resin and resins can be hard on the kidneys. Even in tincture, the resins are present and will stick to the glass, your teeth and your lips. I put drops in hot to warm water, let the resin gather, then swirl it out with my finger or a paper towel tip. I also only use paper cups so I can toss them when they get yucky.

I've seen propolis do some miraculous things in others and I've survived on it myself. I have an extreme sensitivity to poison ivy and found this out by being in a delirious fever for days at a time, over a three month period, after my first and only contact. For over a year I'd awake with chipmunk cheeks (from swollen glands) and twenty minutes after 20-60 drops of propolis, they'd be back to normal.

Propolis gargle has saved my voice after eight hours of clients. It's kicked out flus and colds. It's cleared infections from scratches, killed warts and moles after repeated use internally and externally, and healed blood imbalances.

There's been many medical studies done on propolis, both in the US and Europe. They've reported things from cancer healings to the clearing of acne, the death of Strep and Staph organisms, and a clearing of blood fats. Regular use has not created any negative side affects. As soon as you feel slightly 'off,' start taking some extract. Figure that as soon as you feel out of sorts with yourself, there is an increased stress happening somewhere in your life. It means that you have moved into some level of vulnerability! And if you're vulnerable, then you need to take steps to protect yourself.

On a physical level, propolis is a great protector! With the physical vulnerability under control, you can then turn your attention to what the core reason for this shift and deal with it directly!

Chapter 9
Special People and Their Situations

CHILDREN AND HEALTH

One of the real gifts that we can give our kids is health. But along with this gift we have to give them the training on how to stay healthy. Kids are intuitively tuned into their bodies until we disturb that knowingness by feeding them unhealthy foods, by teaching them to connect emotional reactions to foods, and by 'teaching' their minds to take over this naturally intuitive function.

It's a well known 'fact' that kids don't generally like vegetables. With the first twenty kids I worked on, I saw an obvious pattern developing; the percentages of fruits and veggies that most kids need is just the OPPOSITE of their parents. Most adults need from 70% fruits and veggies in their diets with 30% being proteins, starches, sweeteners and oils.

KIDS NEED 70%-90% PROTEINS, STARCHES, SWEETENERS and OILS in their diets with only 10%-30% fruits and veggies! I'll never forget these two sisters, six and eight years old, who literally flew out of their chairs and hugged me repeatedly, as I told their mother to back off pushing them to eat their vegetables!!!

We adults have been taught that 'kids need their vegetables' but the kids have been right all along!!! The things kids love, the pastas and cereals and crackers and peanut butter, are full of the building materials that their bodies need to develop into adults. And the amounts of nutrients they need from fruits and veggies are minimal, at least until they reach basic adult size and until their hormones start to click in.

Somewhere between twelve to sixteen years old, a transition begins and kids' bodies need more and more fruits and veggies and fewer and fewer of the building block foods. Unfortunately by the time kids reach this point, we have usually set some negative patterns in their heads about veggies. And we wonder why they go into patterns of resistance!!!

It's time that we change this whole scenario and let our kids stay in a 'trust' relationship with their bodies and foods. And we can start doing this by trusting their instincts and intuition. Stop pushing the need for them to eat their veggies and let them taste and sample them when they are interested, not before! By making tasty veggie dishes for yourself, you can entice kids into wanting to try them, but don't push. Whenever you try to push something onto someone, you can be guaranteed you will create RESISTANCE!

When kids start to become interested in the adult world, they start to hang out around adults. They listen to us in a new way, not necessarily to what we are saying to them, but definitely what we are saying to each other. They start to emulate the people they respect and the people they want love from. They are open to all kinds of new things. And THIS is where the introduction of vegetables can start on a positive footing. The discovery of food can be very exciting if all the "shoulds" of eating vegetables has been dropped.

The Diet Approach and Kids

All kids, from the healthiest to the sickest, can greatly benefit from following this diet approach. Because their bodies are growing and changing so quickly and because they usually don't have the same high levels of deficiencies as their adult counterparts, they tend to heal more rapidly than their parents. But because of these considerations, it is also important to restrict their diets with care and to make sure that they take adequate amounts of supplemental vitamins and minerals.

I recommend that children use Basic Diet #1 or #2 no matter what health group their symptoms put them in. With more serious health problems I recommend that they follow the first two basic diets for longer periods of time instead of eliminating more foods, unless they are obviously having stress, mucus or emotional reactions to specific foods.

The following schedule will give you an idea of how long children in different health groups may need to do a particular diet approach.

FOR CHILDREN (12 & under)				**MONTHS ON EACH APPROACH:**			
	Basic 3	Basic 2	Basic 1	Phase 2	Getting There	Core Diet	Semi Final
Group 1			1	1 to 2	1 to 2	1 to 2	1 to 2
Group 2		1	1 to 2	1 to 2	2	2	2
Group 3		2	2	2	2	2	2
Group 4	2 to 3	2 to 3	2	2	2		

Watch your kids closely for stress, mucus or emotional reactions to specific foods. Third and Fourth Group kids may have additional foods that need to be removed from their diets. When you notice a reaction, remove the difficult food from the child's diet for one or two months, then try reintroducing it. If there continues to be a problem, the first thing I suggest, besides continuing to avoid the food, is increasing the vitamin and mineral intake. The second suggestion is to treat the food as having a possible emotional reaction attached to it. Go through the process of removing emotional food connections (see page 68 in Chapter 7, How Do I _____?) then try reintroducing the food.

Remember, even though kids seem to heal and rebalance quickly, if your child had a deficiency from the womb, it will take longer to heal the problems created from the lacking nutrient. As long as you are seeing improvements, be patient.

HORMONE CHANGES AND TEENAGERS

When our bodies make their first changes into adulthood, there are major changes in the amounts of nutrients we require. Look at the First and Second Group symptoms in the Health Assessment;

listed are acne, craving sweets, nervousness and anxiety, self-judgment and vulnerability, B.O., irritability, and mood swings. Doesn't that sound like most teenagers?

Years ago, I had a mother call me, literally out of desperation when her twelve year old son, David, had had a mid-level to severe headache every day for over a year. They had gone the doctor route, had every test possible, and after a year, they were told there was 'nothing wrong' and to basically go away and learn to live with it! Serious medication temporarily stopped the pain, but they knew this was no way to deal with what was happening.

Well, we put the kid on a diet that he called 'inhumane' because it excluded McDonalds and ice cream, but within three days, his headaches stopped. In the first six weeks of the original work-up, he experienced two headaches that were directly related to eating something off the diet and that were controllable with aspirin.

Over the next year we gradually added all foods back into his diet with no return of the headaches. A year and a half after he was back to eating everything, I got a letter from Mom. She just wanted me to know that even though David was eating at McDonalds more regularly than she liked, his headaches had not returned and he seemed to be a healthy teenager.

Most teenage problems stem from the relatively sudden need for more and more nutrients. Getting these building blocks in the diet allows the hormonal transitions to move forward with ease. Teenagers have enough change on their plates; they don't need physical imbalances adding to their already challenging lives. Being a teenager means you are starting to separate out who you really are; having that picture clouded up doesn't help them or their parents.

A WORD TO PARENTS OF TEENAGERS

I realize that getting teenagers to deal with proper nutrition can be hard sometimes. I usually find kids will listen to common sense if you or some other adult can be straight with them. If that doesn't work, just tell them that pimples are directly tied to Vitamin B and zinc deficiencies! Just adding kelp and alfalfa tablets to their diets can eliminate the unsightly sores; so what could be easier?

Don't try to get your kids to eat healthy until you do it first! When teenagers see their parents getting healthy, having new levels of energy and becoming more tolerant because they are eating right, the kids will be much more receptive. Forcing anything on them will only meet with resistance and alienation, so what's the point? The best thing you can always do for your kids and the world is to be true to your own life. What you DO is always more important to kids than what you SAY.

PREGNANCY

IN THE WOMB

Fetuses are little survival thieves. If they need a nutrient they will take it from the mother; there is no concern for the mother's need for that nutrient. The baby MUST have all the nutrients it needs, when it needs them. Its development can't wait for vitamins and minerals to just show up, so it will rob the mother, if need be.

If the mother has plenty of nutrients available in the bloodstream, then she and the baby will be healthy. But if the mother is lacking in some nutrient, then both she and the baby can develop some deficiency problems. Frequently the general health of the kids in a family will go down with each birth, as the mother becomes more deficient with each pregnancy.

So, it is absolutely essential for a pregnant woman to get both a large amount of nutrients and a wide range of them. Unfortunately, with the current health trends, many mothers are going through pregnancies with deficiencies intact and children are being born with concurrent deficiencies.

The vitamins and minerals frequently lacking in children are the B-complex, Vitamins C and E, and the minerals iodine, magnesium and zinc. These deficiencies are not acceptable in adults, let alone a positive way to start life!

BEFORE GETTING PREGNANT

If you are thinking about or planning to get pregnant, the first thing you need to do is get healthy! Literally, put your plans a little further out into the future and make the first step getting YOU as healthy as possible. You want to have a healthy kid, but you also have to do it for yourself!

If you are going to be able to enjoy the experience of motherhood, you better be healthy right from the start because it will be the most physically demanding job you can imagine. Forget that! It's not possible to imagine it!

When you get pregnant, first you go through an intense chemical transformation in your body that requires huge amounts of nutrients. Through the pregnancy, you grow a child that demands its share of vitamins and minerals. And then in labor, you do the hardest physical and emotional work your body can endure. After the birth, your body goes through another set of chemical changes, your whole life changes, your emotional stress increases and now you are getting a whole lot less sleep!

If you weren't in tip-top shape before you started this process, you could quickly be in trouble!!! So, carefully go through the program and get yourself healthy so you can enjoy your choice.

SO YOUR PREGNANT!

One of the interesting things I've observed about pregnant women is the speed with which their bodies heal! I am always reminded of that scene with Barbara Streisand in the movie *Come Saturday Morning* where she is watering some flowers and immediately they grow six inches just from her love. That's exactly how pregnant bodies feel as they go through the diet and healing process. The speed of healing is twice as fast, though I don't recommend women use this as a way to get healthy! Still, it is a joy to witness!

Being pregnant doesn't mean that you are eating food 'for two' but in quantities of vitamins and minerals needed, it IS true. As the baby grows, the squeezed, squashed and kicked digestive system usually won't let you eat food enough for two, anyway. It is a good idea to start getting used to eating small amounts of food every one or two hours now.

One 'food' you need to be especially careful with when you are pregnant is salt. You need natural sodium in your body and will get it with the addition of seaweeds as a mineral supplement, and from your food. While you are pregnant, cut the table salt out completely or use it VERY sparingly! Over use can result in water retention.

So, which diet do you do, now that you're pregnant? Check which Health Assessment Group you are in and use the following chart.

FOR PREGNANT WOMEN ONLY				**MONTHS ON EACH APPROACH:**			
	Basic 3	Basic 2	Basic 1	Phase 2	Getting There	Core Diet	Semi Final
Group 1			1	1	1	1	1
Group 2		1	1	1	1	1	1
Group 3	1	1	1	1	1	1	1
Group 4	1	1	1	1	1	1	1

There are a couple of ways you can do the program even if you are already months pregnant.

First, start taking the suggested amounts of supplements at your current level of pregnancy. See the 'Needed Nutrients' section below. Second, work out a schedule that you feel you can live with.

There is one thing you want to be careful about; that is, you don't want to create a healing crisis by trying to hurry up the healing process. It will be better for you and your baby to do a slow and consistent healing; if you go too fast you may release too many toxins in the bloodstream. This is not a time in your life to create a situation that overloads your body! If you are already over five months pregnant, there are numerous ways you can still benefit from following the program. Say you are five months pregnant and you are in the Third Group, you could cut each program phase down to two and a half to three weeks instead of a month. Or if you are in the Second Group and six months along, then you could do each diet for two weeks instead of four weeks.

Or you can do the Basic Balancer and the following two phases for the remainder of the pregnancy and still be assured that you are getting all the nutrients you need.

NEEDED NUTRIENTS

Food-type vitamin and mineral supplements are really important to add to the diet right from the beginning of the pregnancy. The need for nutrients dramatically increases as the baby grows which means that you have to both eat foods that are highly concentrated sources of vitamins, minerals, proteins, and other nutrients and take plenty of extra supplements.

Just the grams of protein you need goes from twenty grams at the beginning of the pregnancy to sixty plus grams at the end. An egg has six grams, a cup of yogurt has eight, a quart of milk has thirty-two, a 1/2 lb. of fish has approximately fifty-five plus. Cottage cheese is one of the foods that I suggest you work into your diet, once you can digest it; it has thirty-two grams of protein per one cup! You can blend it into salad dressings, add it to smoothies, blend it for making white sauces or ice cream.

The following chart gives some suggestions for vitamin and mineral and protein needs through the nine months. As you can see, the levels go steadily upward over the nine month cycle.

SOURCE MONTHS THROUGH PREGNANCY

	1-2	**3-4**	**5-6**	**7**	**8-9**
Grams of Protein	25	35	45	55	60+

SPLIT THE DOSE, TAKE 1/2 IN THE MORNING AND 1/2 IN THE EVENING

	1-2	**3-4**	**5-6**	**7**	**8-9**
Alfalfa					
juice powder (tsp)	1 1/2	2	2 1/2	2 1/2	3
juice capsules	10	13	15	17	20
tablets	10	13	15	17	20
AlphaPlex					
Barley Green					
powder (in tsp)	1 1/2	2	3	4	5
tablets	6	8	12	16	20
Bee Pollen					
capsules	4	6	8	12	16
loose (in tsp)	1	1 1/2	2	3	4
tablets	4	6	8	14	16
Blue-Green Algae					
Cell-Tech's Alpha	6	8	12	16	20
Chlorophyll					
powder (in tsp)	1 1/2	2	3	4	5
liquid (in tsp)	1 1/2	2	3	4	5
Flora-dix formulas					
Herbs & Iron (tsp)	2	3	3	4	5
Multi-Vitamin (tsp)	2	3	3	4	5
tablets	6	8	11	13	16
Green Magma					
powder (in tsp)	1 1/2	2	3	4	5
tablets	6	8	12	16	20
Km (in tsp)	2	2	3	3	4
Nettles					
capsules	4	7	11	15	18
Spirulina					
powder (in tsp)	3/4	1	1 1/2	1 3/4	2
tablets	3	4	5	7	8
Wheat Grass					
juice powder (tsp)	1 1/2	2	2 1/2	3	4
juice capsules	6	8	11	13	16
tablets	6	8	11	13	16

HERBS AND PREGNANCY

Remember that herbs are powerful plants that have concentrated nutrients within them. They have an immediate affect in the bloodstream, whether you feel it or not. Now, when you're pregnant, you already have lots more activity going on in your bloodstream, like peeing for two! So, it makes sense that you have to be careful about what you add into this busy and sometimes overloaded system.

There are certain herbs that will give you added nutrients and are known to be helpful for pregnant women and there are others that can cause some serious, negative side effects. I have a friend that took Blue Cohosh six weeks before her baby was due and it sent her immediately into labor! Both the Black and Blue Cohoshs have been used to tone the uterus five to six weeks before labor, but some bodies can overreact. So to be extra cautious I suggest:

POSITIVE HERBS FOR PREGNANCY:
Alfalfa, Kelp, Parsley, Raspberry Leaves, Strawberry Leaves.

NEGATIVE HERBS:
Black Cohosh, Blue Cohosh, Dong Quai, Echinacea, Ginseng, Mistletoe, Pennyroyal, Rue.

Remember to trust your own knowingness when deciding what diet to follow and what nutrients to take. Your sensitivity levels are way up when you're pregnant; use them!

LIFE AFTER THE BIRTH

NURSING MOMS

Now you are REALLY eating for two! But there are a few things you need to be aware of:

1) There are certain foods that will travel through your body and into the milk. Unfortunately for my kid, no one warned me that eating garlic might affect my milk and might give my newborn colic. I figured it out the hard way; from months of walking a colicy baby through the night! It finally dawned on me that there was a connection between what I was eating and the nasty look my kid gave me when he took a suck of milk that tasted yucky! So, stay away from:

VEGGIES: cabbage family: cabbages, broccoli, brussels sprouts, cauliflower, kale, kohlrabi, collard greens, garlic, onions, peppers from mild sweets to hot chilis.

DAIRY PRODUCTS: strong-flavored cheeses including mild cheddars, Brie, colby, longhorn

NUTS & SEEDS: harder to digest nuts and seeds: walnuts, Brazil nuts, macadamia, sunflower seeds, sesame seeds, pinenuts

OILS: nut oils

MISCELLANEOUS: brewer's or nutritional yeasts, chocolate, large amounts of parsley or sage, vinegar

2) Since you are eating for two, you have to continue to supply your infant with all the nutrients it needs, so 50% of your diet should be fruits (including quinoa) and veggies (including potatoes, corn,

cornmeal, sprouted grains, and sprouted beans and legumes.) 50% of your diet needs to be proteins (dairy, meats, fish, nuts and seeds,) starches (grains and soy products,) sweeteners, and oils.

3) Be sure to eat enough food!

My own experience of nursing was wonderful and for the two years I nursed my kid, I got to eat like a pig! But the first month or so was pretty intense. When I left the hospital I was right back to the weight I had been before I got pregnant (but with very saggy tummy tissue!) Within a week of nursing, though, I had dropped another 13 pounds! That is dangerously thin for me.

I started eating two to three helpings at each meal, followed with one to two helpings of dessert and in-between snacks consisting of quarts of yogurt! It took a couple of weeks to bring my weight up to 120 which is still too skinny for me. But no matter how much I ate, my weight stayed there for the next two years.

Our bodies are very different in the way they react to the hormones that create milk. You may or may not have a similar experience as mine; the point, though, is to be prepared for whatever changes your body indicates. It is preferable to put on a couple of extra pounds by 'overeating' than to 'under eat' and have to try to make it up! With a little extra weight, you can always eat lightly for a day or two and let the energy needed for your milk production burn it off.

4) I'm sure you've all heard *"If you want good milk production, drink beer."* Well, that statement is actually partly true. But we're not talking about Bud or Miller's Draft! The old, time-honored way of making DARK beers left many of the Vitamin B's from the grains in the beer. Of course, it's the vitamins that increased the milk production! I don't recommend drinking any alcohol while you are nursing, at least until the child is a year or so old. At that point small amounts of alcohol in the milk probably won't have any negative effect on your kid, but watch for them anyway. If you do see any reactions in your child after drinking possibly spiked milk, don't continue with any alcohol products.

There are other ways to increase the quality and quantity of milk. Obviously, the first way is to eat high quality foods and to take an abundance of nutrients. You can also include regular servings of Fennel and Marshmallow teas. They are both reported to increase milk production as well as help the baby sleep better and longer (something all new mothers definitely need!)

5) It's a good idea to remember your baby may need and actually like some just plain water on a regular basis. Use a plastic dropper until the baby is old enough to take liquids from a spoon or cup.

This is also a good time to add additional vitamins and minerals if you want. If your baby is manifesting any ill-health symptoms or you suspect that you may have passed on nutrient deficiencies, add a few drops of a liquid vitamin source and liquid mineral source to the water.

6) TO STOP MILK PRODUCTION — When you and your baby are ready to stop nursing, there are a number of things you can easily do.

a) The addition of parsley and/or sage to the diet will help.

b) Taking 10-30 mg. of manganese daily will also dry you up.

Stopping milk flow is much easier than knowing when is the appropriate time to stop nursing. If you have the luxury of staying home with your baby, then you can nurse them for as long as they need. But you do need to make some judgement calls here. Generally, up to two years old, kids use nursing to get food and security. But there's a point where they can start using it to manipulate you.

Don't let this happen! If you find your kid constantly asking to nurse when you are right in the middle of something, this is a clue. Years ago, I had a friend who nursed her son until he was three and he had her doing somersaults! He may have needed security from her, but he learned to get it through manipulation. Not okay!!

When my kid had just turned two years old, I realized that I was tired of the nursing. I told him, *"You know what, I think it's time to stop giving you a tit."* He responded with a curious look on his face like, *"I think I know what you are saying, but I'm not sure I want to believe it."*

Then I told him that from that point on, when he asked for a tit, I'd race him to the fridge and get him a glass of milk. And that's what we did. It only took four days for him to start asking for a glass of milk and to never ask for a tit again!

INFANTS, BABIES AND INTRODUCING FOODS

ABOUT A FORMULA

I guess I've always been a fan of 'the natural method,' since even twenty-five years ago I nursed my kid for two years. And I had a kid who flourished on mother's milk. But I am practical enough to know that nursing just doesn't work for everyone. (We need to change the male/linear-oriented business world into a more spherical/user-friendly place. But, in the meantime . . .)

If you need to use a formula to feed your baby, do some doctoring on the product you choose. Try to find a formula with the least amount of chemicals. Remember, that the more processed a food is, the harder it will be for the body to deal with it. Boost the digestibility by using diluted yogurt (1 part yogurt and 3 parts water) to mix in the formula. You can also add drops of liquid vitamin and mineral sources.

If your baby is lactose intolerant and cannot have your milk, there are a number of things that you can do. First, you can try a formula using yogurt as the base, adding olive oil, liquid children's vitamins and liquid seaweeds for minerals. Remember, the milk molecule is very difficult for bodies to break down, but the culturing process does it for you.

Many lactose-intolerant children can handle diluted yogurt. I worked on a baby with a 'disease' that listed him as protein-, fat- and sugar-intolerant. He weighed thirteen lbs. at a year and a half old and hadn't gained any weight for almost a year. He was a sweet, smiling baby but was lethargic and jaundiced yellow. We started him on yogurt and quinoa, vitamins and minerals. Within a month, he started to gain weight and to explore his world. In a year, he was a normal, healthy kid.

Second, you can use a soy milk product that you doctor. Use a brand of soy milk that is made from totally organic soybeans. You do NOT want to doctor soy products with dairy products, but still need to boost the acidophilus culture in your baby's intestines. So, twice a week, dilute an acidophilus tablet in some water and dropper feed your baby ONE-HALF of it. Put your formula in the blender and add liquid vitamins/minerals and vegetable oils by drizzling them into the whirling mix. When you introduce foods into a lactose intolerant baby's diet, it is a good idea to wait a few months before you try yogurt in their diets. Lactose intolerance is linked to vitamin and mineral deficiencies, so as you heal these levels in your baby, they should become tolerant of dairy products.

If you want to add drops of herbal extracts into the formula, like drops of Echinacea to fight off a cold, you will need to first deal with the alcohol in the extract. Simply add the herb drops to a 1/4 c of hot water and let that sit for five minutes so the alcohol can evaporate off. Then use the water as part of the formula-mixing water.

INTRODUCING THE FIRST FOODS

Let your baby be the person who decides when he or she is ready for real food. This can happen from four months old to ten months old. My kid was always very precise with his interaction with the world, so when he could feed himself, he finally got interested in food (at ten months old.) At six months, the pediatrician suggested I start giving this quick-growing kid some food. So I mashed some cooked carrots and, with a few other delicacies, tried 'feeding' for a few days. After three days, he showed his displeasure with this whole procedure by spitting each mouthful back at me!

So, let your kid show interest first, then start offering them easy-to-digest foods. Also, let your children decide if they are vegetarians or not! My kid refused to eat fish or meats until he was six and outside pressure caught up with him. On the other hand, I've seen some kids go for meats right from the start!

It's important to understand that a baby's digestive system is not fully developed at birth! It usually takes about three years before that change is complete. (Actually, the digestive system changes throughout our lives.) So the introduction of foods needs to correspond to the changes in the baby's body, otherwise, your baby may develop an allergic reaction to indigestible foods.

Body development takes huge amounts of vitamins, minerals, animal and vegetable proteins, sugars, and fats, so make sure you keep the diet high in these foods.

Check out the information on Mucus Reactions, Emotional Reactions, and on 'How Do I Reintroduce Foods'. Watch for any of them after you introduce a food. Watch for later reactions like napping out of normal rhythms, nighttime crankiness, gas and bloating, and bad dreams.

If and when you have a sick child, cut back on the variety of foods they are eating. Just as you should do for yourself, feed only the easiest-to-digest foods when any extra stress is present.

Within each food group, the lists run with the 'easiest-to-digest' foods at the beginning and the 'harder-to-digest' foods at the end. But don't expect your kid to stick to any order. If they are drawn to a particular food, let them try a small amount and check for reactions. If there are none, try larger amounts and watch again.

Once you have confirmed the body's ability to proper digest a food, then you can start mixing it with other confirmed foods. There are some restrictions that go with mixing foods together though. Pay special attention to them in the Nutritional Rules section on the following page.

FOODS FROM 5 TO 12 MONTHS

<u>FOOD GROUP</u>	<u>YES FOODS</u>
FRUITS-----------------------	dates, bananas, guava, papaya, mango, persimmons, apricots, kiwi, peaches, pears, figs.

FOOD GROUP	YES FOODS
VEGGIES----------------------	fresh peas, carrots, winter squash and pumpkin, potatoes and yams, parsnips, summer squash, greens, jicama, Jerusalem artichokes, celery, cucumbers, arrowroot, corn/cornmeal, beets, wild rice
DAIRY-------------------------	yogurt and eggs
MEATS------------------------	fish and chicken (but no shellfish)
NO NUTS AND SEEDS	
GRAINS-----------------------	quinoa, millet, oats
SWEETENERS---------------	maple syrup, malt syrup, rice/rice bran syrup
OILS---------------------------	butter
SOY PRODUCTS----------	soy milk
NO SPROUTED BEANS OR LEGUMES	
HERBS-------------------------	catnip, fennel, mints, minute amounts of other herbs & extracts
SPECIAL ITEMS------------	carob powder

SUPPLEMENTS:

See the information in the last section of this chapter.

NUTRITIONAL RULES:

1) Food should only be offered in a calm and peaceful environment. As you introduce foods, you are also introducing food-eating habits. Make these habits as healthy as the food!

If your kid is needing hugging, cuddling, and reassuring, don't give them food instead! Suckling a breast or bottle for security is natural, but using food in the same way is a destructive pattern that can screw up eating patterns for life! Create a calm environment. Teach your kid to take a pause to think about the food in front of you BEFORE you feed them. Talk to them about the FOOD as you are preparing it, like where it comes from, what it tastes like, what its texture is like, what it does for your body and how it got to your table. All this talk about food actually gets the body ready for it even before it passes the lips!

2) Offer food only when your kid is obviously hungry. Let your kid decide when they are hungry. You can ask them throughout the day, but don't push it. Follow your schedule through the day, explaining situations to your kid so they can make choices. For example, if your kid hasn't eaten, but you need to go do the laundry, then you can explain that and ask for some choices of what foods to take with you to eat there or on the way.

3) Serve only one fruit at a time. As in adults, mixed fruits can confuse the pancreas. Separate fruits by one-half hour.

4) Serve fruits and veggies separately, as you introduce them. After your baby starts eating at least one half of its diet from food, then you can try combining one fruit and veggies. I'm not sure exactly why this combination can be a problem for some kids, though I think that it has to do with the developing state of the digestive system. But I have seen babies with diaper rashes, stomachs and headaches from eating fruits and veggies together!

5) Never combine proteins (dairy, meats, nuts and seeds) with starches (regular/unsprouted grains and soy products.) Read the Nutritional Rule on this in Chapter 12, page 169. As you will read there, you can combine proteins with other proteins, fruit, veggies, sweeteners and oils OR starches with other starches, fruit, veggies, sweeteners and oils. So, you could add diluted yogurt to cornmeal as a protein/veggie combination or rice milk to oatmeal as a starch to starch combination.

6) No shellfish. As for adults, shellfish are very difficult to digest and should not be introduced to kids until they are five years old or more.

FOOD PERCENTAGES:
10-20% fruits and veggies, 80-90% everything else, and NO raw veggies.

FOODS FROM 12 TO 24 MONTHS
By now you can probably see food habits developing in your kid. I know I was amazed as I watched my kid eat. He'd usually do two or three days of mostly the same foods throughout the day, then he'd switch to a different group for two or three days and then do another group. For him, over a seven to ten day period, he chose an overall diet that was totally balanced. Remember to continue to watch for mucus reactions and/or Emotional Reactions as you introduce foods.

YES FOODS	NO FOODS
FRUITS: all fruits but-----------------	citrus fruits: oranges, lemons, limes, grapefruit, tangerines, tangelos, pineapple
VEGGIES: all veggies but--------------	asparagus and horseradish
DAIRY:	
Up to 18 months: all dairy but-----	cheese and cow's milk (goat is OK)
From 18 - 24 months: all dairy products	

<u>YES FOODS</u>	<u>NO FOODS</u>
MEATS: all meats but--------------------	pork and beef

NUTS AND SEEDS: after 18 months:
       Hazelnut butter-------------   all other nuts and seeds

GRAINS: all grains, sprouted grains
       and quinoa but-------------   spelt, kamut and wheat

SWEETENERS: all natural sweeteners

OILS: butter, olive oil and grapeseed oil only

SOY PRODUCTS: all soy products but soy powders

SPROUTED BEANS & LEGUMES: all

HERBS: all herbs and spices

SPECIAL ITEMS: carob powder, vinegar and condiments only

NUTRITIONAL RULES: Same as for 5-12 month group

SUPPLEMENTS: See the information in the last section of this chapter.

PERCENTAGES OF FOOD:
    10-20% fruits and veggies, 80-90% everything else, and NO raw veggies.

FOODS FROM 24 TO 36 MONTHS

Well, you've got a full-blown kid on your hands, now. Right around two years old, my kid announced that he was no longer a small kid, but said, *"I'm a big kid, now!"* So, it's time to introduce the rest of the foods into these big kids' diets. It's still important to watch for Mucus Reactions and Emotional Reactions as you try a new food. Remember, you don't want to aid the development of any allergic reactions.

<u>You can now add the following:</u>
    FRUITS: all citrus fruits: oranges, lemons, limes, grapefruit, tangerines, tangelos, pineapple
    VEGGIES: asparagus and horseradish
    DAIRY: cheese and all milk
    MEATS: pork and beef
    NUTS AND SEEDS: all other nuts and seeds

GRAINS: spelt, kamut and wheat
OILS: all other oils (but use sparingly)
SOY PRODUCTS: soy powders
HERBS and SPICES: salt
SPECIAL ITEMS: chocolate, brewer's and nutritional yeast

NUTRITIONAL RULES: Same as above

SUPPLEMENTS: See the chart at the end of this section.

PERCENTAGES OF FOOD:
10-30% fruits and veggies, 70-90% everything else, and all the veggies can be raw, if desired.

SUPPLEMENTS FOR INFANTS, BABIES AND BIG KIDS

Because of the development of the digestive system in the first three years, it is important to make sure that added supplements are VERY easy to digest and utilize. I suggest using liquid supplements since they basically take no digestion and go right into the bloodstream. There are a number of food supplements you can buy or make into liquid forms. Here are the most common ones:

Alfalfa powder, for vitamins and minerals
Bee Pollen, blended in water, for vitamins
Blue-Green Algaes, for vitamins
Chlorophyll powder or liquid, or vitamins
Dulse liquid extract, for minerals

Kelp liquid extract, for minerals
Liquid Multi-Vitamins
Spirulina powder, for vitamins & mineral
Sprouted grass juices, for vitamins

Children's Flora-dix and Dulse Extract are the vitamin and mineral sources that have been most commonly asked for by babies bodies, but any of them will boost your baby's nutrient levels.

Use the directions on the bottle if it is listed for children or use 1/8 of the adult dosage for infants under twelve months and 1/4 the dosage for children over twelve months.

Chapter 10
Dis-Ease and Dis-Comfort and
How to Move Them Into Ease and Comfort

ABOUT DIS-EASE IN GENERAL

All serious dis-eases and dis-comforts are the body's and spirit's way of crying out. Something within is NOT in harmony and is demanding attention NOW.

It is very important to take care of the physical health of the body when there is a serious problem, if only to get the body symptoms out of the way or under control so you can see what the deeper level of the dis-ease is. But getting to the core of the situation is the only sure way of healing. You must move the dis-ease into ease and the dis-comfort into comfort.

Once you realize what this core NEED is, address it and take care of it. I mean, if you stand back from most dis-eases and look at the obviousness of the problem you will be able to see what this core problem is. Heart and lung problems create contractions in the physical area and represent the contraction of self-love within the person. When someone experiences, say, a heart attack, their choices become obvious. They HAVE to take care of themselves or else they will die! And most serious dis-eases are this obvious! Cancers are all tied to deep-level fears focused through some body and spirit function. AIDS is about denial. EBV is linked to needed changes in life direction.

There is a great book out there, *The 12 Stages of Healing,* by Donald M Epstein, D.C., that takes you through the different stages of moving dis-ease and dis-comfort into ease and comfort. The techniques are clear and concise, with physical and visual exercises to help you recognize Core Needs and appropriately deal with them. Epstein's approach is clearly nonjudgemental and teaches you to love yourself through your dis-ease.

Less serious problems also have their ways of calling for balance. Hay fever is tied to not wanting to fill the lungs and body with the life-force of Spring! Herniated disks, like most back problems, are linked to needing support or being tired of being the one who supports others.

Louise Hay has a number of books that will give you more information on the spiritual, emotional, or mental aspects of dis-eases and dis-comforts. In some of the following sections, I will discuss emotional, mental or spiritual connections I have repeatedly seen linked to a specific dis-ease or dis-comfort.

I also want to talk to you about one of my pet peeves. The medical profession has latched onto this concept of RISK as a way to . . . I don't know what! I mean, it's a scare tactic that most people respond to, but 'risk' has been blown way out of proportion.

Don't get hooked into the fear pictures that are created around 'risk.' Remember, what the allopathic profession leaves out of the equation: the emotional, mental and spiritual aspects of dis-ease and dis-comfort.

Also, watch out for the belief system of direct cause and effect. If it was true that smoking 'caused' cancer, then why doesn't everyone who smokes get cancer? Only about a third of the people who die of lung cancer ever smoked at all!!! If high cholesterol 'caused' heart disease, why doesn't everyone with high cholesterol develop heart disease? I could go on forever with a list of these kinds of questions, but I think you get the point.

There are two other systems I like to discuss with you, they are the ideas of 'entrainment' and 'contagious.' The first I remember hearing about the theory of 'entrainment' was listening to a Deepak Chopra tape. He explained this phenomena as the body's natural pattern of aligning itself to the flows of life and nature. Examples of entrainment are: women who live together all start having their periods together; mothers and babies develop heartbeat and breath patterns when they hold each other; girlfriends in Hawaii will all have periods when volcanos go off.

After listening to this and looking at the world in a new way, my friend, Trudy, had a great realization, 'contagious' is actually 'entrainment.' When one person picks up a virus or bacteria from someone else, what they really have done is resonate with the energy vibration of the dis-ease!

I couldn't believe the obviousness of this realization when she told me about it! I can't remember a time when I picked up a cold or flu from someone, because I never really believed that germs were the problem. Unconsciously, I just shielded myself from a sick person I was talking to. When Trudy explained 'contagious' I realized what I had been doing. I was just keeping the vibration of the dis-ease out of my body, so I never got sick! And when I have experienced a flu or cold, it has always been clear it was my own creation of overwhelm.

So, if you meet up with a 'contagious' dis-ease, don't let yourself take on the 'feel' of it. Remain in your own center and don't resonate with the 'sick energy.' If you do 'pick up' the vibration and you do get sick, then look for what it was you resonated with, clear the feeling and its issues, and get yourself well. This is a good place to also chuckle at yourself!

HEALING SUGGESTIONS

ABOUT MEDICATIONS

If you are taking medications when you start following this approach, don't change anything about that practice. Keep taking the same number of pills at the same time of day. You want to keep the chemical levels of medications in your bloodstream and body the same as you take yourself through the healing process.

But, be aware. As you heal your body, your need for medications may change. Your medication can actually work better when your body works right! Ask your doctor what symptoms you might experience if you are taking too much of any medicine, then watch for those symptoms. If you start to experience any of them, talk to your doctor about adjusting your prescription.

If your goal is to get off a medication, or get it within controllable limits, wait until your body is obviously getting healthy. I suggest at least a six month wait. Then coordinate the reduction program with your doctor. When your body is healthy, medicinal herbs, that stimulate functions in your body, will also work better and can frequently be used instead of corresponding medicines.

One of the things that happens as you reduce a medication, is you give your body the opportunity to readjust itself and take functions back upon itself again. Just remember that this process takes some time, so work with your body when it is ready; don't push your desire and will upon it.

ABOUT HERBS

Herbs can be taken in either capsules or tinctures. When you decide to take an herb, try it in both forms. Any herb you use for balancing the endocrine system should be taken in capsule form.

Like all supplements, it is always preferable to take herbs in both the morning and the evening. This gives your body more opportunities to use the herb in the healing process.

Start with a small amount (1-2 caps. or 10 drops) and increase them over a week or two. It is safe for most herbs to be increased to 5 capsules or 20 drops of extract, all taken at one time, and to be taken two to three times a day.

High levels of herbs can push people into "a healing crisis," especially cleansing herbs, so be aware of feeling flu-ish, overtired, or off-center. If you push your healing into an overreaction, stop taking herbs for a week or more and let your body catch up with the healing process and toxin release.

Remember, bodies almost always prefer slow gradual healing rather than overload. Gently pace your healing by watching your body's reactions.

AIDS

AIDS is a virus that is worthy of the computer age; the way that it is mutating is like a high-speed computer. There is no way that medicine will be able to keep up with the changes because of the way that it encodes destruction into cellular memory.

The initial way to stop AIDS is to be very careful about your sexuality and to be careful about what enters your bloodstream. If you are concerned about blood transfusions, have your own blood stored for future use.

The 'official' word is that AIDS is incurable; but there are numerous recorded cases of people going from HIV-positive to HIV-negative! NEW AGE magazine had a great article, *"Why I Survive AIDS"* (September/October 1991) written by a woman who beat the infection.

Her conclusion of the energetic basis of the syndrome is the same as the response I have got from AIDS infected bodies. The energetic fields that pull HIV into the body is the energy of DENIAL.

If you have AIDS, the first thing you have to know is that this infection can be cured IF and ONLY IF you release all denial from your life. You have to make every experience in your day to day life totally and completely joyful. You have to see yourself as the universal perfection that you all are. All guilt, judgments, 'shoulds' and 'have to's' need to be dropped into the past and left there. And if you want to avoid this virus, you also have to live with complete joy!

On a physical level I have consistently seen high level vitamin and mineral deficiencies. It is the only group I have consistently seen with ALL their mineral levels deficient! This definitely indicates that the virus is using all the different minerals, diverting them from other body uses and leaving the body deficient. I also have seen AZT deplete minerals.

PHYSICAL SUGGESTIONS: Start with the Super Cleanser Diet and do it until your overall energy and health are at a high level. Then move on through the program to the Basic Balancer. I suggest that you stay on this diet approach until you clear the virus.

Take two or three times the amount of vitamins and minerals listed in the Supplement Charts. Taking Propolis, which is antibiotic, antiviral, antifungal, anti-microbal and antibacterial, in large quantities, say twenty to thirty drops three or four times a day, can help ward off other infections and problems.

SPIRITUAL SUGGESTIONS: Change your life and life-style. Get happy. Whether you beat this virus or not is beside the point. Your inner self has clearly put the warning sign out and it says *"You can't go on the way things are!"* Don't worry about whether you 'know' what direction you should go or not, just change what you know DOESN'T work. As you let go of one thing that makes you unhappy, the next thing will become obvious.

ALCOHOL AND ALCOHOLISM

Alcohol has been around for a long time and I seriously doubt it is going to disappear from our lives. There's no way around the fact that alcohol is a body stress, though in minimal amounts it can actually have some body, mind and soul benefits! For most people, once their bodies are balanced, taking some extra vitamins and minerals will clear the negative side affects of alcohol. You can then use alcohol as a tool to remind you to relax, to chill out from life's stresses.

Alcoholism is not necessarily the same thing as alcohol intolerant. I separate the two like this. Alcoholism is the abuse of alcohol as a way to numb yourself to life and its pains; it's an emotional, mental and spiritual abuse. Alcohol intolerance is a physical imbalance that can lead to alcoholism or total allergic reactions to it.

ABOUT THE PROPER USE OF ALCOHOL

If alcohol is one of those delicacies you wish to have in your life, then you need to take responsibility for the stress that it creates in your life.

Personally, I'm a beer lover. I usually have a beer a day, not for the alcohol content, because I rarely feel affects from it, but for the ph balance it creates in my body. But I have to always be aware of the energy and nutrients it uses in my body. So I compensate by supplying extra vitamins and minerals for to remove the stress.

I have friends that are wine experts and deal in importing wines and beers into New Mexico. They have taken my suggestions on dealing with alcohol, and always compensate their alcohol intake with extra supplements.

One of my friends has put together a combination of herbs to help deal with other negative effects connected with alcohol intake! If alcohol is a regular part of your life, then I suggest you check out the herb combination, Imbibers Sanity, from Delights in Alchemy. It was originally formulated to take the edge off emotional reactions that alcohol can bend out of proportion, especially the disharmony it can create within a couple.

Just make sure that you take a vitamin and mineral food supplement like alfalfa and kelp to both give your body nutrients to deal with the stress and to help your body flush the alcohol. For each beer or shot of tequila, I will take one each of kelp and alfalfa.

I also like to repeat the story of really tying one on a few New Year's Eves ago. I rarely have ever done this because I'm such a sensitive lightweight, but there were four of us on this New Year's Eve. We did alot of mixed alcohols, which is a real no-no, and assorted other indulgences. Around 4 a.m. we all headed off to bed, but my partner and I took hangover precautions. I took a dozen kelp tablets and a bunch of blood-purifying and liver-cleansing herb extracts. I slept like a baby for four hours and then was cheerfully up and ready for the first day of the New Year! I went for a two hour walk and still no one else was up. Hours later, our host and hostess stumbled out of bed. One of them was very gray and the other was a sickly shade of green. They took one look at my smiling face and almost tossed their cookies! I quickly scooted out the door for another walk!

Now, I'm not suggesting that you can stress yourself like this and get away with it. I am saying that if you occasionally do go overboard, you can compensate your body for it by giving your body the tools it needs to deal with the stress.

ALCOHOL INTOLERANCES

But there are those people who just can't do alcohol, no matter how balanced their bodies get! I have seen a strange pattern in some bodies that makes me understand this inability to tolerate alcohol. Outside of the body, fermenting foods create alcohol as a by-product; inside the body, fruits and vegetables ferment in the intestines but the completed process of making alcohol is stopped.

Somehow, in some bodies, this 'uncompleted' fermenting process creates a desire for alcohol to 'complete the process.' And in other bodies, I have seen a total intolerance for not only alcohol, but anything that quickly ferments in the intestines. I don't understand the mechanics behind this situation, but I have worked with a number of people trying to get the body to reinterpret this fermenting process and correct their bodies desire or repulsion for alcohol. It is a difficult, and long-term blueprint to reestablish.

Obviously, if someone with this digestion disorder follows their body's craving for alcohol, they can quickly become addicted to the pattern. When you throw in any other physical imbalances like hypoglycemia and any emotional imbalances like lack of self-esteem, you can have someone physically NEEDING alcohol. Since humans are addictive personalities, these imbalances can quickly create a pattern of indulgence. When the mind, body and emotions are all screaming for alcohol, it's a combined effort few people can refuse. I think this is partly why alcoholism runs in families. Both the physical and emotional patterns are passed on to the children. Just ask any child of an alcoholic!

To work with alcohol intolerances, do the Deep Cleanser Diet for several months and the Basic Balancer for three to four months before you think of moving on through the approach. Be aware that even the fruits on this two diets may be too much for your system. Cut them out, if necessary. Remember that dates are usually the easiest fruit to deal with.

ABOUT ALCOHOLISM

Numbing pain with alcohol obviously works, at least as a way to stay numb. But it's obviously a way to stay stuck in the pain instead of moving through it and out the other side.

By the time you've moved your life into a pattern of alcoholism, you have also set your body into some real vitamin and mineral deficiencies and physical and emotional imbalances. So, it's important to get your body healing, no matter what your relationship to alcohol continues to be. You will find that as you bring your body into a physical balance, your overall desire for alcohol will lessen.

Start by doing the Deep Cleanser for several months and double the amount of vitamins and minerals suggested for that level. Then carefully move through the rest of the program.

Take care of the emotional, mental and spiritual aspects of life with whatever support you need. The twelve step programs work for some people, but not everyone. Look for alternative support groups that have similar philosophies to your own. Self-abuse is not the way to clear yourself of whatever pain you are dragging around. Self-love is really the best revenge!

Use the Temporal Tap technique, Chapter 16, as a tool to change the desire for alcohol and to replace it with patterns of self-love.

ALLERGIES

I use the word 'allergies' to describe a wide range of conditions in the body. An allergen is any out-of-body substance that causes the body to go into a defense reaction when it is brought into the body, either through ingesting it through your mouth, inhaling it through the lungs or absorbing it through the skin. Allergic reactions can range from simple mucus reactions to flu-like symptoms, itchy eyes, sneezing, hives, rashes, digestive distress, diarrhea, constipation, hay fever, asthma or anaphylactic shock.

Having any allergic reaction means that certain levels of nutrients, especially free-radical eating Vitamin C, are deficient in your body, so the first two things you need to do is get your overall toxin levels down and get your overall vitamin and mineral levels up.

Following this diet program will usually take care of most minor level deficiencies without you having to do anything else. But it you have more intense deficiencies, you can do additional things to speed the healing up.

First you need to follow the appropriate level of Basic Diets for a minimum of three to four months. This time frame will give your body a chance to get balanced by removing certain allergens from your diet, by taking the suggested nutrients so you can start bringing up your vitamin and mineral levels and by giving the body the time for the overall toxin level to drop. Then, and only then, should you think about taking extra measures to deal with the problem. Check out the suggestions below.

FOR OVERALL ALLERGIES

Try any of the following, one at a time, for several weeks at a time, to see if your symptoms respond. If they do respond, you can continue with them for six weeks at a time, then take a week or two break and then you can repeat the process.

**Extra Vitamin C. Always do CHEWABLE Vitamin C, as it needs saliva to be properly used in the body. Try adding 500-1500 mg. initially. For intense problems like mercury poisoning, 5-10,000 mg. may be helpful. Increase your C level for a month and then back off it for week or more. Always take Vitamin C with a food that is also high in C, like potato, fruits, and yellow veggies.

**Take Blood-Purifying and Cleansing Herbs. Try any of the following herbs in capsule or tincture/extract form: Burdock, Camomile, Comfrey, Dandelion, Echinacea, Hyssop, Myrrh, Red Clover, Oat Straw, Slippery Elm, Yellow Dock, Yerba Santa.

**Try homeopathic remedies that are especially made for allergies, in general, and specific stuff like reactions to cat and dog hair, feathers, molds, and dust.

**For lung distress, pour a few cups of boiling water into a sink or bowl. Add a few drops of eucalyptus oil and a few drops of one of the following flower remedies: Rescue Remedy, Emergency Mix or Liquid 911. Put a towel over the mix. Now, put your head under the towel and breathe deeply for a few minutes.

ABOUT HAY FEVER

Follow the above suggestions for overall allergies, concentrating your efforts one to two months before your allergy reactions usually start.

Physical-level reactions to pollens is totally understandable. Pictures of pollen granules look like small Sputniks! They have hooks and spikes protruding from them so that they will stick to the flowers they are meant to pollinate. If levels in the air get higher than normal, EVERYONE will react to them. But with high toxin levels in the body, people will just be overloaded by small amounts of pollens in the air.

Also, by aware that hay fever and overreactions to plant pollens are definitely emotional and spiritual reactions to increases of life-force. Spring is budding forth with life and sexuality.

Usually people with hay fever are living their lives way below their joy potential so when joy levels increase around them, they go into reactions to block the flow from coming into their bodies and lives.

If you are having this happen in your life, start repeating, *"I deserve joy in my life. I need to allow more joy into my life. It is my birthright to have high levels of joy in my life."* Then, let your life become more joyful, put your foot down about allowing non-joyful things to continue in your life, and start laughing more!

ABOUT ASTHMA

There are serious allergic reactions linked to asthma, the most recent realizations are for asthmatic children and their smoking parents. Obviously, the physical irritants need to be removed or the person needs to be removed from them (like moving an asthmatic kid out of L.A. smog,) but there are issues of the heart that must also be dealt with!

On a physical level, it is very important to get any and all toxins out of your body, so start with the Super Cleanser and do it for several months before moving onto the Deep Cleanser. Do that diet for two to four months before moving onto the Basic Balancer. Make sure that you follow the supplement suggestions to build up your nutrient levels. After moving onto the Basic Balancer, try some of the additional aids listed above in About Overall Allergies.

As you heal, watch for any change in steroid needs. Be sure to ask your doctor what these might be. I've worked with a number of people as they slowly lowered these levels to nothing. But it takes lots of work and healing time, on all levels.

As far as I can tell, from the various people I've worked with over the years, the real issue behind asthma is letting the inner child come out to play. And that can only happen when an environment of total safety is created in your life. I think there is a direct correlation between the doubling of asthma in this country in the last ten years, especially in children, and the level of violence that is happening on our streets and on our air waves!

The answers to the spiritual causes of asthma present themselves just before the attack. I've always thought "attack" was an interesting word to call a constriction in the lungs. But I think it accurately describes the emotional triggers that are the real base of the problem.

Watch for what sets off the reaction and explore all the aspects of it; all the emotional, mental, spiritual and physical pieces of the puzzle that will eventually give you a clear picture. Fear is one of the basic emotions that operates; it's a little hard to not get fearful when you can't breathe! But, it's more likely that fear of love is the real underling emotion.

Remember that when you are dealing with a chronic problem like asthma, the answers are not always immediate, easy or clear. Don't let that deter you from looking at them.

And also, remember not to judge yourself in your pursuit of answers or the pace with which they come! Just take it on as a part of your growth process on this planet and keep at it. Try using the Temporal Tap, Chapter 16, to release the emotional patterns and to relax the lungs.

ARTHRITIS

Arthritis has become a catch phrase for any pain that happens in the joints. Fortunately, this label is frequently wrong. Many times joint pain is directly related to toxins getting stuck in the joints because the level in the body is just too high. Frequently, lowering this toxin level clears the pain out of the joints.

One of my most recent 'arthritis' clients reported no pain or swelling in her joints after one month of following the right diet plan. She also said that she blew the diet off one day, ate a hamburger and could barely walk up the stairs an hour later! The pain and swelling subsided with 24 hours as the toxin level cleared. And she reported that she won't do that again! The toxin reaction was just too clearly related to her problem.

For more serious arthritis problems, I have seen both quick and slow healings or no healing at all. Arthritis is emotional and spiritually linked to rigid attitudes and sometimes people just don't see them in themselves or they don't want to let go of them. Years ago I worked on a woman who had had rheumatoid arthritis since she was nine years old. We worked on a number of spiritual levels and hit upon a deep issue she needed to release. For several weeks her intense daily pain was gone, but the realizations of this change scared her to her core.

She called me one day to cancel a session and apologized. She said she knew what she needed to do, but she just didn't feel that she could handle the changes it required in her life. It was easier for her to have the pain and concentrate on it than to make the changes. Years later I realized what the core issue around arthritis really is. It is the expression of ALL of the pain in the world! True arthritics are sensitive people who feel all that pain and are overwhelmed by it, understandably! But to clear their body pain, they have to become the pain and then release, the release being the hard part.

Spirit took me through an experience when I was twenty-seven where they had me tune into all the pain that exists on this plane and to feel it in my body. It was one of the most intense three days I've experienced and that's an understatement! At the end of this experience, Spirit said, *"Now, you never have to experience pain again, unless you choose to. Create a pain box in your aura and stuff all those experiences into it. Know what pain is but hold it separate from you."*

Arthritis is the holding of the pain in the body and as it bounces back and forth in the bones, it eventually destroys the joints. So, create a Pain Box, feel your own pain and the pain of the world around you, then push, stuff, shove or move the pain out of your body and be done with it. Pain, whether it's from the rape of the planet or from starving children, is all the same thing. It's an intense reaction that you can feel and then release.

Only when you release your own pain can you stand back from the pain of others and become truly compassionate. Then you can use your love and compassion to change the pain in others.

ATTENTION DEFICIT DISORDER

As of March, 1995, I have only worked with one kid stuck with this new label, and I have 'looked at' two other people who also had a 'diagnosis' of ADD. In all three cases, there were two underlying problems these people exhibited, high levels of hypoglycemia and hormonal imbalances. Both are linked to high levels of vitamin and mineral deficiencies.

The one teenager I worked with throughout the diet program definitely had improvement over both his control and attention. We worked on balancing his teenage hormones and his life got on a more level keel. And then, he still had to wait for time to move forward so he could get on with his own life!

If you or one of your kids is diagnosed with ADD, follow through the Basic Diets, as directed in the Health Assessment and work with the information on Hypoglycemia and Hormone Imbalances in this chapter. Healing yourself in these areas may not totally move you out of the ADD category, but your overall health and stability should improve and this should, in turn, increase your clarity. I just haven't worked with this situation long enough to give you more suggestions than this.

Except for one thing. Once you feel better, look for areas of boredom in your life and change them!

BACKACHES

People experience backaches for a number of reasons. Most of the pains are related to a phenomena linked to muscle-response testing. One of the things Dr. Goodheart discovered as he developed applied kinesiology was the relationship between the condition of an organ and the weakness of corresponding muscles in the body.

The actual muscle tests are based on this connection. When the organ gets sick, it reflects that weakness back into muscle. Since your muscles hold your bones in place, a weakened muscle creates a real problem in the body's structure. But once you heal the organ in the body, the muscle usually automatically readjusts itself and your backaches clear up.

If you are still experiencing backaches or other joint aches after four months on the diet, then I'd suggest you check out someone to help you. The problem may be that you keep holding daily tension in your body or that your muscles have 'forgotten' how to hold the bones properly.

Try a massage, some Shiatsu, or a chiropractor. My own favorite technique is called Ortho-bionomy. It's a technique that gently retrains the muscles to hold the bones properly without traumatizing an already traumatized area. I've seen people walk into a session in pain and walk out pain free, which is hard to beat.

If part of your back problem is linked to a disc, still the best thing you can do is eat well as you relax. Cutting the toxin level down and getting the healing level up can only help. Of course, disc problems usually do tie to more deep level emotional reactions. Watch how you structure your life and look for the weaknesses within it. Look for how your life is out of balance, like taking care of everyone else and not yourself; people with disc problems are always givers. Then change the structure to a balanced pattern. Remember, no one will take care of you, but you!

PHYSICAL SUGGESTIONS: Doing yoga or a stretching program on a regular basis is one way to keep tension from building up in your back.

Any of the Betony family of herbs are great for releasing toxins out of the muscles. I especially like White Betony, a New Mexico herb.

SPIRITUAL SUGGESTIONS: Since the spine is the major bone structure in the body, when it hurts, it's always indicating an imbalance in how you are moving energy through your body.

BLOOD PRESSURE

High blood pressure is directly related to Vitamin B and E deficiencies and high sodium intake. The second problem, salt, has been recognized by the media and the medical profession and rarely is a problem because the knowledge is out there. The Vitamin B and E problems, unfortunately, haven't been recognized and are much harder to deal with.

On a physical level, follow the appropriate diet programs and vitamin and mineral levels. After four months of working with this approach, consider adding a Vitamin B or Stress Tab into your regime, a Vitamin E tablet or two, and/or start taking any of the following herbs: Cayenne, Garlic, Hawthorn, Scullcap, Passion Flower, or Valerian.

If your problem is low blood pressure, follow the above suggestions, but try the following herbs: Brigham or Mormon Tea, Dandelion, Hawthorn, Parsley, Rosemary, or Shepherd's Purse.

The spiritual aspects of blood pressure problems is linked to 'shoulds' and the cultural pressures that go with them. Work with getting your judgements of what 'should' and 'shouldn't' be out of your life. Stop pressuring yourself!

CANCER

Talking about Cancer hasn't gotten easier over the years, because people are facing a life and death situation. It's not a place where you want to be heartless, and yet, like any serious dis-ease, it's a time in someone's' life where pussyfooting around isn't going to solve anything, either.

I've already made comment in this book about cancers being fear-based dis-eases. It is the one common element I have seen in all my clients who have been dealing with cancer.

Cancers in different areas indicate where the fear is based and how it is spiritually connected to your body. This is such an individual 'creation' that no one but the cancer person can truly identify what their base-fear is, but these examples will give you an idea of how to look at the problem. Pancreatic cancer is usually related to imbalances in personal power, throat cancers are usually related to lack of communication or creativity, colon cancer can be the pattern of hanging onto your 'stuff,' lung cancer may be not breathing in life.

Anyone who has been through a cancer experience will tell you that you REALLY have to want to be well to get well. You have to deal with alot of issues, you have to face your death and all your bugaboos, you have to deal with all your family interactions, you have to deal with power issues about your body and the medical profession, and the list can go on and on.

To grow past the cancer and to maybe beat it, you have to take the best care of yourself that you have ever done. You have to follow your heart and take on all responsibility for your life and decisions. Sometimes you have to cut people and situations out of your life to find out who you really are. And you have to do all your growth guilt-free.

All this growth is possible! Find people who will support your growth and change, whether it's to cross into the next realms or to heal your body. Find people who can help you work on all aspects of the situation, physical, emotional, mental and spiritual. You've already pushed yourself to the edge and no longer have the luxury to deal with all the aspects over a long period of time. You have to do all of them at once. You have to let go of your 'stuff' and get ecstatic about life all at the same time.

I had a glorious life experience with a wonderful woman, who also happened to be my mother-in-law. She had ovarian cancer and her body died from it. But I got to live with her the last year and a half of her life and got to watch the healing and dying process right up close and personal.

Grace was a fiercely independent person but accepted love and caring. I was blessed with the opportunity to counsel her on many levels and as we talked, it became apparent guilt was her underlying life-motivator. She felt guilty about being born, about her relationships, even about being happy. She was able to come to terms with her feelings and when she did that, she 'knew' it was time to go.

We were talking one day and I felt her drop a huge, thick curtain between us; it was like she'd gone as far as she could go with her changes, and that was that! I watched her create a situation that sabotaged the healing progress she had been making. She proceeded to clean up the ties with living relatives, and when those were complete, she crossed over. I was also blessed with the opportunity of helping her across, on the psychic plane, which I count as one of the more beautiful experiences I have had in this lifetime!

So, whether your choice in your healing is to stay or go, get on with the process. Rush headlong into it and open to the experience.

On a physical level, there have been 'cancer cures' that have been available for years, though the medical profession actively denies this. I have a friend who cured himself of melanoma, a medical impossibility. He did it with intense cleansing, lots of herbs and homeopathic remedies and, of course, totally changing his life!

I suggest that you follow the Deep Cleanser diet until your cancer goes into remission, then move to the Basic Balancer. Stay at this level until you are free of the cancer. Then start moving through the rest of the program.

I suggest regular use of Propolis tincture to keep you free of other complicating problems like flus and colds. And I've heard great things about Essiac tea; it seems to work on many levels. But, remember, once you deal with the issues behind the cancer, it hardly matters what you do to heal yourself; almost everything or anything will probably work!

CANDIDA, EPSTEIN-BARR VIRUS, CHRONIC FATIGUE SYNDROME

I lump these three problems together for two reasons; I've repeatedly seen the same diet needs with this group and, I swear I could pick a person with any of these problems out in a crowd. They all have a very similar vibration about them and they all have the same personality characteristics!!!

One of the first things I like to say to candida, EBV or CFS people is that they have to recognize these personality traits and the situations they are creating. It's not that the traits are a problem, it's just the way they have been turned internal. The negative aspects of the traits are turned inward and are used to beat up on the inner child. This internal punishment is the core emotional, mental and spiritual aspect of candida, EBV and CFS.

One of these 'positive' traits turned negative and internal is a deep desire 'to do the right thing.' Unfortunately, since we are all human, it doesn't always LOOK like we choose the right thing to do all the time. When a candida, EBV or CFS person comes to a point in their lives where they reach a fork in the road, the deep desire to 'do the right thing' becomes very strong. The fear that they will make a mistake grows within them and they become paralyzed. This is usually where the dis-ease jumps up and grabs them!

A second personality trait is a very high level of sensitivity, awareness and power. I mean, these people are very in tune with the vibrations around them. They understand the subtle emotions of others, all the un-proclaimed nuances that pass between people, all the unspoken feelings. They are some of the most powerful people I ever meet! They have a natural force and command that they are totally out of touch with, though everyone around them clearly sees it.

Unfortunately, a third trait is not believing in themselves, so they ignore their sensitivity, awareness and power and the free-floating information it gives them access to. But, because of the sensitivities, they REACT it!

An underlying trait that keeps bobbing in and out of these scenarios is judgement and self-judgement. The more you start looking at there being a right and wrong way, the less tolerance there is for making 'mistakes.' So, another trait emerges. And that is a convoluted way of looking at things that creates great Catch-22's!

Feeling dizzy from following all this? Well, that's just the energy that candida, EBV and CFS people create in their lives. Funny thing is, they usually gasp in total surprise as I discuss these points with them. I frequently hear, *"That describes me perfectly!"*

As far as I can tell, changing these dis-eases must be accompanied by changes in these traits. They all must be transformed into their positive sides. The idea of 'doing the right thing' must be opened up so that everything they do is conceived of as the right thing. There must be acceptance and development of the sensitivity, awareness and power. They must learn to believe in themselves. All patterns, habits and forms of judgement and self-judgement must be turned into acceptance and self-love. And the cycle of developing Catch-22's must be broken open so their lives can start 'going forward' rather than around in circles.

I know none of the above changes are simple. I've had lots of clients and friends over the years who have been dealing with the problems of candida, EBV and CFS and the changes healing these dis-eases demands. I know the difficulties. But, I have seen alot of people work through these changes, release the dis-ease, and get on with their lives. I know it can be done. Just concentrate on one issue at a time and get on with it.

On a physical level, there are a number of things you can do along with the right Basic Diet:

1) Severe allergic reactions can develop over time. It seems at certain points, as the dis-eases progress, the body will turn in on itself. If you eat a carrot today and there is any resemblance of carrot in your system the next day, when you ingest another carrot, the body can start treating the second carrot as an allergic and toxic substance.

Rotating foods is the major way of stopping this body reaction. It's a real pain in the butt, at least until you get use to the eating patterns and your body moves out of the reaction.

Divide the foods you can eat, food category by food category, into different days. Some people need two day rotations, more severe cases need three day rotations. It usually means that you have to eat simply. If you are following the Super Cleanser Diet, you could eat something like the schedule on the following page.

DAY ONE	DAY TWO	DAY THREE
dates	apricots	avocados
1/3 veggies	1/3 veggies	1/3 veggies
eggs	yogurt	fish
quinoa	sourdough bread	1/3 cooking herbs/spices
maple syrup	stevia	
1/3 cooking herbs/spices	1/3 cooking herbs/spices	
carob powder		
butter		

It's a good idea to keep eggs, quinoa, and maple syrup on the same day so that you can make cookies and cakes. Also, divide the veggies up so there are greens, winter squash, and root veggies each day. Keep some variety in each day.

Be careful with fruits and sweeteners. Severe cases of candida, EBV and CFS sometimes can't deal with any fruits or sweeteners at all. If you know you have problems with these, try liquid stevia extract.

2) Some people run into the same food allergy problems with their supplements, so it is a good idea to take two or three different ones and rotate them also.

3) Another problem with herbs, remedies and medications is that if they don't clear the problem, if you use them some, stop taking them and then use them again, you may develop an allergy to them! If you decide it is time to take an herbal remedy or medicine to clear the underlying virus or yeast problem, be prepared for intense emotional reactions. I've seen people who take, say Capastat or Nystatin to kill candida, go into emotional nose-dives, sometimes getting suicidal. These intense reactions are the dis-eases fight to stay alive and active.

4) I suggest regular use of propolis tincture as a protection against other problems and to work on the viruses involved. Myrrh is a herb that helps clear odd toxins out of the body and can help clear things like dead yeast cells. Chamomile should be avoided.

CHOLESTEROL

Most of you probably know more about what the medical profession has to say about cholesterol than I do. I stopped listening to them after they first issued their warnings about high cholesterol because their ideas didn't jive with what I heard from bodies. It wasn't that they were 'wrong' about their warnings; high levels of cholesterol are a problem. Americans were eating way, way too much meat in their diets, especially because we'd also become so sedentary. But cutting out everything in the diet that contains cholesterol isn't the answer to correcting this imbalance.

When I first started seeing clients, I had an older couple come to me as a last resort. They had been on a no-cholesterol doctor's diet for two years without any changes in their cholesterol levels. Their doctor wanted to put them on some medication, which was against their belief system, so they wanted to correct the problem naturally. They had not eaten eggs or butter for over two years, yet we put them on a diet similar to the Basic Balancer, which allowed them each to eat 1/2 lb. of butter and a dozen eggs a week. Within two months, their cholesterol levels started going down and within six months, the levels were within normal range.

I'm convinced, from seeing this same result over and over again over seventeen years, that balancing the body with the proper diet, vitamins and minerals will let the body to balance its own cholesterol levels.

There are a number of things you can do in conjunction with following this diet approach to help regulate your cholesterol levels.

PHYSICAL SUGGESTIONS: Oat bran is out of the diet for many months, but there is a better food that lowers cholesterol levels. That food is eggplant! Studies show that three small servings of eggplant a week will lower cholesterol 20%!!! The best oat bran studies only show an 8% decrease. So, include steamed eggplant into diet. Don't saute it and add all that fat. Make dips for baked corn chips or veggies, use it in soups and stews, or barbecue slices (this is the best!.) Another approach is to include lecithin capsules into your vitamin and mineral regime. Try one capsule morning and evening.

Both these additions will take some time to manifest results, so be patient for several months. Remember, balance is the ultimate goal.

COLDS AND FLUS

One of the fascinating things about viruses is they cannot go into a healthy cell. They don't have the mechanisms to do that, but they can go into an unhealthy cell. So, it looks to me like viruses are body cleansers.

It's normal in this country for people to have two to four colds or flus a year, which confirms we are not a very healthy people. People are creating too many toxins in their bodies and viruses regularly come along and clean them out. Obviously, once you get your toxin level down to just dealing with day to day clearing, you will be able to avoid picking up viruses. If you do get a virus running around in your system, wreaking havoc, there are numerous things you can physically do to minimize the effects.

1) At the first sign of a cold or flu, start taking propolis tincture. One of propolis's properties is it is antiviral. I usually take twenty drops in warm water several times a day when I feel 'down.' I've seen propolis speed overall healing up in numerous friends who let a virus get active in their bodies.

If you have a sore throat, gargle with the propolis/water mix. When I do eight to nine hours of counselling and straight talking, I will frequently gargle with propolis water to soothe my throat. A number of professional singers I have worked with also say it helps keep their throats.

2) Up your Vitamin C level. Make sure you take chewables and ingest some food or juice naturally high in Vitamin C to make the vitamin more usable.

3) Try adding capsules or tea of any of the following herbs: Echinacea, Myrrh, Comfrey, Mormon Tea, or Fenugreek. Of course, if you entrain with their energy, you may still run a virus through your body. But, you know, this only happens when you are desperately in need of a break from work, family or life!

It's a much better course of action to realize you are stressed and reaching that 'over the edge' point BEFORE you get sick. Let yourself take a few days off and recoup your energy before getting sick. This is usually faster and definitely saner! Remember, it's not that you can't cope with life, it's just that the life we are all leading is relatively crazy!

COLITIS AND OTHER INTESTINAL DISTRESSES

ABOUT GENERAL DISTRESS

Most intestinal distress, from constipation to diarrhea, is directly tied to what you put in your mouth. Then you expect your digestive system to cope with the foods, even if you know the they are a problem for you.

But, what you get and can expect in this situation is that the food is going to rot and putrefy. You are going to get gas and bloat. Most people will get stopped or bound up and experience pain. But some people's bodies will react by pushing the toxic mess through the system at full speed as a way to protect the body from picking up toxins. This can also create spasms and cramps in the intestines themselves. Remember the intestines are strong muscles.

Use these reactions as indicators. They are body messages that say, *"You are eating something the body can't digest properly. Stop!"* Obviously, following a diet that removes these foods, removes the reaction. Sometimes this change is immediate, sometimes it takes some time to get rebalanced. Watch for reactions tied to eating too much of a particular food, like too many dates or dried apricots!

Aloe Vera juice is a great intestinal soother. I know, if I stress my system (usually with too much popcorn or chocolate,) a 1/4 cup of aloe juice twice a day usually straightens my intestines right up.

Massaging the intestines can also be helpful. I have dealt with a number of people with 'impacted' bowels by doing hours of gently massage that gradually goes deeper and deeper until the constriction lets loose.

ABOUT COLITIS

Colitis is the reaction of constant stress and trigger release that develops when the intestines are treated badly over time. One of the more intense cases I worked with was a woman who had been having 'colitis' for twelve years. Within a few weeks on the right diet, her system relaxed and stopped the reaction. Now, it's not always this fast, but be patient. Your body will straighten this reaction out as long as you stop eating the foods that create it.

Follow the Deep Cleanser for a couple of months, incorporate aloe vera juice into your diet and take what prescription or over-the-counter medications you need until it is obvious the trigger reactions have stopped.

ABOUT CROHN'S DISEASE

Crohn's is a condition in the intestines that creates a more intense healing crisis. There is usually a narrowing of the lower intestines, bleeding or pus build up and drainage in the rectum and out the anus. There's pain and cramping from these fistulas. Usually people are placed on steroids to help their bodies deal with the problems and the body stress. Physically, Crohn's needs to be dealt with as a serious problem that needs a doctor's care as well as a very cleansing diet. Do the Deep Cleanser or Super Cleanser until the more intense symptoms subside. Then stay with the Basic Balancer.

Do aloe vera juice regularly. Slippery Elm seems to be a helpful herb. When you are choosing your vitamin and mineral sources, choose a liquid or powdered-made-to-liquid form. Or choose capsules instead of tablets, since some of the binders can be irritating.

Once your doctor can see progressive healing, ask about lowering your steroid use. Work together to get those levels down to zero, but don't attempt this until you've been free of problems for six months or more.

Like all serious conditions, Crohn's indicates emotional, mental and spiritual constrictions that have to be dealt with. Look at what situations in your life find to be 'a pain in the ass.' It's likely that you may experience a flare-up around these situations. Look at how you constrict the flow of love and energy through your life. Look at the pain you feel when you have to 'let go' of a belief, a person, or a situation. Work on 'letting go' with grace.

ABOUT PARASITES

We are in animal bodies and animal bodies are hosts for parasites. Most of the creatures we carry around with us don't cause any problems, but there are some that can cause minor to severe intestinal distress. Symptoms you may experience are gas, bloating, diarrhea, itchy anus, a nauseated stomach (especially in the morning,) or continuation of intestinal problems even though you are eating right.

The most commonly known 'bugs' are amoebas. Take a trip to any tropical or subtropical place and you are likely to run into these fun guys! But there are other parasites or worms that can also be problems. You can pick up parasites from food, water, pets, dirt, or from other people (for pinworms.)

If you suspect parasites, you can treat them safely with herbs. You can have stool tests done to check for parasites, but just like with cats and dogs, you need to keep doing testing every week for at least four weeks. Parasites have life cycles that prevent them from showing up in your stools daily or weekly.

To treat parasites, I suggest the following. In general, take parasite herbs last thing before you go to bed. Herbs need to be taken for anywhere from three to fourteen days, depending upon the severity of the intestinal distress. After doing the first dose of herbs, wait two weeks and repeat the process. Sometimes this needs to be done in three or four cycles.

1) FOR AMOEBAS or Montezuma's Revenge. I like to use Black Walnut Leaves or Hulls to clear amoebas. I have had friends go to places like Mexico, take daily doses of Black Walnut and eat food from venders and drink the regular water without any intestinal reactions. Personally, I don't think I'd try that one! But, using Black Walnut capsules as an amoeba preventative is a good idea.

Most of the other parasites will stay in the intestines, but amoebas can work themselves back up into all the digestive organs. There, they can cause all kinds of organ malfunctions.

Try anywhere between three to eight capsules at night, to clear amoebas. Black Walnut increases the HCL level in the stomach, so sometimes taking over five capsules or more at a time can be irritating. Try taking half the dose at dinner and the second half before bed.

For travel, I'd take two capsules twice a day and still be careful with what I ate.

2) FOR TAPEWORMS. I've had numerous clients see the white, flat-ish sections of tapeworm pass out with their stool. Cute. When they die, they will sometimes look like off-white or brownish raisins. Also cute. You can have tapeworms for a long time without them causing any obvious symptoms. Cute, cute. But once you see them in your stool, get a diagnosis you have them, or get bloated from them, Black Walnut is the herb I use to take care of them.

Dogs and cats are more susceptible to tapeworms than humans. And they will pass them in their stools and get diarrhea when they get overloaded with them. Black Walnut also works great for them. I worm my animals with Black Walnut and Blackberry leaves every six months to keep them clean.

Try capsules of Black Walnut, from five to ten capsules for up to fourteen days. Be sure to do at least one repeat to catch all the eggs.

3) FOR ROUNDWORMS. Domestic animals are more susceptible to roundworms than humans, but if you have animals, it's one to watch for in yourself or your family. Roundworm eggs can circulate in the bloodstream for weeks or years. When conditions are right, when you are depleted, the eggs will settle into the lungs. They hatch into larvae there and irritate the lining. Then, they get coughed up and swallowed, so they can land back in the intestines to grow into adults.

One of the problems they can cause in humans is serious and attacks infants and toddlers. The eggs can circulate in the bloodstream and settle into the eyes. Several hundred U.S. children a year go blind from this happening. If you have young children crawling around where you have dogs and cats, be sure to check your animals regularly for roundworms. Treat the animals away from the play area or change the play area to another part of the yard. And check your kids for roundworms.

To clear roundworms, I use Blackberry Leaves. They can be done in capsule form, but it's actually better to use loose-leaf tea that you soak in water and eat the leaves. Watch out for thorns in the loose tea. Try between three to six capsules or one to three teaspoons of loose leaves. Usually a week is enough time for the Blackberry leaves to work. With my animals, it's obvious; they poop out wiggly, little worms. I just keep giving them herbs until that stops, then repeat the process two weeks later.

4) FOR PINWORMS. Pinworms like to live at the end of the intestinal tract. When they lay eggs, they crawl outside the anus, deposit the eggs in the outside skin, and crawl in again. They cause intense anal itching. Adult pinworms and eggs can get on your bed sheets and clothes and be spread to others. If one person in the house has pinworms, treat everyone, since they are highly transmittable. I treat pinworms with Blackberry Leaves, using the same method listed under Roundworms.

5) If you are concerned about getting parasites from eating raw fish and sushi, you can take hydrochloric acid tablets just before you ingest the fish. High levels of HCL kill parasites, so increasing this level will usually take care of any problem. As you go through the diet program, your HCL levels should increase to high levels, but in the meantime, extra HCL should help with raw fish concerns.

THE ILLEOCECAL VALVE AND PARASITES

Whenever you get parasites in your system, they irritate the illeocecal valve, a one-way bypass valve between the small and large intestines. The valve should be closed except when you are eating and for a short time after. But parasites irritate the valve and make it hang open. This can cause pain around the valve when you exercise or move in certain ways; it can cause constipation or diarrhea, pain in the low back, shoulder area and around the heart; and it can add to any of the following problems: dizziness, bursitis, tinnitus, nausea, faintness, sinus infections, headaches, thirst and an off-look in your skin.

If you've had indications of parasites, you also want to treat the illeocecal valve. A chiropractor can manipulate the valve directly to close it, but the valve really needs to be exercised to get it to work on its own again. Look at the following illustration and exercise. There are acupuncture points that you can activate that will actually open and close the valve as you touch them.

Do the exercise twice a day as you do herbs or medications for parasites. DO NOT OVER EXERCISE! Three or four openings and closings at a time are more than enough to stimulate the valve to work on its own. Over exercise will make the muscles sore, which is a really odd feeling, and doesn't really help the valve function properly.

1) Place your hands around the outside and side of both legs just below the knees.

2) Run your hands down the leg until the little finger is at the bottom of the calf muscle. You may want to flex your toes upward to tighten the calf muscle. We call this hand position the Bobby Sock level.

3) When both hands are in this position, see illustration 1, the illeocecal valve will be CLOSED.

Illustration 1, Closed position

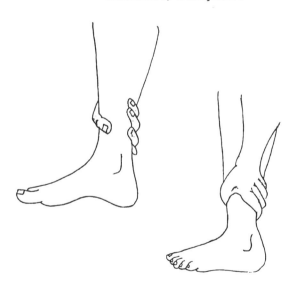

4) To exercise the valve, pick up the RIGHT HAND ONLY and move it into the second hand position, as shown in illustration 2 on the following page.

This will actually OPEN the valve. If you tune into the area of the valve, you may experience a 'fluttering feeling' in the area.

Only hold this position for a slow count of five.

Illustration 2, Open valve

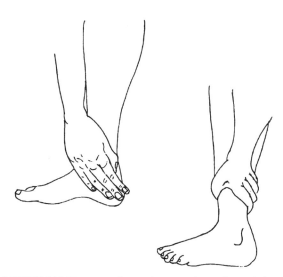

5) Now, pick the RIGHT HAND up again and return it to the original CLOSED valve position, matching the left hand. The left hand never moves from the original position, but must be in place (illustration 3.)

Illustration 3, Closed position

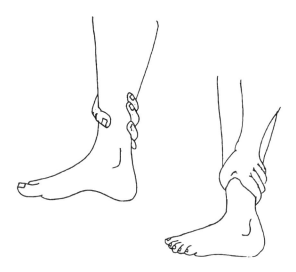

6) Repeat the procedure of opening and closing the valve by picking the RIGHT HAND up and placing it in the OPEN position for a count of five and then back to the CLOSED position.

7) ONLY OPEN AND CLOSE THE VALVE THREE TO FIVE TIMES.

8) ALWAYS LEAVE VALVE CLOSED, with both hands placed in the same position on the legs.

I'll never forget the time I was showing this technique to someone, took my hands off my legs in the OPEN position to show them proper placement, and forgot to go back and close my valve. Later that day, I went for a couple-of-mile run, but didn't get a couple of hundred feet before I had an intense pain in the illeocecal region. A picture flashed up in my mind of my hands in the OPEN position. So, I reached over, did the exercise a couple of times, leaving the valve CLOSED, and the pain stopped. I went on with my run with no further pain.

COMPUTER STRESS

There's something about the vibration of a computer that just puts people into 'automatic pilot,' which is the same thing as putting yourself into a trance. I mean, computers are totally spiritual tools. If you know any programmers, you know they are all intuitive people. It's great that the world is getting connected through an instrument that induces spirituality! But the physical vibrations, noise, eye strain and muscle strain are problems that require more vitamins and minerals in the body.

There is a pattern here (that isn't a pattern) when it comes to what people need to compensate for computer stress. The pattern is different people need very different nutrients!

When I first took a computer class at the community college, I had a very unpleasant experience. I loved the class and working at the computer, but one afternoon I started feeling some eye strain. It quickly moved to the weirdest pain I have ever felt. My eyeballs ached! And the pain rapidly became so bad that I couldn't open my eyes at all. Thank goodness I hadn't driven myself to school that day!

My first stop on the way home was the health food store, where I bought Vitamin A. I took about 80,000 IU's right there and another 20,000 every hour for the rest of the day. The pain started subsiding right in the store. From then on, I've had to take extra vitamin A or else the eye strain begins. I take about 10,000 IU's of vitamin A for every hour I work at the computer!

PHYSICAL SUGGESTIONS: I have seen bodies needing extra vitamin A, B, C, and/or E and a wide range of minerals from computer stress. Taking extra simple food supplements like alfalfa or kelp will give you a wide range of extra nutrients that will counterbalance the computer stress.

Or you can watch for symptoms that you might manifest more intensely after working at the computer for an hour or more. Check with Table 4 in the Appendix for information on what symptoms correspond to what vitamin and mineral deficiencies. Then you can increase those specific nutrients with herbs that are listed in Table 5 in the Appendix.

Watch to see if you have a lessening of symptoms with this change. From that point you can decide whether to continue with the herbs or try something else.

ABOUT DIODES: Diodes are energy transformers. The negative electrical energy that radiates from any technical device, be it the telephone, the copier, the adding machine, or whatever, can be stressful on the body's health. I seriously suggest you invest in a device to change this condition. I use a Wayne Cook 'equipment diode.' They are wonderful (beautiful copper-looking wafers,) inexpensive (under $20,) natural materials (minerals/homeopathic/herbs) and powerful (I love the energetic protection it puts around my telephone)! See the Appendix, Table 3 for diode sources.

DIABETES

One of the functions of the pancreas is to produce and secrete insulin into the bloodstream. When the pancreas malfunctions and stops producing consistent insulin, a person becomes diabetic.

This can happen from infancy to old age, but diabetics can be divided into two basic groups. Juvenile diabetes is the condition that occurs in people under the age of twenty-five to thirty. This problem requires daily shots of insulin or the person will die. Obviously, this situation is serious, but getting the appropriate foods into the body can lower the amount of insulin needed. Over a few months on the right diet, I've seen people drop their insulin levels from seventy units down to ten!

Adult-onset diabetes is the condition that occurs in later years, when a person's pancreas has started to sputter to a stop. This condition usually happens after someone has been hypoglycemic for a number of years. The image that came to me years ago about this explains it all. I saw a fifty year old body with an eighty year old pancreas. The image continues with the pancreas apologizing to the body. *"You may only be fifty, but I'm overworked and quitting!"*

Adult-onset diabetes can usually be controlled with diet and other medications. I have a friend with this condition who has gotten in touch with his body enough to control his insulin levels with diet and herbs. He eats desserts and drinks wine, with care, of course.

Symptoms of diabetes are excessive thirst, low energy and intense hunger. Check with your doctor if you are experiencing these symptoms.

If you already know you are diabetic, check with your doctor before you begin a new diet program. I have worked with many diabetics from both categories and know that when they start to shift their diets around, their insulin levels are definitely affected.

If you are going to be working with this program, you need to be checking your blood sugar at least twice a day, though three times a day is even better! Checking urine ph is not accurate enough.

You may find that you need to give yourself varying amounts of fast-acting and regular insulin than you have been already doing. You may want to try taking several shots through the day instead of one shot in the mornings. Discuss various ways you can do this with your doctor.

I lived with a diabetic friend for a year and got up close and personal with diabetes. She only checked her urine for ph and sugar imbalances, which had worked well for her for twenty years.

One day she came down with a terrible flu. I asked her several times about her sugar levels because she didn't look or feel right. She was concerned, too, and had been checking her urine every time she peed. Everything was fine on that level.

She was up all night, vomiting and coughing. In the morning I listened at her door and was relieved to hear her resting easy. Two hours later, before I left for work, I had the intuition to wake her and see if she needed anything.

Shock of shocks, she was in a diabetic coma! We rushed her to the hospital where her sugar level was in the 400+ range! They were able to bring her out of this coma within a few hours, but it was a scary experience all around!

PHYSICAL ASPECTS AND EATING PATTERNS

When you are diabetic, the pancreas usually doesn't totally stop producing some insulin, even if it's only 10-20% of what it should be doing. The time of day it does secrete its insulin affects what a diabetic should be eating and when.

I've seen a basic pattern. You may either need to eat your proteins in the morning, fruits in the afternoon only, veggies anytime and starches after 6 p.m. Or you may need to eat starches in the morning, fruits in the afternoon only, veggies anytime and proteins after 6 p.m.

I suggest you do the Super Cleanser for one month before trying one of the above patterns. Let your body get adjusted before you start playing around with more change. Watching your insulin levels will be enough to deal with at first. Then try one of the patterns. Since more diabetics I worked with needed to follow the proteins-in-the-morning pattern, I suggest you try that one first, for a week. If it feels good, gives you lots of energy and/or your insulin needs drop, continue with this pattern.

If you don't notice any changes, continue to try this eating pattern for another week or two. Then try the eating the starches-in-the-morning pattern and watch for changes in how you feel. If there is obvious improvement, stay with this pattern.

If neither eating pattern seems to improve your health after several weeks on them, then go back to eating any of the foods at any time. You might also want to play around with only eating veggies at certain times or eating fruit any time and see if these change your energy, insulin levels, sleep, or overall health.

ABOUT INSULIN

I worked with a number of people who tried to change the kind of insulin they used when 'human' insulin became available. Some of them had no problem; most of them also saw their insulin amounts drop. Other people had blatant reactions to this transition, most of which seemed to be emotional reactions! It seemed the more natural form of insulin stirred up the emotions that were the basis of the diabetes.

If you do want to change over to this form of insulin and had troubles in the past, wait awhile and then try again. But wait for at least six months, doing the diet and getting well. Then work with your doctor and a therapist as you start to introduce the 'human' insulin. Start with only two units and deal with the changes, both physical and emotional, that result. Then, gradually increase the amounts, two units at a time, until you are only using this form of insulin.

No matter what form of insulin you take, you have to deal with 'side effects' from the insulin. It seems to put stress on both your Vitamin B and E levels and it is wise to give your body extra sources of these nutrients. You might want to try additional herbs high in vitamins. (See Table 5 in the Appendix for this information.) or additional multivitamins. I think that at least some of the other body problems associated with diabetes, like blindness, are related to these deficiencies.

CHANGING DIABETES

With Adult-onset diabetes, changing the diet and getting healthy frequently brings the body back into balance. Using small doses, a capsule or two at a time of goldenseal is another technique. Goldenseal is a great antibiotic and it also acts as natural insulin in the body, so it lowers blood sugar.

Once you get your body in balance, after at least three to four months on the diet program, try taking a capsule of goldenseal when you feel your sugar level is going up. Check your blood. If it's high, try a capsule and check your blood again, twenty to thirty minutes later or when you feel it dropping.

The friend who drinks wine and enjoys his desserts has learned to keep his sugar levels even with Goldenseal. His life is his!

Juvenile diabetes has an inherent problem. When kids or young adults develop diabetes, they are taught that their lives must revolve around this dis-ease. It becomes so much a basis of their lives and life-styles that it's almost impossible for them to remove it.

I had the opportunity to work with a thirty year old man who had just developed the dis-ease. He and his sweetie were on vacation when he landed in the hospital. From that experience, they went to a mutual friend, who directed them to me. They planned to pass through town and connect with me and ended up staying for five days. One of the first things we worked on besides diet was changing the belief systems that were already in place after only two weeks of his 'being diabetic.'

This patterning became obvious the first time I asked them to go for a walk with me. Instead of following their hearts, they looked at each other and when into a decision-making pattern they had been taught. They checked the clock, discussed when he had eaten last, did a little math and told me they couldn't go because it wasn't 'the right time for his insulin level.'

I was shocked! Within such a short time, their lives were revolving around this dis-ease! It had them under it's thumb and it was scary!

I immediately talked to them about living their lives and then dealing with what it meant to his insulin levels and food instead of the other way around. They were shocked to see how easily they had adopted the medical view of dealing with diabetes and how it had invaded their lives. They promptly gave up this approach and got back to their lives.

After five days of sanely living with diabetes, they went home. We worked together a number of times over the next few months and then I got a call. He had decided that it was time to accelerate his healing and did just that! He was totally off the insulin and doing just fine, thank you! His doctor called it a 'honeymoon' period, but he had healed himself and never had another diabetic reaction or response! I love it!

THE SPIRITUAL ASPECTS OF DIABETES

The core spiritual issue linked to diabetes is power. The 'head' of the pancreas is right smack in the middle of the third chakra, the energetic center of your physical and spiritual power. Now, 'power' is a charged word. Most people relate to it as a sense of force, but I think it has more to do with the energy created when one is in universal flow and joy. All the diabetics I have known are very powerful people who don't understand and relate to that underlying power.

A diabetic friend related a dream to me when we were working on healing her diabetes. Up to this time, she had been fighting the dis-ease from many directions. Then she dreamed she was standing in a factory in front of a conveyor belt. Passing by her on the conveyor belt were many different dis-eases and body problems. She saw herself reach out and pick diabetes off the belt and draw it to her.

When she awoke, she realized that she needed to start embracing the dis-ease because she had chosen it as a way to learn her life's lessons! For awhile, we had her walk around saying, *"I'm diabetic and proud!"* As she got into working with the diabetes instead of fighting it, she began to let her power flow with ease. Her physical healing also began to flow and she 'got a handle' on many of the issues related to the dis-ease.

Obviously, these power issues also relate to the way diabetics are taught to center their lives around the dis-ease.

Another issue related to the lack of insulin in the body also means that you are not allowing 'sweetness' to flow into your life. Especially with juvenile diabetes, the ability to bring sweetness into your life is something a parent needs to demonstrate and teach. The lack of this teaching is manifested in the child in a blatant development of dis-ease. Once this lack of allowing sweetness into your life is understood, then the diabetic needs to learn ways to make their lives sweet!

DYSLEXIA

Dyslexia is usually thought of as a learning disability, but I tend to think of it as a very different way of viewing the world. People and children with dyslexia are creative types, not that all creative types are dyslexic.

For some reason dyslexics never got the brain/body connections that let them naturally see the world the way 'regular' people do. Of course, they see the world in a way that 'regular' people usually don't either, and this other way is more spherical, creative, full and spiritual.

The physical problem is linked to the flow and connection of energies between the body and the brain. We are bilateral animals which means that one side of the brain controls the opposite side of the body. With dyslexics, this brain-to-body connection doesn't totally flow to opposite sides, but sometimes flows within the same side. When this same-side energy flow is operating in the body, people will literally see things 'backwards.'

The real problem dyslexics have in the world is that the world is set up to accommodate a linear way of thinking, where one word or letter, follows another. Since the dyslexic brain doesn't work that way, they are put at a disadvantage.

I am really happy that over the last twenty years, this situation has been recognized and is being dealt with with understanding and love. I know too many creative, intelligent adults who were told they were stupid, in some way or other, because they couldn't read well or listen well.

There are physical manipulations that can be done to move a lateral energy flow back into the appropriate bilateral flow. One of the techniques is called 'cross crawl.' It is a simple technique of 'crawling' on your back to stimulate opposite arm and leg movement. Of course, you can actually get down and crawl around on the floor to stimulate this brain flow, too.

I had one dyslexic kid walk around in a heavy march stance, beating on a drum for ten minutes. He loved it. Then we'd sit him down and let him read. The cross-crawl action moved him out of dyslexic patterns and he had no trouble reading, at least for awhile. We started him out with ten minutes of bilateral exercise, then read for five minutes. Any reading had to follow the exercise so that positive flow patterns were created in the body. A week later we started increasing the reading time, following the ten minutes of exercise. This process is slow and gradual, but finally sets bilateral flow patterns into the body in a permanent way.

Use of the Thymus Thump and Sternum Pressure Massage, which immediately create bilateral flows in the body, and the Temporal Tap techniques are useful in creating non-dyslexic brain flows.

One of my ex's was really dyslexic. He is brilliant but basically couldn't read when we met. We used the Thymus Thump and Sternum Pressure Massage to correct his constant lateral energy flows. It took two years to really get the patterns set in motion, but by then he had become an avid reader!

EATING DISORDERS

ABOUT THE CAUSES

Eating disorders like bulimia and anorexia are not simple issues to deal with, especially with a 'diet' program. The emotional patterns that lead to this dis-eased state are a paradox of simple and complex issues. If you've got an eating disorder or are dealing with someone with anorexia or bulimia, the underlying causes are probably already obvious, though I want to briefly discuss them.

The personality types that tend to develop these problems are usually natural givers who don't normally need support. But when they do need support, they really need it. People around them usually expect that they are strong and don't see the need for support, so don't offer it. An imbalance ensues.

The obvious, underlying issue is a simple, yet deep-seated need, as in all of us, to be loved and nurtured and to be accepted for who we are. Everyone I've dealt with who has an eating disorder is still trying to get that love, nurturing and acceptance from someone, frequently a parent. Sometimes more obvious abuses are involved in these situations, but the simple truths still stand.

The hard and complex truth is that this means changing someone else, which is a rare occurrence. Instead, you need to learn to love and nurture yourself and to accept yourself for who you are. Easy to say, I know, but possible.

Withholding food or binging on food are ways to say you don't deserve to be nurtured. Unfortunately, this is a belief you were taught from someone who also believes it. Beating yourself up with a serious eating disorder gets their attention, but doesn't necessary change the pattern. Don't let someone else's lack of love make you feel powerless. Don't let their misunderstandings of your needs continue into your life. Stop trying to please them and start pleasing yourself.

There are plenty of books, techniques and support groups out there to help deal with these problems. Just remember that you are already running victim patterns so look for help that changes these patterns instead of blaming someone else for what they did or didn't do to you.

STRAIGHT TALK ABOUT FOOD

Just the thought of following a 'diet plan' can send terror into anyone with any level of eating disorder. Remember, it's okay to be scared of a change. You just can't let fear paralyze you. You have to act.

As you consider following this diet approach, realize that you probably won't follow it the way someone without an eating disorder will follow it. Most of the eating-issue-people I've worked with tend to start and stop the program numerous times before their bodies and issues level out. They can get beyond them but it takes some time.

If you start the program and reach a point where your eating issues overwhelm you, stop the program, eat whatever and deal with the issue that has arisen. See a therapist, get some counselling help, get some detachment from the issue. While you go through the issue, continue whatever aspects of the diet you can, like continuing the vitamins and minerals or keeping with the right fruits or keeping the percentages of foods in order.

Once the issue and emotional upheaval has passed, start the program again. If you go back and forth like this for a year or more, that's okay! There's no way that following this approach won't push your buttons. It will! But if you stick with it and work with the issues, you can change the eating patterns. And you can learn to love, nurture and accept yourself.

Try working with the Temporal Tap technique to change the desire to throw up, an overwhelming need to stuff some emotion down, a desire to binge, or a pattern of self-hate.

EXERCISE

What can I say about exercise? We are animal bodies that need it! Our bodies were made to move, to express ourselves through movement, to release tension and toxins through movement and to feel joy through movement.

But we have become a sedentary group of spectators on the whole and it just doesn't help our bodies work properly. We have learned a prejudice that associates hard, physical work with less intelligence. We've learned patterns of watching instead of participating. We've learned to apply our minds instead of our bodies.

It's time to change all these patterns around and make exercise into adult play! Find different things to do that are fun. I love to fly my stunt kites, and in the New Mexico wind, that can be some intense upper body exercise!

Along with the diet program, I suggest starting a regular walking time. You don't want to start a more intense program until you are sure that your toxin level as been lowered. Intense programs, before your body is ready, can release a high level of toxins that can end up making you sick.

I also suggest that you find ways to incorporate some movement into your life. In your eight to nine hour work day, take fifteen minutes every two hours and walk around the block. Not only will you get some exercise, but you will get in touch with what's happening in the natural world around you. You'll find out what the rain feels like. Or that it's warm and sunny out. And you'll release the connection with work so that when you come back to it you will have a new perspective.

Always park farthest away from the store entrances instead of as close as you can get. Walk to work. Always carry a pack of some kind when you hike or walk. Work in the garden using hand tools. Look for a more strenuous way to do something rather than the easiest like hand sanding the paint off a dresser rather than using chemical paint removers.

Once you have been on the diet program for a few months and you are feeling good, start adding in more intense exercise. But remember to make it fun. Try new things. Dance. Play racquetball. Do yoga. Lift weights. Bicycle. Remember that moving your body and enjoying yourself is the point. As soon as you get bored with the activity, change it to something else. It's a rare person that finds an activity that will satisfy their physical and emotional needs forever.

If you get sore muscles, try any of the Betony herb family. They all help release toxins from the muscles and release soreness. Work out a stretching program to release tension, too.

Work with the Temporal Tap technique in Chapter 16 to change the patterns of non-movement you may have learned.

EYESTRAIN AND EYESIGHT

ABOUT EYESTRAIN

The eyes need a number of vitamins and minerals to maintain good eye health. Vitamin A is the major nutrient. Lack of Vitamin A can cause all kinds of eyestrain, night blindness and poor vision.

When you work around florescent lights or technical view screens like computer monitors, you definitely stress the Vitamin A levels in the eye itself. The visual purple, the liquid inside the eye, is made up of mostly Vitamin A. Other vitamins, like B's, are needed for eye health also. A lack of B's will cause bloodshot eyes, a combination of deficiencies is linked to glaucoma, mineral imbalances can cause edema around the eyes. Try taking Eyebright tea. It can definitely help the overall eye health and release eyestrain. The times I've stressed my eyes, Eyebright has helped. It has cleared my vision to the point where the edges of doors seem to appear sharp!

There are eye exercises that can release tension and improve the vision. Deepak Chopra talks about a number of them in *Magical Mind, Magical Body* and the Bates Method exercises are great.

ABOUT EYESIGHT

Changing your poor vision is definitely possible, though you usually have to work at it consistently for some time to make permanent changes. To really change your eyesight, you have to get to the root cause of your vision blurring in the first place. Spiritually and emotionally, poor vision is linked to not wanting to see some aspect of the world just too hard to look at. I'll never forget the experience I had one day when I put on a pair of sunglasses. As I slipped them on, I felt a barrier develop between me and my world. Wearing glasses is a great want to keep pain on the other side of the barrier.

This is especially true in children. I can't forget the numerous clients who have said that they saw fairies, elves and other creatures, until they were told they weren't REAL. They frequently experienced a negative shift in their vision after these 'revelations.'

Whatever the reason behind your vision shift, you have alot of brain cells that have repeatedly been told that you can't see. They all need to be shifted into a new memory of being able to see. The Bates Method glasses are great to use for this change. They are blacked out lens with small holes all over them. One of my ex's, who had terrible vision (20/400,) put them on and could see perfectly! It actually scared him silly and within two weeks the glasses were broken and not replaced!

Which brings up another point. If you are going to work on your vision, you have to be ready to really see, on all levels, or else your work will be futile. Years ago a friend went to the big city to have her cornea cut and molded to correct her vision. She returned with 20/20 vision. When she walked in my door, it was like meeting the real her for the first time.

But, she wasn't ready for what she saw with her new vision. Her life scared her and now it was staring her in the face. Within six months her vision started fluctuating, some days it was perfect, some days it was awful. Slowly, it slid back to the old patterns until it was like the change had never happened!

Another friend has had the cornea molding done with complete success, but we worked on all the issues around her poor vision before and after the work. She was truly ready to stop hiding truth from herself and her vision has not wavered at all.

If you are going to pursue any of the cornea molding techniques, be sure that you are really ready to see your life clearly on all levels. Then increase both your vitamin and mineral intake a week before the work and several weeks after.

ABOUT THE GALLBLADDER

There are three major functions of the gallbladder. First, it stores bile produced in the liver, second it concentrates the bile, and third, it 'squirts' bile out when oils are present in the duodenum (the top of the small intestines.)

Bile is a soap-like substance that breaks fats and oils down so they are usable by the body. Remember that you need a couple of tablespoons of good quality oil on a daily basis to maintain good health and to utilized fat-soluble vitamins.

When I first work with clients, most of them are exhibiting low bile production and low quality bile. Straightening up the diet allows the liver to make good quality bile and for the gallbladder to properly concentrate and release it. But, remember, the concentrated oils that most people use are not natural and definitely stress the body. They should only be used in very small quantities.

LIVING WITHOUT A GALLBLADDER

Obviously, you can live without your gallbladder, lots of people do. But you lose two important functions, the concentration of bile and the release triggered by the presence of oils in the duodenum. This means the liver squirts thinned-out bile into the intestines as it makes it without regard to the actual need for oil and fat digestion. This means that you need to keep oils and fatty foods to a real minimum in your overall diet, since you won't be able to break them down most of the time. They will only create toxins without the bile present.

But there is some time during the day that the liver will do most of its production and release of bile. This is the time that you want to make sure that you DO eat some fatty foods and oils.

For most people this production and release happens between one and three o'clock in the afternoon, through it could happen at any other time. Try eating the majority of your oils and fatty foods between those hours and see how you feel. Watch for Mucus Reactions that day and extra mucus in your stools the next day.

Try this routine for a week, then switch the time around and see if you notice any differences in the mucus buildup in the throat and stools. Once you feel you have a handle on the lowest Mucus Reaction time, then work it into your life to eat the majority of your oils and fats at that time period.

ABOUT GALLSTONES

Gallstones, like many body problems, relate to imbalances in vitamin and mineral levels. Bringing the nutrient levels to balance will both clear them out of the system and stop the reoccurrence of them in the gallbladder. But the healing in this area is very slow. The body is going to repair many other systems including the proper bile levels before it starts to dissolve gallstones.

After six months on the diet program, you can introduce some capsuled herbs like Barberry, Burdock, Vervain or Willow to your vitamin and mineral regime. Start with two capsules each time you take other nutrients. Continue for three to four weeks, pause for a week and repeat the herbs.

Most bodies prefer this slow healing, but if you are really sick from gallstones, having pain and passing them anyway, you might want to consider doing a gallbladder flush. Remember, bodies like moderation, so you only want to consider this if you are really sick or extremely healthy.

To do a gallstone or gallbladder flush, you need to fast, doing only apple juice for two or three days. Don't do this if you are hypoglycemic or you will throw that whole healing process off. On the second or third morning, drink 1/2 cup olive oil and 1/2 cup lemon juice. This will make the gallbladder squeeze itself empty, pushing out the gallstones. It's also a good idea to follow this oil/lemon 'drink' with an enema or colonic. I know it doesn't sound appetizing. It's not! But if you are still in gallbladder pain after months on the diet, it's a quick, nonmedical way to clear the gallbladder.

HAIR LOSS

I see two major physical reasons for hair loss.

One, it's just written into your genetic and cultural coding. Get over it or do something about it. But know that it's true, bald men are more virile. High levels of testosterone is what kills certain hair follicles!

If you want to pursue any of the transplant, surgery, or other options, I suggest that you first get yourself healthy so your body can help you maintain healthy hair growth. Check out the suggestions for Surgery Preparation.

Two, hair loss is a direct result of vitamin and mineral deficiencies, especially Vitamin B levels. Remember, this is the stress vitamin and is needed for almost every function in the body. It takes six months to a year to bring these deficiencies in line.

But the deficiency problems can be dealt with. Adelle Davis, in one of her books, talks about a bald, grey-haired man who's black hair returned after a high Vitamin B diet. And one of my ex-husbands had his bald spot grow new hair after a few months on the right diet and nutrients.

The physical levels usually take some time to turn around, if they are going to change at all. Remember, your body doesn't feel that the loss of hair is a life-threatening problem and it will heal alot of other more important body problems before it ever gets to your hair.

PHYSICAL SUGGESTION:

1) Hair is made from proteins. Some bodies use animal proteins but others use vegetable proteins to make hair, so you must make sure that you supply first one, then the other to check out which your body uses.

If you've had trouble with your hair thinning and you have been eating proteins, it may be you just weren't digesting them properly. This problem usually corrects itself as you go through the diet approach. If you've noticed your hair thickening, great. But you still may want to add higher levels of vegetable proteins to see if this increases the growth and condition of your hair.

If you've been doing the diet for six months or more and notice no change in your hair growth, then it's time to try increasing your vegetable protein levels. One of the best and easiest ways to do this is to increase your intake of sprouted beans and legumes. You can increase your quinoa intake, also, though sprouted beans seem to work better for most people.

I suggest that you start eating 1/2 c. of sprouted beans or legumes daily. Lentils are one of the easiest legumes to sprout (it usually takes a day to soak them and a day or two in the colander,) so sprout, cook and freeze a bunch of them and just defrost a daily dose. Whatever bean source you choose, make it fun to eat so you don't get bored! Try a bean dip or taco filling!

2) Stimulation of the scalp is also important. You need to get the blood flowing to the scalp so it can carry nutrients to the hair follicles. Try a five minute yoga technique where you grab handfuls of your hair and you gently pull it back and forth. Do it every day. Or, gently massage your scalp for five to ten minutes each day.

3) If other techniques fail, you might want to try some chemical stimulant. The companies who make these hair-growth stimulants claim they cause no side effects, but I have worked with sensitive people who got dizzy and experienced headaches after using them. I have also worked with people who had no negative reactions at all.

Just make sure you are healthy before trying this route. Use the stimulants for a week or two, stop for a week or two and then use them again.

HEART PROBLEMS

I'm not sure what to say about 'heart dis-ease' and 'heart attacks,' because I think that says it all! The heart is in dis-ease on all levels, physical, emotional, mental and spiritual.

The physical aspects of dis-ease come from following poor living habits, like not eating right, no exercise and lots of stress. Following a healthy eating pattern, getting exercise and releasing stress are known 'cures' for all heart problems. The other aspects, the emotional, mental and spiritual imbalance, come from years of believing and following taught patterns that do not honor the self or others with love.

I've got a friend in the sixty plus age range in the hospital right now, getting open heart surgery. He and his wife of thirty years fought like cats and dogs for years. Just recently they were ready to examine the way they responded to each other and started getting counselling separately and together.

He and I laughed together that it had taken years of pain, of running the same old tapes their parents had taught them, before they realized that there was another way.

At the same time they realized this, one of his heart valves gave out. So, he's physically having his heart 'opened' as he is emotionally, mentally and spiritually opening to a new level of love. I love the obviousness of the situation and I find most 'heart problems' to be this obvious!

Get healthy and learn to love yourself. Learn to accept others for who they are. If you don't like an aspect of someone, keep it out of your life, or keep them out of your life altogether. Loving yourself means you have to place clear perimeters on what you will and won't except into your life!

HEADACHES

Common headaches are created from a number of situations, from vitamin and mineral deficiencies, from tension, noise, and environmental stresses, from the re-absorption of toxins from the intestines, and from sugar imbalances.

Taking care of the above problems by removing and correcting the causes is the first step. But while you are doing that, don't just suffer silently. Do what you need to do to move yourself away from pain. Take an aspirin or capsules of willow bark, if you need to. And definitely try the following technique.

The following chart shows a suture line, a connecting line between the bones in the head. This particular suture line, the temporal-sphenoidal suture, has healing points located along it that are miraculous for relieving headaches.

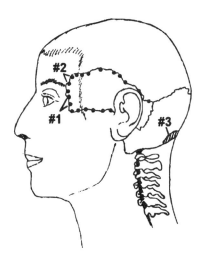

Most headaches will start changing after rubbing all three points, on each side of the head, for thirty seconds each. The sinuses will open up and start draining and the pressure in the head will start moving. Frequently people can feel the tension flow right down the spine.

I've rubbed hundreds and hundreds of heads that are aching from small tension headaches to 4-day migraines. And they all quickly became nonexistent headaches! Kids are so responsive that just hitting the six points one time will usually relieve most of their headaches.

The young man who had the 4-day migraine was in alot of dis-comfort when he arrived at my door. He hadn't eaten or slept since the migraine had hit, his eyes were totally bloodshot, and he was on the verge of collapse. As I worked the points along the suture line and points at the back of the skull, tears rolled down his face. It took a half hour of going back over and over the points, but it worked. The pain stopped, his eyes were totally clear, nausea was gone, and he was totally energized.

The points themselves almost always hurt just to the touch. That's how you know you are on the right spot! You can go back over the points repeatedly until the headache is gone.

There was only one headache I worked on that I couldn't totally release with these points. And that was from a woman who had been having migraines from the day she ovulated to the day her periods started for many years! I felt good that I was able to help by lessening it with this technique.

There are two other uses for this suture line. There are actually points along this suture line that correspond to all the different organs in the body. Rubbing a corresponding point can aid that organ in its healing process. Stimulating the points acts much like hand or foot reflexology.

There is another aspect to this suture line that you might also want to check out. It's like a self-hypnosis technique for changing habits, desires and patterns and is one of the easiest and most powerful techniques I have ever seen. See Chapter 16 under the heading Temporal Tap.

SUGGESTIONS: Relax!!! Don't take life so seriously. As people who live through disasters know, life and love is what's important.

HERPES

Herpes is a virus and can be controlled in the bloodstream. I have worked with numerous people who have regular outbreaks of herpes, either cold sores or genital herpes, and have got them totally under control.

On a physical level, getting all the vitamin levels up, especially the B-complex, getting the minerals balanced and taking the amino acid lysine can keep the body out of the stress zone that herpes loves. There are things you can do like eating foods high in lysine and avoid foods that use alot of lysine in the body.

But, there is another side to the herpes issue. It is directly linked to a certain kind of stress. An imbalance of personal power creates the environment for herpes to exist in the body.

When you have an outbreak of herpes, look back a day or two. Somewhere in that time frame, there will have been an incident where you either got aggressive or passive, where you felt your power slip away, or where you overpowered someone or something. Whatever it was, there was an imbalance of power created. It's this imbalance that triggers herpes to erupt!

The energetic imbalance looks like this to me. There is a blockage, tension, or holding of energy somewhere in the body that starts to build up pressure just like a volcano. The energy needs to be released, but you are holding it static instead. And, like volcanic pressure, the energy needs to escape. So it finally explodes outward and travels 'exit paths' to the surface where a herpes sore erupts.

When I first moved to New Mexico, I got a sunburn that left my chest full of deep blisters, the skin a dusty purple color and my lips exploding with cold sores! I'd never had one in my life and now I had a multitude of them! Thereafter, every time I got a sunburn on my lips, I got a cold sore. You can believe I protected them VERY well after that, but with New Mexico sun, I still experience an occasional outbreak.

One day, though, I felt the tingles on my upper lip and heard an internal voice instructing me on what the problem was. I was given the volcano visualization described below and did it on the spot. That particular cold sore never erupted, but I had to keep going back and sucking the energy out of the pathway until the whole energy shift became a new pattern.

Fourteen years later I will still occasionally get a twinge on my lips when I start to work in the garden in the spring. I just use the visual and clear the energy out and no cold sores! And if I don't catch it in time, at least I can keep the size and duration within limits.

PHYSICAL SUGGESTIONS:

1) When you have a herpes flare-up or you feel a sore coming on, you will probably experience some symptoms. They range from sore or stiff muscles, tiredness, and itching in an old eruption site to out and out flu-type symptoms.

2) Eat foods high in lysine like yogurt, kefir, sprouted beans and legumes, eggs, fish, chicken, turkey, lamb.

3) Avoid foods that use alot of lysine like nuts and seeds, beef, pork, milk, cheese, wheat, rice and most other grains.

4) Take tablets of lysine. Usually 500 mg. to 1500 mg. on a daily dosage is all the body can utilize in a 24 hour period.

SPIRITUAL SUGGESTIONS:

As soon as you recognize an eruption pattern there is a visual you can use to deal with the herpes energy.

1) Note old spots where the herpes has come to the surface in the past or some new spot you feel developing.

2) Visualize following the internal pathway back to the core, where the energy is blocked.

3) Once you find that core, find another way to release it. Breathe it out or scream it out. Jump up and down and throw a tantrum. Or sit down and have a good cry. But whatever you do, release the energy!

4) Suck all the energy that was going out the pathway back into the core and make sure it goes out with your emotional release.

5) Visualize the pathway between the core and the sore collapsing in on itself.

HORMONE IMBALANCES

ABOUT HORMONES IN GENERAL

Hormones are the chemical transmitters in the body that tell different organs and glands to do different functions. Most problems related to them, like infertility, imbalances and depletions, are the result of deep vitamin and mineral deficiencies.

If you are experiencing any level of imbalance in the endocrine system, first, get your diet cleaned up and your nutrient levels increased. The more intense the problem the longer it will take to clear, but anything is possible. I've seen numerous women struggling to get pregnant, who became healthy and produced a number of children.

FEMALE HORMONES, BECOMING A WOMAN

Anyone who thinks that being a kid is fun and games must have skipped being a teenager. It can be such a great time, but it's never easy. The hormonal shifts a young body deals with can send emotions swinging from one end to the other.

When a young woman's body starts to shift into womanhood, it needs a huge a amount of daily nutrients, especially minerals. I think part of the body's ups and downs during this transition also related to the switch in food needs that happens between twelve to sixteen years old.

By this age range, the body has usually grown to its basic adult height and size. Though there will be filling out, the main growth starts to slow and the body's needs move into a maintenance pattern where more and more veggies and fruits are needed and less and less proteins and starches are needed. There's more information about this transition in Chapter 9.

With both the hormonal and food shifts happening at the same time, it's no wonder teens sometimes exude chaotic and intense energy!

Because of their youth and resiliency, it usually doesn't take long for teenagers to rebound into health. They just need to following the diet program and double up on their mineral intake. They need to watch the amount of junk food, making it a once a week treat instead of a daily indulgence.

PREMENSTRUAL SYNDROME (PMS)

There are two major contributors to all PMS problems; the first is definitely nutritional and the second is emotional. Physical level deficiencies will create stress in your system resulting in emotional mood swings, cravings, swelling in the abdomen and breasts, skin breaking out, heavy or prolonged bleeding, and, ultimately, cramping.

A week to ten days before your cycle changes (and this is both for men and women!!!) your body's mineral NEEDS start to increase. You need alot of minerals, it seems, to make hormonal switches; that is basically what happens to make a woman's period start.

Now if your mineral needs are balanced and nothing is deficient, you will probably have some cravings for high mineral foods about a week before the end of the cycle. I know as a teenager, I craved tuna for the whole week before my period without really ever putting the two together!

You might find yourself craving salty foods, seaweeds, and seafood, or you just can't get enough milk or yogurt, or you want more and more green veggies.

On the other hand, if you are already deficient in any of the minerals when your body starts demanding more of them, you may also experience cravings of the uncontrollable kind. You know, those cravings for sweets and those turns around the kitchen, grazing on this and that, never finding the thing that satisfies.

The trick, obviously, is to make sure that you get enough minerals in your body before, during and after this peak increase. As with all natural healing processes, this takes some time, but most women start feeling the differences within two cycles.

The only change in the body that is normal is a fluctuation in temperature. A few days before the end of the cycle, you will probably feel cold and need some extra clothing. A day or two before menstruation your body temperature will go back up to normal.

Any other body indications, like breasts getting tender, negative food cravings, a pimple here or there, are all signs for you to start getting some extra minerals into your system.

Besides the physical reactions, there can be PMS emotional stress. At the same time your mineral needs go up, you may experience a sense of vulnerability or overwhelm. This is NORMAL. What I psychically see is a woman's aura or energy field expanding. It gets 'loose' and more open. And this time can be wonderful.

It is a time when we see very clearly what we may have otherwise been able to overlook!!! When I was about twenty I realized every relationship I had ended had corresponded to the end of my cycle! With this realization, a feeling of guilt swept over me. *"Whoa! Am I, just one of those women who lose it before my periods?"* I asked myself.

A reassuring internal voice answered me, *"No, take a closer look. None of those past decisions were irrational. All the reasons for doing what you did were valid. Up to that point in the relationship, though, you were able to say to yourself things like* 'He doesn't mean to be rude.' *Or* 'He's just having a bad day.' *Or* 'He'll learn to change.' *You were being patient and that's okay to a point. But before your period, you actually see situations for what they are. The 'polite' blinders come off and situations that had a fog around them become crystal clear."*

As I listened to this voice, I knew it was true. In all those situations I had reached the outer limits of what I could tolerate without even knowing it. When I was faced with those situations and the fog was gone, I acted from the clarity that remained. From that time on, I have become friends with this 'time of opening and clarity' that happens just before my periods. I have learned to trust the emotions and thoughts I experience as clear guidance that I can act on with a clear conscience.

Once you clear the mineral deficiencies out of the body, you can learn to more clearly befriend this extraordinary time at the end of your hormonal cycle. It may be helpful to set aside a day or two around this time to get away from kids and hubbies and heavy responsibilities. Give yourself a little time to honor your ties with Mother Earth and with your body. Give yourself a little time to reflect and redirect.

I know this can be hard to do sometimes, with all the demands of daily life in this insane culture, but just do it! You will find that the renewal you do on yourself will quickly filter down through all your connections and contacts with others. Eventually, everyone will thank you for it! After a few months of incorporating a retreat into your life, you may find the rest of the family shoving you out the door in support of this 'break from each other'!

PHYSICAL SUGGESTIONS:

Seven to ten days before the start of your period (and the end of your cycle) start increasing your intake of minerals depending upon how intense your PMS symptoms are.

Since I had my tubes tied and don't need to monitor my periods, I usually take extra kelp tablets as soon as I experience an extra pimple or breast tenderness. I have seen women using anywhere between six to twenty tablets of kelp or dulse daily to bring these PMS symptoms under control.

After several menstrual cycles on this diet approach, most women will find their cycles becoming normal. But I suggest that you continue the higher levels of minerals for some months after you are through the whole plan. Then you can try dropping the amounts of extra minerals in the 'seven to ten days before' period.

Don't be surprised, though, if you find that you always need to supplement minerals in your body before your periods. Remember, just general stress will eat up minerals.

IRREGULAR PERIODS

Irregular cycles are directly related to vitamin and mineral imbalances that make the endocrine system fluctuate. Getting the body and nutrient levels balanced is the key to getting the menstrual cycles flowing on a regular basis.

Follow the appropriate diet programs for three to four months and see if your cycle straightens itself out. If it does, great! If it doesn't straighten itself out in this time frame, then consider taking a hormone herb to aid the body to find a balance.

The first herb I suggest trying is Blessed Thistle. It's a very mild hormone herb that gently nudges your cycle into balance. Hormone herbs work best if they are only taken in the morning.

So, try a couple of capsules of Blessed Thistle every day for two months and see how it affects your cycle. If your irregularity has been long term, it may take a few months to get balance. Be patient.

If Blessed Thistle doesn't do it for you, you may want to try Damiana or Dong Quai. The Damiana is a stronger female hormone herb and the Dong Quai is a good male and female hormone balancer. Also try only one or two capsules of herbs on a daily basis. And take them in the morning.

Remember, you want to gently move your body back into balance, not send it bouncing all over the hormonal range.

If you have had trouble getting your hormonal cycles balanced, I also suggest that you be very careful about eating animal products that have been fed hormones, which is most commercially-raised chicken, turkeys, lambs, pigs and cows. Go for free-range and organically-raised meats.

I worked with a friend for months on getting her cycle balanced. She had three months of regular cycles and then it went haywire. We traced the problem to a commercial chicken she had eaten! The hormones in the meat had thrown her right out of balance and it took several months to get it back in line again!

MENOPAUSE

Stopping the menstrual flow causes the same kind of stress in the body that starting the menstrual flow does. The emotional aspects are quite different, but the physical need for high levels of minerals is the same.

Most women, if they have kept their bodies balanced, can go through menopause with no physical symptoms at all. If you are in the menopausal phase as you are starting the diet program or if you are having body difficulties through this transition, start taking double doses of minerals.

Many women who are showing early menopause signs frequently get back into their regular cycles when they start the diet program, so don't be surprised if this happens. If, after following the diet for four plus months and doing extra minerals, menopausal symptoms have not cleared, then consider taking some herbs to help the body balance. You might want to try a capsule or two of Dong Quai or Blessed Thistle each morning for a month or two.

If you are still having symptoms after trying these suggestions, consider having some acupuncture, doing Chinese herbs, doing homeopathic remedies or taking allopathic hormones.

You will also need to look at the spiritual aspects of menopause, to see if these changes are having an negative affect on your body.

For thirty-five plus years, the female body is in constant "heat." We can get pregnant at any time and our hormonal messages are programmed to achieve just that. It wasn't until after I had my tubes tied that I felt fully free enough to allow my body to feel how 'in heat' it was all the time! Once I couldn't get pregnant, I could get into the 'heat' space without fear!

When this ' constant heat' pattern changes, a large part of our innate interests change. The hormonal messages push us to seek mates, to nurture the children that result, and to focus our attention onto the needs of others.

When menopause arrives, our focus turns to the next part of our lives where we can focus more of our energy onto ourselves and our own interests. This can be a scary proposition, especially for women who haven't pursued interests outside the home before this time.

I had one client tell me that menopause represented a step into freedom. She was relieved that the first part of her life was behind her, that she related to men totally differently, and that she was able to get back to some interests she'd put aside for a long time!

Remember, women are natural givers and this doesn't change with this hormonal shift. The focus of it may shift but it's still there for you to draw your energy from.

MALE HORMONES

Men have hormonal cycles just like women, though they seem less obvious. That is, they seem less obvious until you identify them. Then they can become very obvious. Their cycles are anywhere from eighteen to forty days long, are marked by temperature shifts, pimples, low energy and general weirdness. Start watching for your own cycles and mark them off on a calendar. Also, there is a temperature shift in the middle of the cycle that is matched by a higher sperm count!

BECOMING A MAN

Usually around nine to ten years old, boys start to go through their hormonal shifts. Usually you can see this in their attitudes toward all the women in their lives.

One of my woman friends came to me freaked out, saying, *"I think I'm starting to hate my kid!"* When I looked at the situation, it was obvious that the boy's hormones were starting to shift. He just needed some information at that point that his viewpoint was shifting but that he needed to learn how to properly and respectfully approach girls and women. Both mom and boy understood the information and shifted their interactions.

Just like with girls, male hormonal shifts require large amounts of minerals. If you have a young man in the house, have him take double the recommended amounts of minerals, have him work through the diet program and, if needed, get him to take an herb for balancing male hormones.

ABOUT ALL MALE HORMONES

First, the male body needs large amounts of Vitamins B and E and the mineral, zinc, to keep a proper balance of hormones. Getting these levels balanced through following the diet program and vitamin and mineral suggestions is very important.

Years ago I had a forty year old client who had married a sweet young thing and promptly developed some sexual problems. He actually had a pain in his hip and leg for two years that no one could nail down. He came to see me for both problems without realizing the problems where connected!

The pain in the hip and leg were connected to a Sex-Circulation muscle problem, his Vitamin E levels were almost nonexistent, and his zinc level was struggling. Within a month on the right diet, the pain subsided and his sex drive soared. He was a very happy man, to say the least!

Sometimes male hormones are more difficult to balance than female hormones. Rarely does a woman need male hormones to balance her body, but men may need female hormone herbs as much as they need male hormone herbs to bring them into balance.

One of my ex's had experienced a lifelong hormonal imbalance without knowing it. Over the first few months we lived together, I saw him go through a cycle of weirdness that was really out there. He suddenly became a stranger. He wouldn't know where he was or what he was doing. He was a total space cadet. And nothing seemed to penetrate this weirdness.

This imbalance continued for three to five days, always before a full moon, and then suddenly be gone. He'd be back to his normal, sweet self and have almost no memory of the previous few days. When I saw him going into this for the fourth month, something snapped ON in me. This was all too regular. It happened in connection with the full moon. It was cyclical!

I asked his body what hormonal herb he needed to bring him into balance and heard, "Damiana." So I slipped him a cup of Damiana tea. Ten minutes later, he shook himself, just like a dog waking up, and asked, *"What happened?"* He was completely there!

For the next year, a week before the full moon, he drank a cup or two of Damiana tea every day and the weirdness didn't come on at all. After a year of this, his body learned to make shifts within itself and he no longer needed aid of the herbs!

So, if you are dealing with a male hormone imbalance, try taking a capsule or two of the hormonal balancer, Dong Quai, the female hormone herb, Damiana, or the male hormone herbs, Ginseng or Sarsaparilla.

A word of caution. Just because Ginseng has been used for eons to increase male virility, doesn't mean that it will do that specifically. I had a friend years ago who thought he'd increase his virility by taking Ginseng. He'd been having a problem, but the problem just persisted. When he finally got around to asking me about the problem, his hormones were zinging all over the place. I told him that his male hormones were way out of balance and he finally confessed up to taking alot of Ginseng. With female hormone herbs and diet we were able to get things back to normal.

THYROID

The thyroid gland is located in the throat and needs high levels of Vitamins A, B, and E and iodine, calcium and cobalt to function properly. The gland regulates the metabolism in the body and regulates the use of calcium.

If you are taking thyroxin in some form, continue to do so as you start the diet. But, be aware that as your body and thyroid heals, you may need to lower your dosage.

When you are taking or making too much thyroxin, you may experience nervousness, irritability, fatigue, weakness, loss of weight or a rapid heart beat. Consult with your doctor before you decrease your medication.

I have worked with a number of people who have been able to totally heal their thyroids and no longer needed medication. But this total healing usually takes from one to three years. You have to make sure your diet stays very clean and your nutrient levels stay very high. Extra stresses like caffeine and alcohol should stay out of the diet for at least a year AFTER the thyroid has totally healed.

HYPOGLYCEMIA

Hypoglycemia or low blood sugar is in epidemic proportions in the US. From my testing I guess that at least 85% of the population in the US are having minor to major hypoglycemic swings. Hypoglycemic symptoms range from minor levels of fatigue, cravings and mood swings to major levels of depression, headaches and fainting.

The patterns that I have seen are fairly predictable and there is a direct correlation between hypoglycemia and deficiencies of vitamin B's. When a body experiences stress, Vitamin B's are needed in huge quantities. If a deficiency develops, certain organs start to experience problems; the stomach has trouble making HCL, proteins do not get digested well, creating toxins, the large intestines suffer from the increase in toxins, the kidneys get stressed from having to deal with an increase in toxins in the blood and the pancreas is left without enough vitamin B to properly make its digestive enzymes.

When the pancreas cannot make its starch digesting enzymes from this lack of vitamin B's, it also experiences a stress in its other function, that is, the production and distribution of insulin. Insulin is a hormone that pulls sugars out of the bloodstream for storage and later use. I always think of insulin as a waiter, it serves sugar out of the blood and into the cells.

There needs to be a balanced level of sugars in the blood to maintain functioning energy levels. When the body experiences an increase in blood sugars from foods you have eaten, it sends a message to the pancreas to put out insulin. But when the pancreas is stressed, it loses its ability to regulate the amount of insulin that is put into the bloodstream; it overreacts to this message by dumping insulin into the bloodstream. All of a sudden too many waiters are running around, pulling TOO MUCH sugar out of the blood and the sugar levels start to fall.

When the sugar levels fall below a certain point, you will start to experience certain reactions. Below is a basic guide I developed over the years to determine what levels of hypoglycemia people are experiencing. As you can see, the symptoms are cumulative.

Here is a scale from 1 to 10, with 10 being a HIGH level of hypoglycemia, that lists symptoms. The beginning imbalances don't physically manifest until people reach a level of 4.

LEVEL	SYMPTOMS
4 ------------------	**mid-afternoon spaciness, lack of concentration, or fatigue **cravings for food, sugars, or caffeine **possible self-judgment
5 ------------------	all of the above **minor mood swings **irritability or snappiness **self-judgment (*"What's wrong with me?" "Why can't I do this?"*)
6 ------------------	all of the above experienced any time during the day or night and possibly some of #7 symptoms
7 ------------------	all of the above **headaches **dizziness or fainting **depression
8-10 --------------	all of the above **frequent urination **excessive thirst **acetone breathe **a pattern of different symptoms throughout the day, i.e. experiencing levels 1- 6 of hypoglycemia in the morning and levels of 7-10 in the afternoon and evening.

If you have been experiencing levels of hypoglycemia of 5 or more, you know how frustrating it can be. The irritability and snappiness can make you think you are going nuts. You are going along fine, then all of a sudden you turn around and snap at someone and you are as surprised as they are!

What's happened is simple. Your blood sugar levels have just dropped and whatever comes at you next is just TOO MUCH! Of course, this triggers the self-judgment patterns, *"What's wrong with me?"*

"Why can't I control myself?" And the cravings that come with the sugar level drops can also trigger alot of judgments, *"Why can't I control my eating?"*

One of the major reasons I want you to understand hypoglycemia is so I can then say to you *"Let go of the guilt!"* These problems have been a reaction in the body. They are NOT who you are! As the hypoglycemia clears, you will be able to separate reactions from who you are; and you will find yourself again.

Following this diet approach you will find that the hypoglycemic reactions start slowing down within a few days; and within two weeks the reactions will either be 'gone' or they will obviously be getting under control.

Be aware, it will take six months to a year to really heal the pancreas, but you don't need to deal with the symptoms in the meantime. And remember, after a two to four week period, you will find a new level of sensitivity about foods. And if you eat something off the diet, you may find you experience a swift hypoglycemic reaction. The reactions usually pass quickly. Use these reactions to help your resolve to stay on the diet.

Besides hypoglycemic reactions disrupting peoples lives and psyches, I have seen a more serious problem. People can move from high levels of hypoglycemia into diabetes, the inability for the pancreas to make enough insulin to sustain life. When the pancreas is overworked, the picture I get is that it ages faster than other organs in the body. Finally, the pancreas says, *"Look, you may have a thirty year old body, but you have a seventy year old pancreas; and I quit!"*

When people reach this stage, they start fluctuating between the high level symptoms of hypoglycemia and the beginnings of diabetes. Usually there will be a dramatic difference in the energy levels within a day with one part of the day demonstrating hypoglycemic reactions and the other part manifesting diabetic reactions. One friend who developed this imbalance felt pretty good in the morning, then went through sugar drops as the day progressed.

She attempted to bring her sugar levels up but never felt she was catching up to the problem. By 2:00 to 3:00 in the afternoon, she would start really dropping into a tail spin. Her body would start creating acetone as she went into diabetic reactions. Her breathe would stink of acetone, she would be thirsty, and exhausted, emotionally overwhelmed and irritable. Her eyes felt extreme levels of strain, her vision got obviously worse, and her night vision became nonexistent.

PHYSICAL SUGGESTIONS:

Licorice Root is an herb that will help balance the whole endocrine system, which the pancreas is part of, since insulin is a hormone. When the pancreas is the major gland demonstrating imbalance, the licorice will quickly help bring the swings of the blood sugar into balance.

Depending upon the level of hypoglycemia, you might want to try taking anywhere between one capsule of Licorice Root twice a day to three capsules twice a day. Remember that it takes time for the body to heal an unbalanced organ, so you may want to continue taking the Licorice Root up to and through the Final Phase diet.

SPIRITUAL SUGGESTIONS:

Let go of the guilt, the feelings you are out-of-control, the fears you might be 'losing it' and remember that this has been a physical imbalance. Those reactions were never you, they were just reactions.

INSOMNIA

There are many conditions that can induce insomnia from physical imbalances to emotional tension to energetic interference. Causes range from deficiencies in vitamins and minerals, lack of exercise, and hypoglycemia on the physical level, to carrying your emotional upsets, work tensions and overactive mental/creative process into your sleep, to literally let someone else's energy invade your sleep.

Following the diet program usually will take care of most insomnia linked to physical causes. If you are experiencing sleep problems, be sure to take your second dose of vitamins and minerals with your dinner, since they can increase your energy. Eating them with food will slow down their rush of energy and even it out before bedtime.

If you are taking a sleeping aid, continue with it until you feel your body is more balanced, then try skipping it for a night or two. Or try taking extracts of Valerian and/or Skullcap instead.

If you have followed the diet program for several months and are still having trouble sleeping, then start looking at other situations that may be the root cause. If your brain is going a mile a minute, then try some meditation techniques to quiet it down.

One of the visualizations I have always liked works well. Divide your life into different aspects, like your work self, your parent self, and your private self. See each aspect existing within its own separate ball of light. When you go to work, step into your work 'bubble,' leaving behind your personal and other bubbles. When you go home, leave your work bubble and step into your parent bubble or your personal bubble. If work thoughts come up, push them out of your mind and into the work bubble. Tell them you will deal with them when you step back into that energy space, but not before!

Sometimes, lack of exercise causes insomnia. If you need to burn off tension from life or work situations or if you just have more energy than the day has expended, find a creative outlet that will both get your body in shape and clear your mind. Simple walking (or stomping, as the case may be) can work out alot of thoughts so you can go to your bed relaxed and with a quieted mind.

Don't be surprised if you find yourself waking up around the same time each night. Frequently this indication means you are having a body or energy shift at that time. Get up and sit with the energy. Meditate. Relax and feel your body. Release any particular tense place you feel. Then go back to bed. There are planetary shifts of energy around 4 a.m., so if you find you are waking up then (which newborns will frequently do,) take it as a message that you need to feel the quiet around you and meditate on it.

If you are awakened in the night with someone specific in your thoughts, it is possible that that person is thinking about you or dreaming about you! Visualize yourself pushing their energy and thoughts back to them. See a barrier of white light or a mirror between you so their energy is reflected back to them. If this happens repeatedly, you might need to talk to them and ask them to direct their thoughts elsewhere.

The most important thing to remember about insomnia is that fighting it doesn't work. If you are awake, get up. Don't lie there tossing and turning. Work with the energy instead.

Also, be aware as you get healthy, you may need less sleep! I'll never forget the woman who called and exclaimed, *"I'm someone who has always needed eight hours of sleep. Now I only need six and I feel great. But what am I supposed to do with all this energy?"* My response was, *"Remember that list of dream-things you always wanted to do, but never had the time for? Well, pull it back out and start doing them!"*

MERCURY POISONING AND OTHER HEAVY METAL PROBLEMS

Mercury and other toxic, heavy metals will cause all kinds of ill-health. Symptoms range from allergies, memory loss, disorientation, mood swings, insomnia, metallic mouth taste, excessive tooth and gum problems, intestinal problems, chest pains or pressure, irregular heartbeats, headaches, emphysema, asthma, sinus infections, subnormal body temperature, anemia, hallucinations and manic-depression.

This stuff messes with every function in the body! It is possible to clear mercury out of the body, though it takes a long, long time.

You can pick up these 'heavy' metals from a number of sources, from foods, to food additives, to auto exhaust, to chemical products, to water. One of the major places you can pick up mercury is from the fillings in your mouth!!!

Don't be surprised if your regular dentist denies amalgam fillings cause any problems at all. The dental profession is scared stiff that we are all going to start suing them for the problems mercury has caused. They are in denial of the problem, yet suggest that people not rush to have all their fillings replaced because of the trauma it could cause!

After dealing with a number of people suffering from mercury poisoning, I'd never have another amalgam filling put in my mouth. Over time, I have been having my metal filling replaced with nonmetal fillings.

I had the opportunity to help a friend prove to the State of New Mexico Rehabilitation Department that she was sick from mercury poisoning. They accepted her documentation and paid for her very expensive dental work. By the time mercury poisoning was diagnosed, this friend was very sick. She dragged herself to her three hour teaching job, dragged herself home and spent most of her time in bed.

If you suspect a heavy metal problem, have a Hair Analysis done. Most chiropractors will have access to a lab performing this service. If any of the metals are in excess in the body, a hair analysis will show the problem, though mercury vapor from fillings may only show up in your blood or cell structure. If a hair analysis does not show a heavy metal problem, yet you still suspect it, work with someone doing muscle-testing or radionics or microscopic blood work to check out heavy metals in the blood or cells.

If you do have a heavy metal problem in your body, I suggest that you follow the food and diet suggestions listed in the Candida section in this chapter.

If you show positive for high metals or if you wish to remove the metal fillings from your teeth, you must proceed with great caution! Last summer I had three fillings redone. I went to the dentist fully prepared, with a build up of vitamins and minerals in my bloodstream, and still felt body stress for the next three to four weeks!

Unless you are seriously ill from heavy metal poisoning, before you start to work on clearing the metals from your bloodstream and body, you want to get as healthy as you can. You want to get all your vitamin and mineral deficiencies cleared and have no acute or chronic symptoms.

Even when you are healthy and ready to tackle this situation, you must proceed with caution. If you DO have mercury symptoms, get healthy then slowly replace the fillings as you work with a dentist specializing in this problem. I suggest that you find a dentist who has been dealing with mercury poisoning, one who uses a mouth dam, has oxygen and possibly intravenous vitamins available, and has a way to calculate which teeth to work on first. Or, have someone doing muscle testing determine the proper pattern of removal.

Mercury will set up an electromagnetic flow in the body. If this flow is not properly dealt with, numerous side affects can result. I worked, after the fact, with a client whose teeth crumbled apart a year after all the mercury was removed. Her body said that the improper removal of her fillings had interfered with the electromagnetic flow in her mouth and body. It was like pulling all the life-force out of her teeth and they reacted accordingly.

If you have no obvious mercury poisoning symptoms, I suggest you take massive amounts of Vitamin C, garlic and regular vitamin and minerals before, during and for the month following any filling removal. I took twenty grams of C before my last dentist visit and took 1/2 cup of bee pollen daily for months after!

There is scientific information out there, if you are interested. Some of it differs with what I've seen in bodies and some of it backs up what I have seen. You can send a self-addressed stamped envelope (a #10 size) to the Foundation for Toxic-Free Dentistry, PO Box 608010, Orlando, FL 328060-8010 for more scientific information on books, dentists in your area, and a newsletter. They do not necessarily represent my viewpoint.

Also see the information in the TMJ section in this chapter for exercises to clear jaw muscle stress caused from dental work.

MULTIPLE SCLEROSIS

Like a number of serious and mysterious diseases, Multiple Sclerosis is physically related to deep-seated Vitamin B deficiencies. Of course, by the time Vitamin B's deficiencies are deep-seated, all the other vitamins and numerous minerals are also in deep levels of deficiencies.

Obviously, following the Super Cleanser for months and taking the appropriate amount of nutrients is essential for healing to begin. After several months on the diet program, gradually increase your vitamin and mineral intake so that you are taking double the regular amounts.

The first MS client I had surprised me. When I tuned into her body, I saw that running a body was a new experience for her. Now, this was a relatively straightlaced woman and what I saw in her body was out there! But, I couldn't find a way around the situation so I said, *"I know this is going to sound weird to you, but I think that this is the first human body you have been in. Up until this time, you were an elf. The 'reason' for this dis-ease in your body is tied to the fact that you don't know HOW to make it work properly."*

She was a little shocked, but not in the way I expected.

Her reply was, *"I know that."* Now, her husband who was sitting next to her was shocked! She'd never expressed this to him! She went on to say that she'd never related to people but that nature was her best friend. And that she knew that she had come in as a twin so she could relate to a human body in a more connected way.

The next MS client I had heard a similar story, except that the only word I could get for his previous lives was an 'angel.' He also confessed that he knew this!

And the experiences have continued over 15 years!

If you have MS, you need to learn how to run your body! Remember that they are very intelligent and you only have to instruct them as to WHAT to do and they will do it. I've used a technique myself of asking my body to observe the way someone else runs their body around a particular issue and watched my body observe and then repeat the pattern.

Look for people who are healthy and seem to know how to maintain a healthy mind and body. Ask your body to observe how they run these patterns and then to 'try on' the pattern. If it works for you, then you can keep it. If it doesn't work in your body, fine. Release the pattern and try another.

Another thing to remember, if you are connected to your 'previous life self.' You chose to come into this body and you most likely came here with a specific purpose in mind. Relax into this life's experience. It's just another form of perfection. Then get on with your purpose, whether it is to spread a new level of joy onto the planet or to link humans to their care-taking position with the plant realms or whatever. I have yet to see an MS person who didn't have a high goal and the abilities to reach that goal!

SKIN PROBLEMS

There are a number of skin problems like acne, eczema, and psoriasis. There are physical, dietary aspects to all of them and spiritual aspects to the more severe problems.

ACNE

One of the major functions of the skin is release of toxins. Toxins can be released through the bowels and through the lymph system by way of the lungs and breath and through the breathing of the skin. Since different bodies work differently, some people tend to use the skin as their 'first choice' for release of toxins, while others use it as the second or third method of release.

No matter which release method you are demonstrating, if you are having acne, you are creating too many toxins! I am in the 'first choice' group. Since my hormones clicked on, around twelve, I have been dealing with varying levels of acne. If I get into a period of having too much oil or chocolate or garbage, my skin will get rough and I'll have an occasional pimple. I know I can 'get away' with more out-of-balance behavior if I am getting alot of exercise, where I am moving the toxins out in different way or if I am increasing my mineral intake to compensate.

But no matter how you are dealing with the release of toxins, acne still means there are just too many of them in your body! This is more obvious the more severe the acne problem.

So, the first thing you have to do to deal with acne, on any level, is to cut out toxin-creating foods. Following the Basic Balancer is a good place to start. But if you are having really nasty eruptions and cysts, do the Deep Cleanser. Whichever basic diet you follow, if you are having serious or long term problems, follow the diet for two to three times longer than the regular schedule indicates.

Letting the overall toxin level drop in your body means that you may continue experiencing some acne, since the acne is a toxin release. Be patient! Your body's method of release won't change, but as you drop the toxin level, you will see your skin improving and the number and severity of the acne decreasing. If your body does its major toxin release through the bowels or lungs, then you will probably quickly see improvement.

The second contributor to acne problems is from mineral deficiencies, especially zinc. High levels of minerals are needed for all hormonal changes, so as teenagers, many of us start developing deficiencies. If you started breaking out then, you can be assured your mineral levels were low. For people who start having acne problems later in life, it indicates their mineral levels have dropped into deficiencies over the years.

All levels of mineral deficiencies can be cleared by including seaweeds into the diet, either through the use of them directly in your food or taking tablets or capsules of them, or by the use of other complete mineral supplements and other high mineral foods. Even higher levels of minerals are needed for women seven to ten days before their periods.

The third aid to dealing with acne has to do with exercise. Your skin breathes, but if you don't exercise and open up the pores, the skin becomes clogged. You end up with a buildup of particles that were supposed to be release out of the skin. So, get out there and sweat those pores open!

Obviously, keeping the skin clean is important, but do it gently, without harsh soaps and scrubs. Remember, acne is an internal problem that you can't scrub off.

ECZEMA AND PSORIASIS

Eczema and Psoriasis, like acne, are an internal toxic problems directly related to Vitamin E and mineral deficiencies, respectively, and emotional reactions. Actual skin flare ups are toxic release sights and may or may not be related to acupuncture meridians and points and organs associated with them. See a good acupuncture chart to see if your flare up points as related to a specific organ or system.

Because both skin problems are toxic releases, it is very important to lower your overall toxicity. Follow the Basic Diet indicated in the Health Assessment chapter and always to back to it when you have a flare up. After three to four months on the program, you might want to start taking a vegetable (non-oil) based Vitamin E for eczema and extra minerals for psoriasis. Remember to take them both in the morning and evening. Also rubbing Vitamin E directly into the affected eczema area may help.

The emotional aspects of eczema and psoriasis seem to have a direct connection with personal power issues. When you have a flare up, look back a day or two and see if you can find a situation where your power was suppressed.

I recently worked on a three year old who started breaking out in eczema when her child care situation changed. Everything in the situation was the same, but the introduction in the house of a relatively negative person. She reacted by pushing the negative interaction to the surface of her skin. It was a reaction her parents couldn't miss!

I don't mean to make this power suppression sound easy to change. In most teens and adults it is a long-term pattern that goes to the core of the personality. I suggest you work seriously with a therapist on the pattern and learn to stand in your power. Don't let other people's belief systems suppress your own. Learn to accept your right to see the world in your own way.

SMOKING AND OTHER VICES

ABOUT SMOKING

Humans must have been smoking natural plants since they started controlling fire. Smoking tools have been found in all ancient cultures. I mean, can't you just see the picture? There our ancestors were, inhaling smoke from plants thrown on the fire and finding different effects were felt from different burning plants. Certain ones made their lungs feel more open and certain plants gave them visions. The desire 'to smoke' was there then, and is with us still.

I don't think smoking is a bad thing all by itself. And I think our ancestors would agree. There are lots of centurions in the world who have smoked all their lives. Smoking anything however, whether it be herbs, tobacco, or tree barks, IS stressful for the body. Our lungs can only deal with so much smoke before they develop problems, but compensating with the vitamins and minerals needed to deal with smoke-stress can keep the lungs cleared out.

There are two major problems I see with cigarettes. One problem is the chemicals that are added to commercial products. I strongly suggest if you are going to smoke cigarettes that you use natural tobacco. The only source I know for a variety of natural tobacco products is the brand American Spirit. Check out Table 3 of the Appendix for information.

The second problem is the amount of cigarettes that are smoked. Past cultures used all smoking materials with respect in ritual situations, but we have moved the obvious ceremony out of the experience. We have moved smoking into high levels of indulgence and the physical problems associated with it attest to that fact.

Now, one of the things about cigarettes is the way that people use them. There actually is some ceremony in the process, though most people are totally detached from it.

Watch the times when you desire a cigarette. The desire will always come up when you are making an energy transition! Smoking is a way to recollect yourself, pause and refocus your energy in another direction! Whether you smoke after eating, or after sex, or before a phone call, or as a way to separate yourself from your coworkers, you are using the cigarette as a transition tool.

This is a kind of energetic ceremony that you obviously need and that need in itself is not a problem. But using cigarettes to make all these needed transitions is not a healthy answer.

Start watching for these transitions and start finding other ways that are less stressful. Take a walk around the block. Do some deep breathing exercises. Stretch. But recollect yourself, pull your energy in around you like you are giving yourself a hug, and push everyone and everything else from your space. Then refocus your energy into the next step in your day.

If another transition technique doesn't work, then light up! But only take a few puffs. If you're going to smoke, it has to become a pleasurable experience, not a habit.

Then, make sure you let go of the guilt the culture has placed on smoking, use it as one of your transition tools, and compensate for the stress with extra Vitamin C. Usually for every two cigarettes, people need 500 mg. of a chewable C.

If you want to totally quit smoking, first, get yourself healthy! Work with the diet approach for at least four months before you attempt to release the habit. Work with the above suggestions and establish new transition tools into your life. Then and only then, work on stopping altogether!

Use the Temporal Tap technique in Chapter 16 to help change the desire patterns. Try using LOTS of Chamomile in tea or capsules; it will make the cigarettes taste terrible and work as a blood cleanser to clear the nicotine out of the system.

ABOUT OTHER VICES

I find the cultural attitude toward drugs very curious, to say the least! It condones most of the drugs that numb you out, like Valium and alcohol and condemns mind-expanding or mind-altering things, like LSD and pot.

Unfortunately, another cultural aspect of drugs is abuse and physical or emotional addiction. Like smoking in ancient cultures, drugs were done with honor and respect. They were NOT done to escape from day to day responsibilities. Drugs used as a tool to open and expand are quite a different thing.

Now, I'm not saying that you should rush out and do drugs, but if you are using them, examine the 'whys.' If you are using them as an escape from aspects of your life, then change the aspect! Make your life better instead of giving control over to an external substance.

In any case, if you are using drugs, compensate for the stress they cause in the body. Take any of the food supplements for vitamins and minerals in large doses along with getting your body cleared through the diet program.

SURGERY PREPARATION

Surgeries are one of the greatest accomplishments and tools that the medical profession has given us. But surgeries are still options that you don't want to take lightly. They are major body stresses, so you want to make sure that if you elect to do a surgery, you prepare yourself for it physically, emotionally, mentally, and spiritually.

Obviously, the kind of surgery you are needing or choosing makes some difference in what preparation time you have. Make sure that you grill your doctor for all the options you have available. Get a second and third opinion. Then ask: What will happen if you wait and watch the situation? What symptoms do you need to watch for if you choose to wait? What other procedures are available concerning your problem? Where are these options available?

Research your problem well before you make your decision and then work on your preparations to be ready for action. First, you want to be as healthy as you can be before you go under the knife. Even if your situation is only days away, you can up your vitamin and mineral levels to help your body cope with the stress. Obviously, the longer you have to prepare physically, the better.

If you have time, follow the Basic Balancer for all the time before your surgery. Take double the regular suggested vitamins and minerals. If you include 800-1200 IU's of Vitamin E into your diet, you are less likely to scar and will usually heal faster. Also, up your Vitamin B levels to deal with the extra stress that just being in the hospital brings on.

After surgery, for the first one to three days, depending on the severity of the situation, I suggest you only do veggie and fruit juices, herbal teas and broths, especially miso broth. If you are knocked out, your intestinal tract is 'put to sleep' and it is the last organ to 'wake back up.' Give it a rest.

Start eating again with just cooked veggies for a day or more. Then gradually add fruits, proteins and starches back into your system. Check out Chapter 15 and the information on cleansing diets. Following those patterns are a great help. Continue the extra nutrient intake for a week to a month after the surgery, again, depending upon its severity.

Second, deal with the emotional, mental and spiritual aspects of your surgery need. If you are having a tumor removed, talk to people who have dealt with the same problem. Check out support groups for your specific problem. Talk to a therapist.

When you actually go into surgery, give your trust over to God or the Universe or however you see your fate. Relax. You've done all you can. Now is the time to see what comes next and be ready to deal with it from a place of calm. I've worked with a number of wholistic healers and wholistic-minded people who saw their need for surgeries as a sign of their failure to heal themselves. And I've had to point out to them that surgery is a tool that you can use as part of your healing resources.

Having a problem removed physically doesn't mean you get out of dealing with any emotional, mental or spiritual aspects of it. They will be in your face until you deal with them. Having the physical aspect removed can actually help you deal with the other stuff! I believe everyone is doing the best they can in the moment. If you could do 'better' it's likely you'd do it in that moment. Be gentle with yourself.

TEMPORAL MANDIBULAR JOINT (TMJ)

The Temporal Mandibular Joint is made up by the group of muscles and bones that move your lower jaw upward into the upper jaw. If you squeeze your back teeth together, you will see the muscles in the area tighten. Of course, if you are having TMJ problems, you can probably see the muscles without additional tension because that's what makes it a problem! Tension held constantly in this area can happen during waking hours or manifest itself at night with grinding your teeth. There are alot of fancy remedies for fixing the TMJ, from braces to night retainers, but the underlying problem is the anger and tension that you hold in.

If you've been holding emotions in this area for a long time, it may take years of work to change the structures you created that hold the tension. I suggest, once you have learned to release the tension in the area, that you do whatever method makes sense to you. But, if you haven't dealt with the release of emotions, then physically working in this area may be futile.

One of the TMJ issues we all need to deal with sometimes throughout our lives is connected to the visits to the dentist. These muscles were never made to be held open. They are made for going up and down while you chew your food. But when they are held open for more than a few minutes, the brain wave impulses that tell the muscles to contract and relax get cancelled out.

If you are lucky and healthy, the impulses will resume after about 24 hours. But, for many people, this doesn't happen and the major nerve message flow is affected. I suggest that after a visit to the dentist that you work the TMJ muscles a couple of times as described in the Fix It section below. One of the underlying problems with the TMJ, that I have dealt with, is the blockage of body-to-brain messages. One-half the messages that flow from your body to your brain flow through a nerve that runs right through the TMJ muscles. If this flow of messages is interrupted because of tension, odd things can happen.

I had two sets of experiences that showed me the importance of easy flow through the TMJ area. Twice I had people who had had gallbladder surgeries with no relief in the pain they experienced in their gallbladder area. They were told *"It's all in your head"* which was somewhat accurate. The TMJ never let the message get to their brains that the gallbladder problem was resolved, so their brains continued to run the same message that their gallbladders were sick and in pain. Once we released the TMJ tension and told their gallbladders, through pressure-point stimulation, that they were essentially healed, the pain stopped.

The other client was a woman who was a telephone operator. She started having this problem with her back going out and her arms and legs going to sleep. She couldn't sit for more than twenty minutes before the problem started, which seriously interfered with her work. This had been going on for six months and nothing seemed to make it better. She'd see a chiropractor, have her back put into place and barely hit the door before the bones were going out again. As a last resort, she was scheduled for major back surgery!

After I determined the problem was TMJ related, I showed her how to exercise the muscles. She sat for thirty minutes with no tingling at all and flew out of the chair to give me a big hug! When I started looking for the cause of this problem, I asked her about dental work. Sure enough, she'd had all four impacted wisdom teeth surgically removed just before this started! She needed to rework the muscles for the next couple of weeks, but the problem never returned and her back stayed in place!

TO FIX THE JOINT

There are two simple muscle manipulations that need to be done to relax the TMJ. First, look at the muscles in the figures on the following page. The two main muscles you need to work are the Masseter and the Internal Pterigoid (that's pronounced without the 'P' sound.)

To work the Masseter, put your fingers in a line along the top of the muscle where it attaches to the cheekbone and the thumb along the base of the jaw, at the bottom of the muscle. Squeeze your thumb and fingers toward each other and hold for a slow count of five. Release and repeat this squeezing three times.

Then, work the Internal Pterigoid. You do this by putting your clean finger just inside the lips at the corner. Run your finger back, along inside the cheek until you come to what feels like bone. If you relax your jaw you'll feel this 'bone' relax. It's actually a very strong muscle!

Rub in the center of the muscle, the area between the upper and lower teeth, for a few seconds. It's usually sore if it needs rubbing. Repeat this rubbing 2 more times.

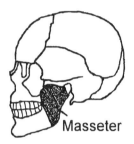
Masseter

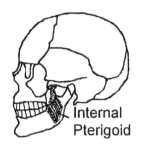
Internal Pterigoid

After a trip to the dentist, I will do this 'joint fixing' several times and feel how my jaw feels as I move it around. If I still feel tension, I'll repeat it every few hours until it feels normal again.

If you have a well-developed TMJ problem, you might need to work the area several times a day for weeks and weeks. I also suggest you massage all the other TMJ muscles pictured below once a day.

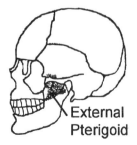
External Pterigoid

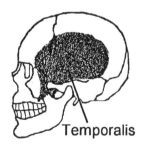
Temporalis

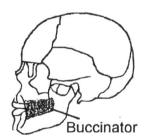
Buccinator

Use the Temporal Tap technique in Chapter 16 to change the patterns of holding emotions here, and especially release the emotions. Most of the TMJ people I have worked with need to scream! And then, they need to change the things in their lives they need to scream about!

ULCERS AND OTHER STOMACH PROBLEMS

One of my pet peeves with the school systems in the U.S. is that, as children, they never taught us about anatomy. I'm always amazed at how few people actually know where their stomachs are!

The valve that goes from the throat into the stomach is called the cardiac valve because it is right next to the heart! The stomach sets behind the left nipple. Of course, if you have been having a problem with the stomach, instead of the intestines (which are located between the end of your breastbone and the pubic bone,) then you know where the stomach is!

ABOUT HEARTBURN

There is no question that heartburn is the direct affect of eating a food or group of foods that you are not digesting properly. And the obvious way to 'cure' it is to stopping eating the offending foods! Remember, that this doesn't mean it will be forever. When you can digest the food without stress, you may to able to eat it again with no mucus reactions or heartburn.

Eating certain combinations of foods may always end in this predicament, though. Eating starch and protein combinations is a case in point. I think 'getting over it' and not eating them is the best solution, but if you do overstep your bounds and indulge, there are a couple of things you can do to minimize the negative affects.

1) Before partaking of a starch and protein combination, take a few tablets of either HCL or pancreatic enzymes. Take the HCL if the bulk of the food is a dairy, fish, meat, nut or seed; or take pancreatic enzyme tablets if most of the food is a grain or soy product.

2) Upon experiencing heartburn, chew on a 1/2-1 tsp. of fennel seeds.

3) Try a cup of catnip/fennel tea before and after.

4) And, as a last resort, take an anti-acid. You'll still end up suffering some for your 'offense' and should remember what this body message means. But there is no reason to continue suffering once the point has gotten across!

ABOUT STOMACH VALVE PROBLEMS

This condition is one of those problems that doctors have a pat answer for: *"Here. Take this pill. Oh, and by the way, you will have to do this for the rest of your life."* NOT!!!

The problem occurs when the cardiac valve doesn't close the stomach off from the esophagus. Foods are then free to 'come back up,' especially when you lie down.

I have worked with lots of people with this problem. To date, we have never had to do any special work to reverse the condition. Following the diet program for a few months usually reverses this 'irreversible' condition. I have seen a direct connection with Vitamin E deficiencies and general stress, through bringing all the vitamin and mineral levels into line is the underlying answer.

ABOUT ULCERS

Obviously, ulcers are a stomach problem that being more severe, indicate physical AND emotional imbalances. The physical imbalance will take care of itself, in most situations, by following the diet program. But the emotional aspects must also go through major change to really 'solve' the problem.

On a physical level, follow the appropriate Basic Diet for an extra month or two before moving on to the next diet. Try taking either Myrrh extract or Slippery Elm tea daily for immediately soothing of a painful ulcer.

On an emotional level, the need to control or the fear of not being in control have to be addressed, resolved and released. I suggest that you work with a therapist of some kind to address these needs and fears.

I know that control is a culturally manufactured idea that is an impossibility. There is no such thing as controlling your life or lives of others. And, of course, this is where the fear comes from. 'Letting go' is the only answer! Give the control over to your Spirit, Higher Self or God/Goddess and relax! The 'higher' forces have a much clearer picture of what we need in our lives and are responsible for bringing those needs to us.

But they can't do it if you are in the way. Spirit gave me a great picture years ago about control. It said, *"You are supposed to go through life like you are riding in the back of a limo and Spirit is behind the drivers wheel. But when you feel that you need to 'control,' you crawl over the seat, straight-arm Spirit out the door and pull yourself behind the wheel."*

"Of course, as soon as you take the wheel, you realize that you don't know where in the hell you are supposed to drive to! That's because it's not your job to know that!"

Whenever you realize that you have climbed behind the wheel, whenever you find yourself thinking that you should know what to do, whenever you get overwhelmed or whenever feel out of control, climb back over the seat! Apologize to Spirit for overstepping your bounds and relax.

As soon as you do this, you'll be able to see your life moving forward again. I know it's scary, and that's okay. Just don't let the fear run your life. Release it and relax!

URINARY TRACT HEALTH

BED WETTING

Like most problems, there are physical and emotional reasons for bed-wetting to occur. On a physical level, it is directly linked to Vitamin B deficiencies. The emotional specifics for this problem can be widespread, but the underlying reason is feeling or being out of control.

On the physical level, work with the Basic Balancer for several extra months. Increase the vitamin and mineral levels overall for the first two months, then drop them back to the normal suggested level and increase the Vitamin B either with a B-Stress tab or herbs and foods high in B's. Do the obvious: keep the liquid levels down from about 6 p.m. on, use suck-on candies or foods for keeping the mouth moist after dinner, pee before bedtime, and don't make an issue out of the whole thing.

On the emotional levels, ask your kid where they feel powerful and where they don't. Correct the power imbalance and give them new ways to feel in control of their lives.

I'll never forget the day I got this response from my kid, *"You always get to do what you want!"* I sat down with him and asked, *"Does it really look like that?"* and realized even as I said it, that from a kid's perspective, that's exactly how the world looks. So, I explained to him that even though it may look like that, I had to do all kinds of things I didn't want to do, at times I didn't want to do them. He was skeptical about the reality of that, so I pointed out all kinds of 'have to's' that I dealt with throughout the next week. He got the point.

We also discussed ways that he got to make more choices in his day to day living. We implemented these choice-making patterns into our lives, choices like having two or three places he could stay while I was attending a college class, and he felt more empowered.

BLADDER AND KIDNEY INFECTIONS

Urinary tract infections are one of the body's signs of toxin overload. They can also come from bacteria getting up into the urinary tract through alot of sexual contact. Symptoms of an infection are frequent urination, frequent need to pee with little result, burning sensations, back pain around the kidneys (above the waist and around the spine) and pain deep in the abdomen.

At the first sign of an irritation, I suggest trying an herb called Uva Ursi. This herb was used by almost every Indian tribe across this country for bladder and kidney infections. Usually a few capsules or cups of this tea a day will clear infections. But if the herb doesn't clear the symptoms right away, be sure to see your doctor. Sometimes people let infections get away from them and when this happens, herbs just won't do it by themselves. When it's time to use antibiotics, do it. Don't let your kidneys suffer, they are too important to your overall health.

If your kidneys are one of your weak places, doing a cup or two of Uva Ursi weekly is a good way to keep them cleansed. You especially want to do this if you are releasing toxins for any reason.

WEIGHT

First I want to address weight imbalances on the high end. If your problem is not being able to hold weight on your body, skip down to the section, Under the Comfort Zone.

OVER THE COMFORT ZONE

There's so much information floating around out there about weight problems, it's hard to know what to do or think. Hardly a week goes by when there isn't a new flash of information, *"Mexican food is bad for you, it's fattening." "There's good fats you need in your body and bad fats you should avoid." "Obesity is genetic."*

I think the underlying point is that all our bodies are very different in the way we deal with foods and fats, we vary in size and shape, the amounts of exercise we need varies, and the foods and exercise we need change as we go through life. What seems important is for people to get in touch with their own bodies, their own food needs and nutrients and their own needs for exercise.

Stop looking for 'answers' outside yourself and concentrate on getting in touch within. Let go of the emotional and mental 'shoulds' so you can become familiar with your personal needs. And let go of the images the culture portrays as 'perfect'; we all have our own perfect bodies and most of them don't look like models.

The major reasons for out-of-balance weight problems, in descending order, are: 1) Vitamin and mineral deficiencies, which can cause overeating, 2) Eating indigestible foods, 3) Lack of exercise, 4) Overeating from emotions.

As each of these problems is addressed, weight levels begin to balance themselves out. Beginning this diet program, like many diet programs, usually means you lose five to fifteen pounds. On this approach the loss usually comes from taking out indigestible foods and starting to provide daily vitamin and mineral levels.

If your weight comes to balance just following the diets through to a new way of eating, great! But if excess doesn't just melt away, don't get discouraged. Stop thinking of quick cures and start dealing with reality. Sometimes it takes months to bring the body into a balanced state. For some, high body weight won't shift until certain vitamins and minerals are brought out of deficient levels.

Think of your excess as a indicator of imbalance that you are working on bringing into balance. So what if that takes a year or even two? Remember, it took many years for this imbalance to develop. Why should it turn around in a few months? Why should pills and quick cures fix it?

Set yourself a workable 'goal program.' First, you are going to get your body eating right. You are going to bring your deficiencies into balance. And you are going to start looking for emotional, mental and spiritual situations that push your eating buttons.

Second, you are going to continue learning about your body, your food reactions, and yourself. As clarity comes to you and you see emotional reactions, you can start changing them and find ways to express these reactions outside your body. Instead of stuffing your anger down with food, you can learn to appropriately express it outwardly. Instead of swallowing other people's crap, you can learn to stand strong and say 'No.' Instead of beating yourself up by stuffing yourself with food, you can learn to love yourself.

Third, you can ease into an exercise program that fits into your life and is fun, rather than work. Check out the exercise information in this chapter.

Recently, 'exercise experts' have found that intense workouts are not the only way to burn fat. Walking a hundred feet, stopping, walking a hundred feet, stopping, burns off fat in the same way as walking the distance without stopping! Movement is movement no matter what the pace is! This kind of 'workout' may not give your heart alot of exercise, but burning off fat and being aerobic don't have to go together!

Fourth, look for support groups that fit into your belief systems. These can be formal groups or just a good friend who understands you and your problem. Don't let people tell you, in any way, shape or form, that excess weight equals ill-health, either physical or emotional. Remember, your eating habits were taught patterns or reaction patterns to 'shoulds' that belong to other people or the culture.

Find your own balance and get happy with it! If it doesn't fit into other people's pictures, then they are missing the real you and that is THEIR problem!

UNDER THE COMFORT ZONE

Being 'underweight' has almost as much pressure put on it these days as overweight problems. If you are underweight because of an eating disorder, check out that section in this chapter. If you are a healthy eater, but are still underweight, read on.

First, your weight may or may not be a problem. If you are thin but are healthy, happy and energetic, your body weight may be normal for you. You can still 'build up' your body, but first you need to bring any vitamin and mineral deficiencies into balance.

Second, most 'underweight' clients I have dealt with don't have enough 'decadence' in their lives. You know, most of us have to curtail our decadence, especially with food. But, this is a place where you can really go for it! Your body is built to receive a higher level of food fun, so start taking advantage of it!

As you give yourself a second piece of cheesecake, watch for the voices that tell you something is 'wrong' with 'giving to yourself' and start telling them to shut up! We all need to learn to do that, but you get to nurture your self-giving through food decadence as well as through other aspects of your life! So enjoy!

Be sure that you eat alot of food as you go through the diet program. It takes alot of food to keep your weight up when a large portion of your diet is fruits and veggies. Of course, this means that you need to increase the amount of other foods (dairy, meats, nuts and seeds, grains, oils and sweeteners) to keep the proportions correct (70-80% fruits and veggies and 20-30% everything else.)

Once you have worked with the diet approach for six months, then you can start working on building your body and weight up, if you wish.

1) Start an exercise program that builds muscle tissue.

2) Also, increase your overall food intake and the quality of proteins. High quality proteins foods that contain alot of protein in a small package like cottage cheese or nuts and seeds. Continue to eat easy-to-digest proteins as well, but definitely include the more intense foods.

3) Include some of the protein/bodybuilding powders into your diet when you reach the point in the program that you can digest them.

4) Double up on your vitamin and mineral supplements to make sure you have the nutrients to produce any enzymes needed to digest all this food.

5) Give yourself alot of time to see results. Remember, you body has had 'non-building' patterns in it for a long time and it will take time to turn them around. If you don't want to take the time to really work on this building program, then get happy with your thinness!

Chapter 11
Phase Two

This diet workup is the first follow-up phase to the three Basic Diets. Look at following this diet workup only if you are feeling alot better than when you started the Basic Diet series. If you are NOT feeling better, if you are NOT feeling like you are getting on track, then instead of adding more foods into your diet, you should continue with the plan you have been following until you DO feel better.

A PAT ON THE BACK!

At this point it is likely that a number of your symptoms have either cleared or are obviously getting better. Your energy level should be up. Mood swings should be gone or subsiding Your skin should be starting to have a glow of health to it. Your digestive system should be running smoothly. A few pounds will probably have melted away. And you should be feeling more centered, more yourself.

Go back and look at your initial Health Assessment and review it. We humans sort of forget about pain when we stop feeling it. So, you may realize that you are feeling better without realizing that you haven't had a headache for three weeks or your back isn't hurting any more or you haven't had to clear your throat regularly since you can't remember when!

Pat yourself on the back!!! It's taken some concentrated work on your part to set real healing in motion!!! This diet approach isn't necessarily easy to do, because it makes you look at patterns in your life; patterns that are not necessarily working for you anymore.

When you reestablish patterns of health, the negative patterns of your life become more obvious. And with a sense of health you have the energy to CHANGE the patterns that no longer serve you. Patterns like 'eating-to-stuff-emotions' or 'I-wonder-if-I-deserve-to-feel-this-good' start to take on a comic look even if you still get caught up in them!

At this point you probably also have experienced a craving or two for some new additions in your diet. Don't be surprised as you look over this next diet if there aren't additions that you were also craving! I've heard it over and over again, someone will say, *"I just picked that up at the store yesterday and almost bought it!"* If you've experienced this, pat yourself on the back again because it means that you are getting in tune with your body and its needs!

HOW YOUR PERSONALITY AFFECTS HEALING

Bodies and personalities are linked together. Your body will heal itself within the guidelines of the personality, so if you tend to be overwhelmed by life, then you may find that your body gets overwhelmed easily with new food additions. If you find yourself backsliding when you add new foods in, then you are probably getting overwhelmed. Try this: take out some of the foods you were eating within the same food group, i.e. if you were eating yogurt and are adding in cottage cheese then only eat cottage cheese for a week or two and avoid the yogurt. Then reintroduce the yogurt and see if you can eat them both with NO reactions.

A FEW REMINDERS

**It's a good idea, before you add other foods back into your diet, to review the section on 'How Do I Reintroduce Foods' and on 'Emotional Food Reactions' in Chapter 7. You want to pin down any reactions to a new food right away and you want to check out whether it's an emotional food reaction instead of a physical one.

**Now is a good time to review your whole interaction with food. Remember that the foods you can easily digest are also nurturing and loving for your body because they don't cause stress.

**Trust your feelings when you reintroduce a food; just make sure that your taste buds aren't getting into the picture.

PHASE TWO DIET

YES FOODS	NO FOODS
FRUITS: All fruits BUT------------------	citrus (oranges, limes, lemons, tangerines, tangelos, pineapple, grapefruit), pears, apples, kiwi, papaya, guava, mangoes
VEGGIES: all veggies including potatoes and corn/cornmeal	
DAIRY PRODUCTS: eggs, yogurt, kefir and kefir cheese, sour cream, cottage cheese, cream cheese------------	buttermilk, cheese, milk
MEATS: fish, chicken, & turkey--------	all other meats and shellfish
NUTS and SEEDS: hazelnuts only----	all nuts and seeds
GRAINS: 100% sprouted grains and quinoa and their flours---------------------	rice, rye, oats, millet, barley, buckwheat, triticale, wheat, kamut, amaranth, spelt, couscous, and teff, their flours and pastas
SWEETENERS: 100% maple syrup, malt syrups, rice and rice bran syrups	all other sweeteners

YES FOODS	NO FOODS
OILS: butter and olive oil----------------	all other oils
SOY PRODUCTS: miso & tamari-----	all other soy products
SPROUTED BEANS & LEGUMES ONLY------------------------	all regular beans and legumes
HERBS & SPICES: all herbs and spices	NO goldenseal
SPECIAL ITEMS: Carob powder, vinegar and most condiments: (catsup, prepared mustard, horseradish, pickles)	coffee, chocolate, alcohol, brewer's and nutritional yeasts, mayo

PERCENTAGES OF FOODS:

FOR ADULTS:

50% veggies (20% of which can be raw veggies if you want them.)

20% fruits

30% everything else (dairy products, fish, chicken, turkey, hazelnuts, maple syrup, malt syrups, rice/bran syrups, butter and olive oil.)

FOR PREGNANT WOMEN:

40% veggies (20% of which can be raw veggies if you want them.)

20% fruits

40% everything else (dairy products, fish, chicken, turkey, hazelnuts, maple syrup, malt syrups, rice/bran syrups, butter and olive oil.)

FOR CHILDREN UNDER 12:

10-20% fruits and veggies (all of which can be raw veggies if you want them.)

80-90% everything else (dairy products, fish, chicken, turkey, hazelnuts, maple syrup, malt syrups, rice/bran syrups, butter and olive oil.)

SUPPLEMENTS:

See Chapter 8, On Supplements.

NUTRITIONAL RULES:

1) Eat something as soon as you get up in the morning and then eat a little something every two hours after that.

2) Avoid shellfish.

3) Fruits can be eaten with anything except other fruits. Leave a half hour between different fruits.

4) Beans and legumes must be sprouted.

PHASE TWO EXPLANATIONS

FRUITS
All fruits but NO citrus (oranges, limes, lemons, tangerines, tangelos,
pineapple, grapefruit,) pears, apples, kiwi, papaya, guava, mangoes.

Wow! This is a big change from the limited fruits allowed for the Basic Diet. This inclusion of most fruits into the diet happens because bodies quickly work on bringing blood sugar imbalances in line.

At this point in the diet plan, most bodies will be able to handle regular sugar ups and downs in the bloodstream without having hypoglycemic reactions. So, now you can eat all fruits listed in Table 2 in the Appendix except the ones listed above. Fruits that are out of the diet still are too fast in the bloodstream and can still cause some uncontrolled sugar reactions. Stay away from them for now. This is especially true for apples and pears, which are the highest sugar-content fruits.

VEGGIES
All veggies including potatoes, corn and cornmeal.

Of all the food groups, veggies are the easiest foods that bodies can digest. And now that you've taken a break from the cabbage family, you should be able to easily digest all of them.

As you reintroduce broccoli, brussels sprouts, cabbages, cauliflower, collard greens, kale, and/or kohlrabi back into your diet, watch out for any digestive problems, especially gas, bloating or flatulence. And check out saurkraut now.

Remember to try all the different veggies on the market, there's a great variety of taste treats out there! Last year I made a basic salad mix from the garden that consisted of lamb's quarters, arugula, lettuce, endive, anise-hyssop leaves, pansy leaves and flowers, spinach, mustard greens, baby cabbage leaves, chard, baby collard greens and wild prickly lettuce. I bet you haven't even heard some of these things, let alone tasted them! Get out there and play with your food!

DAIRY PRODUCTS
Yogurt, kefir and kefir cheese, sour cream, cream cheese, and cottage cheese.

The additions of cream cheese and cottage cheese indicate an increase in hydrochloric acid in the stomach and an increase in the production of lactose enzymes. This increase is directly related to the increase in usable vitamins and minerals in the body. For proper health the body knows it has to increase the HCL so that it can properly digest proteins. Since they are essential building blocks, you have to have a good supply of proteins available for your body to cleanse, heal and rebuild itself.

This group of dairy products is always much easier to digest than buttermilk, cheese and milk because of the souring and culturing processes they go through.

These dairy product additions can be used in many different ways as well as eaten plain. I've made some great ice cream with blended cottage cheese! Some great grilled cheese sandwiches with cream cheese! Some great quiches with plain and blended cottage cheese! And some great salad dressings with diluted and blended cream cheese!

MEATS
Fish, chicken, and turkey

Turkey is now included in the meat group because of the increase of HCL in the stomach and an increase in quality of bile from the gallbladder. Other meats take much higher levels of protein and fat digestion; these levels will continue to increase but your body needs some time to accomplish this healing.

NUTS AND SEEDS
Hazelnuts ONLY

Here's one of the benefits of the HCL and bile levels increasing; you can add hazelnuts into your diet. Hazelnuts are also called Filberts. They are always the first nut to come back into the diet. You can find them in the shell, ground for nut butter and already shelled. Check out the recipes under "Quick Treats" for a way to make a quick 'candy' with hazelnut butter!

GRAINS
100% Sprouted Grains and Panocha flour, Quinoa and quinoa flour

It always takes the pancreas a long time to start making pancreatic enzymes after it initially gets out of balance. So, even though you need to continue eating only 100% sprouted products and quinoa, the pancreas will have experienced some healing. The pancreas has already done some healing. This is evident from the clearing of hypoglycemic symptoms, the ability to include more fruits into your diet and the increase in concentrated sugars as indicated by the addition of malt and rice syrups.

SWEETENERS
Maple syrup, malt syrups, rice and rice bran syrups.

After two months or more of using maple syrup as the only sweetener, most people don't even want to hear about adding other sweeteners to their diets, they are so happy! But, whether you want to include other sweeteners or not, it's a good idea to at least try them. Remember, part of this diet approach has to do with creating new patterns of digestion in the system. You have to at least introduce the new foods into the body for it to be able to create these patterns. And who knows, you may find a product that you just can't live without!

The words 'malt' or 'malted' mean a grain that has been SPROUTED!!! Usually the grain is barley, though sometimes it's barley and corn together. Malt syrups are made by first soaking and sprouting the grains in water. As the grains sprout the starch molecules are changed back into vegetable sugars which dilute in the water. Then the water is cooked down just like maple syrup. Malt syrup is the consistency of honey, but it doesn't have that biting-sweet taste that honey has. When you first taste malt syrup, it's hardly even sweet; then the sweetness sort of grows in your mouth.

Rice syrup and rice bran syrups are basically made the same way as malt syrups. They are slightly sweeter to the taste. Good old Yinny's rice syrup has been around for ages as well as some great hard candies. One of the nice things about these two products, malt and rice syrups, is their use in a wide variety of health food products. My favorite corn flakes (by Grainfield) are made from corn and malt syrup. I've seen all kinds of candies with one or the other of them. And T and A Gourmet make some incredible rice syrup jams, jellies and fruit syrups.

OILS
Butter and Olive Oil

Besides butter, olive oil seems to be the easiest concentrated oil for human bodies to digest. It usually takes several months for any of the other oils to come back into the diet. But this makes sense to me. When you stop and think about what concentrated oils are, it becomes obvious that they are not in any natural form. Do you think about corn being oily? I don't. Yet corn oil is in common use.

I make my own tomato juice. It naturally separates and a beautiful 'oil' floats on the top of the juice. But this 'oil' isn't ready to just pour off and use. It's still got other liquids in it that have to be cooked off.

So I know veggies can have alot of oil in them, but it isn't anywhere close to what a bottled oil is like. It requires alot of handling and processing to make it into a cooking oil. And the more you process any food, the more difficult it becomes to digest and utilize! All oils usually do come back into the diet, but patience is required. I think the hardest part about giving up oils for a time is the elimination of mayonnaise! But check out the Mayo Substitute in the Recipes section.

SOY PRODUCTS
Miso and tamari only

Remember, soy products are digested as starches, taking pancreatic enzymes in large amounts. Like oils, the other soy products are usually some of the last things to come back into the diet.

BEANS AND LEGUMES
All Sprouted beans and legumes

Remember, beans and legumes are always going to need to be sprouted! Unsprouted beans and legumes are just never digestible by humans. You know, *"Beans! Beans!! The musical fruit....."*

So, if you haven't played with them yet, sprout some beans or lentils and get to it! Read the information on how to sprout them in the Recipes section.

HERBS AND SPICES
All herbs and spices

If you are getting bored with your food, try changing it with herbs and spices. Check out some cookbooks for ideas on directions to go, like what herbs and spices make food taste Oriental or Italian or Indian. And trust your nose! Smell your food and smell the herb or spice. If they go together, you will be able to 'taste' them through your nose. If they don't smell good together, they surely won't taste good together!

SPECIAL ITEMS

Carob powder, vinegar and most condiments:
(catsup, prepared mustard, horseradish, pickles,) coffee, chocolate, or alcohol,
NO brewer's and nutritional yeasts, NO Mayo.

One of the first things the body starts to heal is any ph or acid/alkaline imbalance, so at this point in the program, you should be able to add vinegar products.

The fun and indulgent things like coffee, chocolate and alcohol are still out because of harsh but natural chemicals. Be patient a little longer. The supplemental yeasts take alot of HCL to break down properly; they are like digesting red meats, so they are out for awhile.

And Mayonnaise. It's almost all oil and hard to digest, so it's still out for now.

PERCENTAGES OF FOODS

<u>FOR ADULTS:</u>

After two or more months of doing a cleansing diet, most bodies are ready to move to more of what I call "a rebuild mode." This means that it is time to give the body more building nutrients, especially more proteins.

Also most bodies can now handle some raw veggies with no stress. Remember to chew them well, since opening up the cell walls is the only way you are going to get any nutrients out of them.

<u>FOR PREGNANT WOMEN:</u>

The higher need for building blocks for the baby means you need to be eating more proteins; reread the section on pregnancy in Chapter 9.

NUTRITIONAL RULES

1) Eat something as soon as you get up in the morning and then eat a little something every two hours after that. It is still important to eat frequently to help keep the sugar level balanced in the blood. Some of you may be able to start lengthening the time between foods, but trust your instincts.

If you do find you can start going two and a half to three hours between meals and snacks, remember that if you have any extra stresses added to your life, you may need to go back to two hour time frames until things get back to normal.

2) Avoid shellfish. We'll talk about them again when you are REALLY healthy.

3) Fruits can be eaten with anything except other fruits. Leave a half hour between different fruits.

4) Beans and legumes must be sprouted.

PHASE TWO TIME FRAME

I suggest you do this diet for two months. There are just enough additions in it to keep you from getting bored and enough changes to keep your body moving in a positive, healing direction.

So, after two months, move on to the next chapter, PHASE THREE.

Chapter 12
Phase Three

GETTING THERE

Your healing process should be progressing right along by now. Most symptoms should be well on their way through a healing process; they should be gone, going or in some way, changing if you are moving onto this diet phase.

If you are feeling good, but still have some symptoms that are sluggish in their change, now is a good time to focus specific attention in their direction. Say one of your symptoms was hair loss, but you aren't seeing a change in this area. Now is the time to try different methods of healing this problem. See the Dis-Ease and Dis-Comfort Chapter for information on healing specific symptoms.

This is also a good time to add new practices into your life like exercise, acupuncture or massage; things that help speed up your specific or general healing process.

There are major additions in this diet phase, so take care in adding new foods back in. Reread the section on 'How Do I Reintroduce Foods' in Chapter 7. Also see Table 1 for new ideas on things to eat.

These new additions indicate the typical increases in enzyme production in a healthy and healing body. At this point, you should be feeling more in touch with your body and what you are putting into it. It might be a good time to work with some of the techniques offered in Chapter 16.

Pat yourself on the back for getting this far, enjoy your health and start shouting it to the world that *"Life is Good!"*

PHASE THREE DIET

YES FOODS	NO FOODS
FRUITS: All fruits BUT------------------	No apples or pears
VEGGIES: all veggies including potatoes and corn/cornmeal	
DAIRY PRODUCTS: eggs, yogurt, kefir and kefir cheese, sour cream, cottage cheese, cream cheese------------------------	No buttermilk, cheese or milk
MEATS: fish, all poultry, rabbit and lamb ---	Beef, pork, bear, buffalo, elk, goat, moose, veal, venison and shellfish

YES FOODS	NO FOODS
NUTS & SEEDS: hazelnuts and almonds--------------------------------------	all other nuts and seeds
GRAINS: 100% sprouted grains and quinoa, oats, millet, and their flours---	barley, buckwheat, amaranth, triticale, wheat, kamut, spelt, couscous and teff, all their flours and pastas
SWEETENERS: 100% maple syrup, malt syrups, rice and rice bran syrups, black-strap molasses------------------------	all other sweeteners
OILS: butter, grape seed oil and olive oil--------------------------------------	all other oils
SOY PRODUCTS: miso and tamari---	all other soy products
SPROUTED BEANS & LEGUMES ONLY-------------------------	all regular beans and legumes
HERBS & SPICES: all herbs and spices	NO goldenseal
SPECIAL ITEMS: Carob powder, vinegar and most condiments: occasional tequila---------------------------	other alcohol, mayo, chocolate, brewer's and nutritional yeasts, coffee

PERCENTAGES OF FOODS:
  FOR ADULTS:
    50% veggies (20% of which can be raw veggies if you want them.)
    20% fruits
    30% everything else (dairy products, fish and meats, nuts and seeds, sweeteners and oils.)
  FOR PREGNANT WOMEN:
    40% veggies (20% of which can be raw veggies if you want them.)
    20% fruits
    40% everything else (dairy products, fish, chicken, turkey, hazelnuts, maple syrup, malt syrups, rice/bran syrups, butter and olive oil.)
  FOR CHILDREN UNDER 12:
    10-20% fruits and veggies (all of which can be raw veggies if you want them.)

80-90% everything else (dairy products, fish, chicken, turkey, hazelnuts, maple syrup, malt syrups, rice/bran syrups, butter and olive oil.)

SUPPLEMENTS:
See Chapter 8, On Supplements.

NUTRITIONAL RULES:
1) Eat something as soon as you get up in the morning and then eat a little something every two, two and half or three hours after that.
2) Avoid shellfish.
3) Fruits can be eaten with anything except other fruits. Leave a half hour between different fruits.
4) Beans and legumes must be sprouted.
5) Do NOT eat starches (grains and soy products) with proteins (dairy, eggs, fish, meats, nuts & seeds.)

PHASE THREE DIET EXPLANATIONS

FRUITS
All fruits BUT apples and pears.
At this point the only fruits that are typically problems are apples and pears because of the speed with which they go into the blood stream.

VEGGIES
All the vegetables are fine. Try to eat only the veggies in season.

DAIRY PRODUCTS
All dairy products BUT NO buttermilk, cheese or milk.
This category is the same as the previous diet. There is a big gap between the amounts of HCL and lactose enzymes that are needed to digest yogurt, kefir, cottage cheese, cream cheese and sour cream in comparison to the amounts needed to digest buttermilk, cheese and milk.

If you can see it on a numbers chart, the easier-to-digest dairy products need 5-6 points and the harder-to-digest foods need 8-9 points. Patience and time are needed.

MEATS
All fish, all poultry, rabbit and lamb BUT
NO beef, pork, bear, buffalo, elk, goat, moose, veal, venison or shellfish.
This category of proteins, like the above dairy products, is leaving the hardest-to-digest meats out of the diet. Note that they are all red meats. The list of okay meats now reads: chicken, duck, goose, pheasant, lamb, rabbit, snake and turkey and all fish with fins, tails and scales. Enjoy!

NUTS & SEEDS
Hazelnuts and almonds.

You can enjoy either of these nuts raw, roasted or ground. Both are available in nut butter form. There's a recipe for ground almond pancakes in Volume II of *Creating Heaven ON Your Plate* and you can purchase ground almond pancake mixes.

The increases in the above listed proteins (the meats and nuts) indicate higher levels of bile production, hydrochloric acid and lactose enzymes.

GRAINS
100% sprouted grains and quinoa, millet, oats, and their flours.

The step of adding in the first regular grains is a biggy! After giving the pancreas a rest, it is finally ready to start producing starch digesting enzymes without stress. The easiest of the grains to digest is millet and the next easiest is oats. They can be used in any form or variety, i.e. rolled oats or ground millet.

There is one major consideration to be made now that you can try adding some regular starches into your diet. That is, you can only eat them with other grains, fruits, veggies, sweeteners and oils. Grains can NOT be eaten with proteins that take hydrochloric acid to digest. See the explanations below for the 5th Nutritional Rule.

SWEETENERS
Maple syrup, malt syrups, rice and rice bran syrups, black-strap molasses.

The use of concentrated sweeteners continues to include new forms; with this Diet Phase you can add black-strap molasses. The molasses I am talking about comes from sugar cane, which means that you can also add in anything that's called cane juice or granulated cane juice. One brand name I am familiar with is Sucanat; it's a granulated cane juice that is wonderful.

You will also see a product on the market called Sorghum Molasses. This product is not from sugar cane, though it does come from a plant that is related to cane. It does have a different chemical structure from cane juice and for now Sorghum Molasses is NOT in the diet.

OILS
Butter, grape seed oil and olive oil only.

Grape seed oil is the new addition here. It is a wonderful oil that is becoming more popular. It has a light taste and reminds me of a typical American salad oil. You will probably have to ask for your stores to carry it. The only brand I have seen on the open market is the Trader Joe's brand in California. Wholesale herb companies are also handling it.

SPECIAL ITEMS
Carob powder, vinegar and most condiments (catsup, prepared mustard, horseradish, pickles) and occasional tequila.

ABOUT ALCOHOL
Alcohol is always a stress on the system, but at this point you should be able to introduce a little. And of all the alcohols, tequila is the easiest to deal with in the body. I am sure the fact that it comes from a cactus is part of what makes it different. Whenever you do add alcohol to your system, take some extra vitamins and minerals to compensate for the nutrients it requires to flush alcohol from the body. It's also fine to add tequila and any of the fruit juices.

NUTRITIONAL RULES
1) Eat something as soon as you get up in the morning and then eat a little something every couple of hours or so after that. It's probably time to start lengthening the time between meals. Remember, it takes six to twelve months to totally heal the pancreas depending on how severe your hypoglycemia was. For most of you the time between snacking and meals can probably be more like two and a half to three hours now. But if you go through some extra life stresses, it is likely that you will need to go back to eating every two hours until the stress passes.

2) Avoid shellfish.

3) Fruits can be eaten with anything except other fruits. Leave a half hour between different fruits. Get use to this one, because it basically doesn't change.

4) Beans and legumes must be sprouted. You should also get use to following this rule, because it never changes either.

5) Do NOT eat starches (grains and soy products) with proteins (dairy, eggs, fish, meats, nuts and seeds.) See the Appendix, Table 2, for what foods are starches and what foods are proteins.

WHY NO STARCHES AND PROTEINS TOGETHER
This new rule addition is major! Combining starches and proteins together creates major digestive problems and is so common in all cultural foods, it's scary!

When you eat proteins (dairy, fish, meats, nuts or seeds) they need hydrochloric acid to break down. The stomach needs to hold these foods, mixing them with HCL, for a MINIMUM of one and a half to two hours for this process to begin.

Now the stomach has NO ability to separate foods, so every thing you eat with the protein is also going to be held in the stomach. This is the reason high protein meals make you feel full for a long time. This is not a problem for fruits and veggies, which ferment in the digestive system to break down. Or for oils, which are broken down by bile which is 'squirted' into the system when oils go by the bile duct. Or for sweeteners, which are easily released from foods and absorbed into the system from the stomach on down.

Starches, on the other hand, are digested mainly by pancreatic enzymes which are added to the digestive system below the stomach. When you eat a starch (any unsprouted or regular grain, soy product or flour) the pancreas is triggered to release pancreatic enzymes. But it does this WHILE you are eating the starch and only for a fifteen to twenty minute period after that.

Because the pancreatic enzymes are added BELOW the stomach, the grains are in a 'catch-up' situation. The starches must get quickly through the stomach and into the small intestines so they will be mixed with the pancreatic enzymes and properly broken down.

So, the stomach is set up with a 'release trigger.' When starches enter the stomach, the stomach will empty itself! This is why everyone feels that Japanese or Chinese foods leave them feeling hungry an hour later. People have become used to feeling full or hungry because of the way their stomachs feel. Obviously, this isn't an appropriate gauge!

Remember, the stomach cannot separate foods, so when you mix starches and proteins into the same meal, you create a digestive dilemma. The proteins need to be held in the stomach but the starches will trigger it to empty!

The body's solution is to only deal with EITHER the starch OR the protein. It usually decides this by volume; that is, if the major amount of food is a protein, the stomach will hold the foods for several hours. In the meantime, the pancreatic enzymes are released and work their way down through the digestive system unused! Two hours later, when the stomach starts releasing wheat it has held, the starches never get digested.

And what does happen to the starches? They rot and putrefy! This causes gas, constipation, bloating and sometimes diarrhea.

On the other hand, if the majority of the mixed starches and proteins eaten was a grain or soy product, then the stomach will release all the food quickly. The starches will get mixed with the pancreatic enzymes, the fruits, veggies, oils and sweeteners will all be properly broken down and the PROTEINS will rot and putrefy!

Whenever you mix starches and proteins, you create many toxins in the system from one of the foods not being broken down. This situation creates fat, cellulite, and fatty tumors as well as digestive discomforts!

Now, I realize that eliminating this combination from the diet sounds drastic, but it's not as bad as it sounds. Remember, quinoa is a fruit and can be eaten with anything, And sprouted grain breads and sprouted beans and legumes are digested as veggies and can be eaten with anything. Potatoes and corn/cornmeal are veggies and can be eaten with anything. Quinoa and corn pastas are fruit/veggie combinations and can be eaten with anything!

One of the hardest things to change is the making and eating of pastries. Any time you combine flour and eggs, you've got a starch and protein combination. The solutions are making your own cakes and cookies with quinoa, potato, corn or panocha (sprouted wheat) flours or using wheat flour in making yeast-raised breads, rolls and pastries without eggs or milk products. Check out Volume II, *Creating Heaven ON Your Plate* for recipes.

When I first encountered this rule, I thought, *"I've never had a problem eating starch and protein together."* But through the muscle-testing I was doing, bodies definitely said it was a problem. So I did an experiment. For six weeks I didn't eat any starch and protein combinations; then I consciously ate one of my old, favorite meals.

I combined rice with sauteed broccoli, onions and mushrooms with a cheese sauce. And I thought I was going to die. I couldn't believe what it was doing to me! I felt like I'd eaten rocks! It sat in my stomach giving me heartburn and pain for hours. I was stopped up for three days and I put on three pounds! That was the last time I did that.

Well, sort of the last time. Sometimes there is just no way to avoid mixing starches and proteins, like when you go to dinner at someone's house and they've fixed you 'something special.' I try to eat as little of the combination as possible and still be polite, filling up with veggies or salad. But, these meals are always followed by some digestive upset.

WHAT DO I EAT WITH STARCHES? WITH PROTEINS?

Avoiding this combination is not that difficult. First, eat proteins with other proteins, fruits, veggies, sweeteners and oils. And eat starches with other starches, fruits, veggies, sweeteners, and oils.

You can eat eggs (a protein) with potatoes (a veggie) together, use sprouted breads to make French Toast because the bread is a veggie and the eggs are a protein, and Tuna Casserole with quinoa/corn noodles (a fruit/veggie combo,) tuna (a protein,) sour cream (protein,) corn flakes and peas (veggies.)

Eating out can be a little tricky, but it's not that hard. If you order a fish dish that includes rice, ask for a baked potato instead of the rice. Eating Chinese is easy; if you want to eat the rice then order only veggie dishes. If you want to eat Cashew Chicken, then don't eat the rice or noodles and order other veggie dishes.

WHAT TO EAT WHEN

If you eat a protein in a meal, then you need to wait AT LEAST two hours before you finish off the meal with a piece of cake or other starch.

If you eat a starch first, then you can follow it with a protein after a half hour.

If I go to a restaurant that makes great bread, I ask for it to be served first and to hold my protein-based meal up for a half hour. Then I can enjoy the bread and eat a protein meal later without any stomach upset. And if I want dessert later, I will choose a protein one like pudding or ice cream or I'll get a starch dessert TO GO!

So, it's not all that hard! You just have to be familiar with what foods are starches and what are proteins, then make your choices with wisdom!

Chapter 13
Phase Four and Eating a Core Diet

So, it's probably been six months or more that you've been working with this diet approach and you should be feeling pretty good about your health and your body. Now is the time to do some major rethinking about your overall approach to foods. There are additions you will be making in this Phase, like including coffee back into your diet, but first I want to talk to you about this 'food rethinking.'

ABOUT 'CORE' DIET

After doing this diet work for twelve years and seeing numerous patterns, I started to see some shifts in some of the patterns, beginning around 1990. By 1995, the shifts seemed to have been completed, though I wouldn't be surprised to see shifts similar to this happen again in the future.

Before 1990, I used to see three patterns in bodies; one, totally healthy bodies usually settled into percentages of foods of 60% fruits and veggies and 40% everything else; two, once vitamin and mineral deficiencies were brought into balance, extra supplements were only needed in serious stress situations because people were getting what they needed out of their food; and three, people could literally 'eat anything' within the percentage boundaries.

I was a little surprised when I started to see these shifts. I'd assumed that bodies where more constant than that. Anyway, I started to see the shifts here and there, then they started becoming more common, then they became 'the norm.' As this process of change became more apparent, I started asking bodies why this was happening and the picture became more clear. What I was hearing from bodies was simple. The TIMES were changing and bodies were needing to change with the times.

In 1990, growth and change started to accelerate into an obvious new pace. Growth, to this point, had been at a more comfortable pace; we went through two to three months of change, had a period of time to recuperate, and then some time to incorporate it into our lives. But in 1990, it seemed that two to three weeks was all we were getting to go through a change, with barely time to catch a breath before the next change was arriving!

Bodies had to also accelerate to match this new pace and some of the old eating patterns had to go. Whenever I was explaining food percentages to a client, I would call 70% fruits and veggies and 30% everything else, a "cleanse and rebuild mode." And that makes sense to me. We are in a major time of change, of 'cleanse and rebuild' and our bodies need to aid the change by maintaining a 70%/30% eating balance.

The second shift I observed had to do with vitamin and mineral levels. People used to stop taking extra supplements after their vitamin and mineral deficiencies were totally healed. But after 1990, I started seeing bodies needing MORE nutrients on a daily basis than they could get out of their food! After 1990, when people 'graduated' from the program, I'd suggest they continue to use some level of supplements, adjusting them to seasonal needs and life stresses.

The third shift had more to do with the way we think than the way we eat, though that's affected, too. It's become clear from talking to bodies that we just can't think of 'being able to eat everything.' It isn't that you wouldn't be able to eat 'everything,' it's just that we have to start thinking about many more foods as treats than as foods we can eat all the time.

I started thinking about what my Spirit called 'Core Diet.' Eating to 'keep up with the times' means that we need to eat a high percentage of our diet from the easiest-to-digest food groups. And we need to think of the harder-to-digest foods as treats or embellishments.

I love this concept! It feels good to think about a piece of wheat bread or a steak or peanuts as a treat. So, what foods are part of a Core Diet?

CORE DIET

You want to make 80-90% of your food choices from the Core Diet list. If you are having an abnormal amount of stress or growth in your life, make more choices from this group. Foods listed in parenthesis are choices you should make less often.

There are foods listed on the Core Diet side you cannot actually have right now, like all sweeteners, so don't get excited when you read that. The specifics for Phase 4 follow the Core Diet info.

CORE DIET FOODS

CORE DIET	EMBELLISHMENTS
FRUITS: all fruits	
VEGGIES: all veggies	
DAIRY: eggs, yogurt, (kefir and sour cream)----	all other dairy products
MEATS: fish and chicken----------------------------	all other meats
NUTS and SEEDS:-------------------------------------	all nuts and seeds
GRAINS: sprouted grains and quinoa-------------	all regular grains
SWEETENERS: All natural sweeteners	
OILS: butter, olive oil, (grape seed oil,) all other oils	
SOY PRODUCTS: miso and tamari, all other soy products	
BEANS AND LEGUMES: sprouted only	

HERBS and SPICES: all herbs and spices

SPECIAL ITEMS: carob powder, vinegar, condiments, baking yeast, coffee, chocolate, alcohol, supplemental yeasts

PERCENTAGES OF FOODS:
  FOR ADULTS:
    70% fruits and veggies
    30% everything else
    0-70% can be raw veggies
  FOR PREGNANT WOMEN:
    50% fruits and veggies
    50% everything else
    0-50% can be raw veggies
  FOR CHILDREN UNDER 12:
    10-30% fruits and veggies
    70-90% everything else
    0-30% can be raw veggies

So, on to the new additions you get in your diet.

PHASE FOUR DIET

YES FOODS	NO FOODS
FRUITS: All fruits BUT----------------	No apples or pears
VEGGIES: all veggies	
DAIRY PRODUCTS: eggs, yogurt, kefir, kefir cheese, sour cream, cottage cheese, cream cheese and buttermilk----------	No cheese or milk
MEATS: fish, all poultry, lamb and rabbit---	beef, pork, bear, buffalo, elk, goat, moose, veal, venison and shellfish
NUTS and SEEDS: hazelnuts, almonds, cashews and pecans-----------------------	all other nuts and seeds.

YES FOODS

GRAINS: 100% sprouted grains and quinoa, oats, millet, rice, rye, teff, couscous and their flours, pastas, barley, buckwheat, amaranth, triticale, wheat, kamut, spelt, their flours and pastas.

SWEETENERS: 100% maple syrup, malt syrups, rice and rice bran syrups, black-strap and sorghum molasses, date sugar, fructose, honey.

OILS: butter, grape seed oil and olive oil. All other oils.

SOY PRODUCTS: miso and tamari, and tempeh. All other soy products.

SPROUTED BEANS and LEGUMES ONLY. All regular beans and legumes.

HERBS and SPICES: all herbs and spices. NO goldenseal.

SPECIAL ITEMS: Carob powder, vinegar and most condiments, occasional tequila and coffee, other alcohol, mayo, chocolate, brewer's and nutritional yeasts.

PERCENTAGES OF FOODS:
 FOR ADULTS:
  50% veggies (20% of which can be raw veggies.)
  20% fruits
  30% everything else (dairy products, fish and meats, nuts and seeds, sweeteners and oils.)
 FOR PREGNANT WOMEN:
  40% veggies (20% of which can be raw veggies.)
  20% fruits
  40% everything else (dairy products, fish, chicken, turkey, hazelnuts, maple syrup, malt syrups, rice/bran syrups, butter and olive oil.)
 FOR CHILDREN UNDER 12:
  10-20% fruits and veggies (all of which can be raw veggies.)
  80-90% everything else (dairy products, fish, chicken, turkey, hazelnuts, maple syrup, malt syrups, rice/bran syrups, butter and olive oil.)

SUPPLEMENTS
 See Chapter 8, On Supplements.

NUTRITIONAL RULES
 1) Eat something as soon as you get up in the morning and then eat a little something every two, two and half or three hours after that.
 2) Avoid shellfish.

3) Fruits can be eaten with anything except other fruits. Leave a half hour between different fruits.

4) Beans and legumes must be sprouted.

5) Do NOT eat starches (grains and soy products) with proteins (dairy, eggs, fish, meats, nuts and seeds.)

PHASE FOUR DIET EXPLANATIONS

FRUITS

All fruits BUT apples and pears.

At this point the only fruits that are typically problems are apples and pears because of the speed with which they go into the blood stream. There is only one other thing you might want to pay attention to, especially if you live in an urban area. Since our bodies are mostly water and since they are definitely animal bodies, we are all very affected by the tides, moon cycles and seasons. When you live in the country your body follows the seasonal shifts much more easily than if you live in an environment that makes you less aware of these shifts. But you can help your body stay more in touch with these flows by eating fruits and veggies when they are in season in your part of the world. Read about this in the Miscellaneous Information Chapter 16.

VEGGIES

All the vegetables are fine. Try to eat only the veggies that are in season.

DAIRY PRODUCTS

All dairy products, BUT NO cheese or milk.

You can now try to add buttermilk into your diet, drinking it straight if you like it, or using it to make salad dressings. But your body may still need more time to increase the HCL and lactose enzymes. Check for Mucus Reactions and Emotional Reactions when you try buttermilk. Remember, eggs, yogurt, kefir and sour cream are the dairy products that are part of the Core Diet and should be the major products you use.

MEATS

All fish, all poultry, rabbit and lamb, BUT
NO beef, pork, bear, buffalo, elk, goat, moose, veal, venison and shellfish.

This category of proteins, like the above dairy products, is leaving the hardest-to-digest meats out of the diet. Note that they are all red meats. The list of okay meats now reads: chicken, duck, goose, pheasant, lamb, rabbit, snake and turkey and all fish with fins, tails and scales. Enjoy!

NUTS & SEEDS

Hazelnuts, almonds, cashews and pecans.

You can enjoy all of these nuts raw, roasted or ground and they are all available in nut butter form. Be aware of one possible problem with cashews. They are related to poison oak and poison ivy. Every once in awhile, people sensitive to that plant family can experience rashes from eating raw cashews. I had a client that did get a regular rash every time she came in contact with her cashew tree!

GRAINS

100% sprouted grains and quinoa, couscous, millet,
oats, rice, rye, teff, their flours and pastas.

Four new regular grains are added into this phase: couscous, rice, rye and teff.

It's difficult to find single grain, unsprouted rye products (like good old RyKrisp crackers) because it doesn't have any natural gluten. Gluten is the vegetable protein of grains that will stretch and hold air bubbles. Usually wheat flour is added to rye breads, then, to make them rise, so watch out for that combination.

Rice, in all it's types and forms, is now okay. Noodles made without eggs or other flours are fine. And you can use Rice Dream, which is a rice milk. It's the only rice milk I am familiar with though there may be other brands on the market. Remember, you can't use rice products with protein foods, but you can use them with other starches, like putting Rice Dream on your oatmeal or using rice milk to make a White Sauce for a rice and veggie dish. Couscous and teff can also be added to the diet. They are both African grains, teff being a very new product on the market. Couscous is frequently served with fish in restaurant, but this constitutes a starch and protein combination, so stay away from it.

SWEETENERS

Maple, malt, rice and rice bran syrups, black-strap and sorghum molasses.

The use of concentrated sweeteners continues to include new forms; with this diet phase you can add sorghum molasses. The molasses I am talking about comes from a relative of sugar cane. You've seen the plant growing if you have driven through the Midwest in the summer. It looks much like corn plants, but the leaves are narrower and longer than corn and the tassel at the top turns a beautiful red-brown. Sorghum is grown mainly for cattle feed, but some of it is pressed like sugar cane and the juice is cooked into Sorghum Molasses. It has a slightly different chemical structure than black-strap molasses and is a little more difficult to break down.

OILS

Butter, grape seed oil and olive oil only.

You've probably noticed that changes in the oil department are not happening. Remember, concentrated oils are not natural and they are very difficult to digest. Even though you can now eat almonds, you still should stay away from almond oil. There are natural enzymes in the nuts that help your body break down the oils, but those enzymes are not present in the oil.

I don't even recommend that you use oils ON your body that you can't digest through your digestive system. Your skin will suck up oil molecules because there is ten times more absorption through the skin than through the digestive system. At least your internal system has some safeguards that keep you from absorbing some problem molecules; the skin has none.

SPECIAL ITEMS
Carob powder, chocolate, vinegar, most condiments, occasional tequila, and coffee.

ABOUT COFFEE
Hurrah! Coffee is such a delicious embellishment to add back into your diet. Of course, there is a special way that you have to make it from now on, and you should only do one to two cups a day, but I love to see this point arrive. It means your body is doing really well with handling some of the harsh, natural chemicals in coffee.

The way we MAKE coffee is a major problem! When you add hot water to the coffee grounds, it releases the coffee's oil and acids into the water. These substances are impossible for the human body to digest. But there is a way to make coffee that doesn't bring out these negative substances. Basically you make a coffee extract just like you make an herbal extract. You mix the coffee grounds with COLD water and let them soak for thirty-six hours. After filtering the grounds out from the extract, it only takes a couple of tablespoons of the strong liquid to make a cup of the most wonderful coffee. You know how coffee smells? That's how this coffee tastes. There is no bitter bite, no stomach upsets and for most people no negative caffeine reactions.

I didn't drink coffee until I was thirty-five years old, when I discovered Cold-Processed Coffee. Before that time, I only drank a cup of coffee if I wanted to stay up all night, usually to drive across country. Within five minutes of one cup of coffee, my heart was pounding out of my chest, I'd be shaking like a leaf, I'd spent fifteen minutes in the bathroom emptying my bowels and I'd be wide awake for twenty-four hours. With Cold-Processed Coffee, I have NONE of those reactions. I can have a cup of coffee now and go directly to bed!

The recipe is in the 'How to Make Section' in the Recipe section. And, guess what? Cold-Processed Coffee is digested as a fruit in the body! This surprised me until I realized that coffee beans are the fruit of a tree!

A FEW FINAL WORDS

Enjoy adding in your new embellishments as you work with the ideas around the Core Diet. Now is a good time to start a more aggressive exercise program. If you are having some symptoms that are being persistent, now is a good time to think about new ways to deal with them. You might want to try some acupuncture or counselling or different medicines. Remember that sometimes a method that didn't work in the past, will work when your body is healing itself nutritionally.

Chapter 14
Semi-Final Phase

This diet adds in foods that are harder-to-digest but still leaves out the hardest-to-digest things. You will now be eating almost all foods and should be feeling what real health is. You should be feeling great, feeling very in touch with your body, be getting more and more in tune with other general needs in your life, and be getting some regular exercise. If you are not working with any persistent problems, do it now. This is also a good time to start adding some regular cleansing patterns into your life. Once or twice a month, go back to the Basic Balancer Diet and follow it for a few days at a time. Or once a month do the Deep Cleanser Diet for a day or two. The next chapter has more information about cleansing for longer times.

SEMI-FINAL PHASE DIET

YES FOODS	NO FOODS
FRUITS: All fruits	
VEGGIES: All vegetables	
DAIRY PRODUCTS: All but---------------	no milk
MEATS and FISH: All but-------------------	no shellfish
NUTS & SEEDS: All but--------------------	no macadamia, Brazil nuts or pistachios
GRAINS: All but-----------------------------	no spelt, kamut or wheat
SWEETENERS: All natural sweeteners	
OILS: Butter, Grape seed, Olive, Corn, Safflower, and Soya or Soybean oils but--	all other oils
SOY PRODUCTS: All soy products but--	soy powders
BEANS, LEGUMES: All sprouted beans, legumes	
HERBS, SPICES: All herbs and spices	
SPECIAL ITEMS: All except beers and wines	

PERCENTAGES OF FOODS:
    FOR ADULTS:
        70% Veggies and Fruits
        30% Everything else
        0-50% Raw foods
    FOR PREGNANT WOMEN:
        50% fruits and veggies
        50% everything else
        0-50% can be raw veggies
    FOR CHILDREN UNDER 12:
        10-30% fruits and veggies
        70-90% everything else
        0-30% can be raw veggies

SUPPLEMENTS
    See Chapter 8, On Supplements.

NUTRITIONAL RULES
    1) Avoid Shellfish.
    2) Eat fruits with anything except other fruits. Leave one half hour between different fruits.
    3) Beans and legumes must be sprouted.
    4) Do NOT mix starches with proteins.

SEMI-FINAL PHASE DIET EXPLANATIONS

FRUITS
All fruits.

Sugar imbalances from fruits should be nonexistent at this point in the healing process. Even the fast sugar actions of apples and pears should pose no problems. Enjoy!!!

DAIRY PRODUCTS
All dairy products except NO milk.

Milk is the hardest-to-digest food of the dairy products, so it is still out. The culturing and souring process that all the other products go through help break down the complex milk molecule and you shouldn't have any problem with them. You can also, now add regular cheeses into your diet. Remember that they need to be used as embellishments to Core Diet foods.

ABOUT CHEESE

The first step in making cheese is to make it curdle. This is done by the addition of a curdling agent. The most common agent is called rennet, which is calf stomach, in the form of pills or powder.

The other agents are vegetable enzymes or microbial enzymes. If the cheese doesn't say it's vegetable or microbial enzyme cheese (rennetless cheese,) then it is probably a rennet cheese.

There is no taste difference in the cheeses made with different curdling agents, but there are minor differences in the chemical structures. For some people, because of the chemical structure differences, there can be a difference in the digestion. I have a friend that can eat any of the rennetless cheeses with no problem but if he eats a rennet cheese, he'll experience gas for a day or two.

As you add cheeses back into the diet, eat each different cheese type — rennet, vegetable enzyme and microbial enzyme — by themselves. Wait a day or two between cheese types and see if you have any digestive reactions. Then eat them accordingly.

MEATS
All meats and fish, except shellfish.

Your HCL levels should be high enough now to eat all the different meats and fish. The only exception is shellfish. At the beginning of this program, I mentioned the difficulties with shellfish, and unfortunately, those difficulties don't really get better as you get healthy. Now, this doesn't mean that you can never touch shellfish again. It just means that you want to be extremely careful with them. I eat shellfish two to three times a year, but I only do it when I feel that I am emotionally, mentally, physically, and spiritually balanced and all stress levels are way down. Then I will bless the lobster, crab, shrimp, scallops, or whatever, and enjoy the hell out of it. But for the next couple of days I will do some level of cleansing, depending on how I feel the shellfish has affected me.

NUTS & SEEDS
All nuts and seeds, except macadamia, Brazil nuts, pistachios.

This is a big increase in nuts and seeds. You can now add in Black Walnuts, butternuts, chestnuts, hickory nuts, peanuts, pine nuts, pumpkin seeds, sesame seeds, sunflower seeds, and walnuts. Enjoy! The nuts that are still out of the diet are the hardest-to-digest ones. Remember that nuts and seeds should basically be treated as embellishments.

GRAINS
All sprouted grains and quinoa.
All regular grains except NO Spelt, Kamut or Wheat.

Except for the wheat varieties, which take huge amounts of pancreatic enzymes, all the other regular grains can be added to the diet. This includes: amaranth, barley, buckwheat, couscous, millet, oats, rice, rye, teff and triticale. Remember, you CANNOT eat any of these grains with proteins (dairy, meats, nuts and seeds.) So, no buckwheat pancakes, rice pudding, or chicken/barley soup.

SWEETENERS
All natural sweeteners.

All the natural sweeteners, cane sugars, date sugar, fructose, maple syrup, malt syrups, black-strap molasses, rice syrups, sorghum molasses, and honey are fine to use in the diet at this point. The additions of date sugar, fructose, and honey means that sugar imbalances should be totally under control. Usually at this point in the program, most hypoglycemic levels have dropped away totally.

Fructose can be added to the diet, which opens up many possibilities since fructose is used in alot of health food products. It is a fairly processed sugar from fruits, so I don't recommend using alot of it, but it can be easy to bake with if you are looking for a lighter texture than liquid sweeteners will give you.

OILS
Butter, Grapeseed, Olive, Corn, Safflower, and Soya or Soybean oils.
Yes! Finally, some new oils can be added to the diet! You can see that there are still quite a few that are out, like all the nut oils. But the above oils are the easier ones to digest. I do HIGHLY recommend that you only use 'cold-processed' oils. "Cold-processed' means that the oils are not subjected to temperatures higher than 110 degrees. Most oils are processed out of foods with high heat, which destroys most of the nutrients in them. With the addition of these oils, you can also add mayonnaise made from these oils back into the diet. Also buy mayo made from cold-processed oils. Remember that all concentrated oils are hard for human bodies to deal with and you always want to go light on them.

SOY PRODUCTS
All soy products: tofu, tempeh, soy milk, soy cheese, soy flour, miso and tamari.
Soy products digest as starches, so remember to only eat them with other starches, fruits, veggies, sweeteners and oils. Soy milk can be used on cereals, soy cheese can be used on vegetarian pizza, tofu and rice go great together. Enjoy!!! Because of the high processing of soy powders, they take the highest levels of enzymes to break down. You are almost there, but not quite. A little more time is a good idea.

SPECIAL ITEMS
All alcohols except beers and wines, coffee, chocolate,
vinegar and condiments, carob powder, brewer's and nutritional yeasts.

ABOUT ALCOHOL
At this point tequila and all the hard alcohols are okay. Remember they are hard on the system and you need to compensate for the nutrients they eat up by taking extra vitamins and minerals.

Beers and wines are still excluded because of the high level of impurities in them that cause more stress on the body than the distilled alcohols.

ABOUT CHOCOLATE
Chocolate beans are picked in the fields and fermented for three to nine days. Then they are dried and shipped to the chocolate factories.

The next step the beans go through is a gentle heating and grinding process. Chocolate burns easily so this step is done slowly. At this point, chocolate is 70% cocoa butter and 30% chocolate solids. Once the chocolate is smooth, it is poured out into Unsweetened Baking Chocolate Squares. This is the most pure form of chocolate you can buy and the only one I recommend using.

After this step, all kinds of stuff is added to chocolate that can make it more of a problem than it already is. Cocoa is taken through a chemical process that leaves some chemical residue as it removes the cocoa butter and I don't recommend using it.

Make your own chocolate candies, cakes and cookies with other healthy ingredients and you shouldn't have any problems with sometimes indulging yourself! There are a few health food brands of chocolate that use chocolate liqueurs that are fine when eaten occasionally. And Sunspire Company makes a great chocolate chip sweetened with malt syrup!

BREWER'S & NUTRITIONAL YEASTS

These supplemental yeasts are digested as proteins. They are excellent sources of vitamin B's and numerous minerals now that you can digest and utilize them.

If you want to use them as a stress supplement, try a tablespoon in tomato or grapefruit juice. The off taste of the yeasts is hidden in both of these juices.

My popcorn seems boring without a spoonful of brewer's yeast mixed in the garlic-oregano-cayenne-seasoned butter!

PERCENTAGES OF FOODS

By this time you have probably settled into a percentage pattern that works for you. As an adult you have to remember you are maintaining your body, which needs many more fruits and veggies than building-block foods like proteins and starches.

The amount of raw foods that your body wants will vary with the seasons and where you live. In snowy areas, a raw salad in December is just out of sync with the body's needs.

Usually people find their desire for raw foods starts to increase with the first signs of Spring. Many different healing systems suggest following the body's lead by doing Spring cleanses by eating those first Spring plants like dandelion greens.

THE NEXT STAGE

I suggest that you do this diet approach for two months and then move on to the next chapter when it will be time to add in the hardest-to-digest foods and where you will be back to eating everything!!!

Chapter 15
It's Graduation Time!

Congratulations! You've worked hard for your health! At this point in time, you know how to get healthy and to maintain that state of grace. And I am sure that you have had numerous realizations about yourself, your old eating habits, what you do to yourself when you get out-of-balance and much, much more. Give yourself all the credit for making these changes in your life and in your awareness!

FINAL ADDITIONS

It's time to add the remaining and hardest-to-digest foods back into your diet. Of course, these foods are out of the Core Diet and you eat much less of them, but what treats! Be aware that sometimes the hardest-to-digest foods NEVER work in certain people's systems. I've never seen a clear and specific pattern that indicates who this will happen to, but you must be prepared for that possibility.

Remember to watch for Mucus Reactions and Emotional Reactions as you introduce these last additions. Remember, too, that whenever you are stressed, the harder- and hardest-to-digest foods are the first things you should avoid eating.

So, you can now attempt to add in the following: ☑milk,   ☑macadamia, Brazil nuts and pistachios, ☑spelt, kamut and wheat, ☑soy powder,   ☑all concentrated oils,   ☑beers and wines.

FINAL ADDITIONS—EXPLANATIONS

ABOUT MILK

There's some debate out there about whether adult humans should drink milk or not. Once I started following what my body says to do, I found that sometimes my body wants milk as an embellishment and sometimes it doesn't. Milk takes so much energy and so many nutrients to break it down, I frequently just don't have the ability to do it because of the intensity of the world these days. But when my body wants milk, it breaks it down with no stress or mucus reactions.

MACADAMIA, BRAZIL NUTS, AND PISTACHIOS

These particular nuts contain fats especially hard to digest, so be careful in their use. Pretend they are even rarer embellishments than the other nuts and seeds.

SPELT, KAMUT, AND WHEAT

All three of these grains are varieties of wheat. The spelt and kamut are Old World varieties and have not suffered from the manipulation our U.S. wheat endured. At the turn of the century, wheat analysis showed it contained 50% vegetable proteins and 50% starch molecules. Now is it more like

92% starch and only 8% vegetable protein! This means it takes almost twice the amount of pancreatic enzymes to digest wheat properly. This kind of demand is very hard on bodies.

I had a client born and raised in Sweden who was a bread maker. When she moved to this country, she said that she had to learn to make bread all over again. But it didn't take her long to realize that she was having difficulty digesting this new product. While we worked together, she visited her homeland and reported she had no trouble digesting the bread products there. Hoping that she had gotten past her 'allergy' to wheat, she tried some regular whole wheat bread when she got back to the States. But it didn't work in her body then, and I couldn't foresee that it ever would!

There are new spelt and kamut products coming onto the market all the time, so keep your eyes out for new things. Vita-Spelt makes a spelt flour only pasta, Arrowhead Mills makes a KAMUT cereal, and there are partially sprouted breads with either or both grains.

COOKING OILS

Go ahead and use the different oils, but use them very sparingly. They don't get any easier to deal with and there are times when they are REALLY difficult. One of the changes I started seeing in 1990 had to do with oils. Each time a spiritual growth period got intense, any oil digestion became difficult, even butter and olive oil. By 1995 these intense periods have become more common and don't seem to affect the body with the same level of discomfort. But if you suddenly find you are reacting to any kind of fats, just back off from eating them for a few weeks and let the growth period pass. Also see if you can pin down what else the growth period may mean to you.

SOY POWDERS

I don't recommend extended use of highly processed foods, but they are fine (when you can digest them) to use for specific purposes, like a weight lifter wanting to bulk up or an underweight person using them along with some exercise to built some new muscle. But use soy powders for short intense periods and then back off of them for a few weeks. Watch for signs of mucus reactions, constipation and gas.

BEERS AND WINES

Beers and wines have more impurities in them than any of the other alcohols, so many things get sucked quickly into your bloodstream along with the alcohol. Just make sure that you take a vitamin and mineral food supplement like alfalfa and kelp to both give your body nutrients to deal with the stress and to help your body flush the alcohol. For each beer or shot of tequila, I will take one each of kelp and alfalfa. And as I mentioned way back at the beginning of the book, I use beer as a ph balancer, because it works in my body!

I want to retell the story of really tying one on a few New Year's Eves ago. (The story also appears under the 'Alcohol and Alcoholism' section in Chapter 10.) I rarely have ever done this because I'm such a sensitive lightweight, but there were four of us one this New Year's Eve. We did alot of mixed alcohols, which is a real no-no, and assorted other indulgences. Around 4 a.m. we all headed off to bed, but my partner and I took hangover precautions. I took a dozen kelp tablets and a bunch of blood-purifying and liver-cleansing herb extracts. I slept like a baby for four hours and then was cheerfully up and ready for the first day of the New Year! I went for a two hour walk and still no one else was up. Hours later our host and hostess stumbled out of bed. One of them was very gray and the other was a sickly shade of green. They took one look at my smiling face and almost tossed their cookies! I quickly scooted out the door for another walk!

Now, I'm not suggesting that you can stress yourself like this and get away with it. I am saying that if you occasionally do go overboard, you can compensate your body for it by giving your body the tools it needs to deal with the stress.

I have friends who are wine experts; that's their business and their love. We formulated an herb combination they take BEFORE they do a wine tasting or party. It's obvious from the way their bodies then react to alcohol, the herb combination is working. (See Appendix, Table 3, for more info.)

LAST FOOD WORDS

I'd suggest that your life approach to food continue on the way it is: using the Core Diet as your basis, using the embellishments with wisdom, eating many more fruits and veggies than other foods (at least a 70/30% ratio,) doing some form of food supplement to offset daily stresses and doing some regular cleansing. Enjoy! And you've got this book in hand. You can always go through and do the program from the beginning or anywhere in between!

ABOUT MAINTAINING YOUR HEALTH

As I mentioned in the previous chapter, cleansing needs to become a semi-regular process in your life. Just a day once in awhile, maybe once or twice a month, where you do only veggies for the day. Or maybe a day to two in a row of only fruits and veggies. Once a year I recommend you do one of the Basic diets for a week or two. And when should you cleanse? Watch your body and let it tell you. And signs? You can't make up your mind what to eat. Nothing feels right. Nothing seems to satisfy. Your body feels heavy and clogged up. You've been through a very intense period of work or growth and change. There's been a period of grieving. There's been a period of change, like moving.

A day or two of being easy on your body, of letting it rest and relax, will usually quickly bring it back into a healthy balance. But if you start to eat and it still doesn't feel right, then you may want to consider doing a more thorough kind of cleansing.

JUICE CLEANSING

If a day or two of veggies hasn't satisfied your body's need for rest, then it's time to do a few days of just juices. If you've never done a juice cleanse, it's important for you to know that it's a wonderful and joyous experience. The first day is usually the hard one, because your mouth wants to chew on something. (That desire in itself may present an issue you want to look into further!) But once you get past that initial reaction, eating stops being an issue. And this really isn't about not eating. It's about giving your body a rest. It's important to not go hungry! You should have a glass of juice, miso broth, or tea within reach at ALL times. Every time you are feeling the need to eat, drink something. Keep your stomach 'full' but just not with chunks of food!

By the time you've done three or four days of just juices, you may find yourself wondering why you'd even WANT to eat anything ever again. That's how good it feels! I've had friends who continued juice fasting for weeks because of this wonderful feeling of lightness.

So, it's not that juice fasting is hard to do (once you get past the eating habit,) but coming off the fast can be a little harder. Once you've done three or more days of just juices, you need to carefully reintroduce food so you don't overload your cleansed system.

There's a simple rule to reintroducing foods: if you do three days of juices, follow it with three days of cooked veggies; then three days of cooked veggies and fresh or cooked fruits; then three days of cooked or raw veggies, fruits and simple proteins; and three days of the above along with simple starches. You really end up doing fifteen or more days of a cleansing diet. If you do six days of juices, then follow it with six day increments of food additions. Use the chart below:

NUMBER OF DAYS	JUICES AND FOODS
For fasting days, do:------------------------ x number of days	All fruit and veggie juices, All herbal teas; Veggie and miso broths, Carbonated waters
To introduce first foods, do: ------------- for same number of days	All veggies, cooked only; All liquids listed above
Add second group of foods--------------- for same number of days	All veggies, cooked or raw; All fruits, fresh or cooked; All liquids listed above
Add third group of foods------------------ for same number of days	Easy-to-digest proteins; All sweeteners; Simple oils; All veggies and fruits; All liquids listed above
Add fourth group of foods--------------- for same number of days	Easy-to-digest starches; All proteins; All sweeteners; All oils; All veggies and fruits; All liquids listed above
After cleansing days-----------------------	Add all the embellishments

MY FINAL WORDS

I want to thank you for your dedication in following and learning this approach to eating. I feel that I arrived on the Earth with a clear job description: Spread Joy! And I figure that I can best do this by helping other people feel the same desire! My wish is that I've helped you smile and spread the message of joy through your body and into your life!

HERE'S TO JOY IN LIVING!!!

Chapter 16
Miscellaneous Information

THYMUS THUMP

For a Quick Energizer and To Clear Negativity

The thymus is a gland at the base of the throat (see fig. 1) that has two major functions; one, it is responsible for the supply of Super T-Cells and antibodies in the blood and two, it regulates the overall energy flow in your aura.

There's alot of misinformation out there about this gland and it's functions. Doctors used to think that it's functioning stopped shortly after birth and unfortunately many of them are still operating from that belief.

Figure 1, Thymus Gland

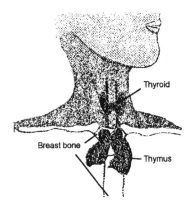

The body is still a great mystery and the thymus is just one of its many secrets. There are medical studies going on concerning this gland and its functions, but there will be alot of controversy around it for awhile longer.

On a physical level, my body philosophy stands: Heal the body and let it take care of healing the thymus (or whatever.)

On an energetic level, we can easily stimulate the thymus and affect the flows in the aura. If you are feeling tired, irritable, grumpy, or just out-of-balance, the energy fields around your body will start flowing in a negative pattern. By simply stimulating the thymus, this negative pattern is reversed and positive energy will again flow in the body and aura.

This simple stimulation is created by 'thumping' anywhere on the breastbone. The thymus is located below the breastbone, at the top end, near the base of the throat. With the first three fingers of your hand tightly pressed together, you lightly thump on your breastbone. You can NOT over stimulate this gland, so thump away until you feel your energy returning and a smile dawning on your face.

HOW CAN I GET MORE IN TUNE WITH MY SENSITIVITIES?

There are a few simply exercises and visualizations you can do that will tune you into sensations that are already happening in your body. The sensations are usually just under our normal observation range, so it is easy to bring them into your conscious awareness.

Sensitivity Exercise

There are natural energy flows in the body that can have positive or negative electrical charges. You can stand in a natural walking stance like the one described below and feel a positive charge; and you can stand in a negative stance that feels very different from it's opposite.

Once you stand in these positions and get a sense of the two different energies, then you can learn to feel the positive or negative charge that different foods create in your body!!! If there is a positive charge, you can assume that your body will easily digest that particular food and if there is a negative charge when you hold the food, it's a message from your body that is saying, *"Nope. Not that. Not Yet."*

You just need to do these exercises for a few minutes every day and then you can practice them as you choose what foods to eat through your day.

1) In a quiet room where you won't get interrupted, stand with your feet together and your hands relaxed, at your sides.

2) Step forward on one leg and balance yourself.

3) Swing out the opposite arm, just like you were walking down the street.

4) Close your eyes or lightly stare at a point in front of you. Just feel how you feel in this position for a minute or two.

5) Now step back with the outstretched leg, leaving the arm swung out in front.

6) Take a step forward with the second leg. You should now have the same arm and leg extended out in front of you.

7) Again, close your eyes or relax, and feel how this energy is different from the energy in the bilateral stance.

So, did you feel a difference? I know it may be very subtle, but as you practice the stances, the difference will become more apparent.

The position of opposite arm and leg in #3 is a natural walking stance which is a positive energy flow in the body. When you walk in this opposite arm and leg position, you recharge your positive energy flows; not a bad thing to do as a break from work every couple of hours!

Also, this walking stance is the result of our being bilateral animals; that is, one side of the brain operates the opposite side of the body. So, again, exercising this opposite arm and leg swing, whether it is from walking, running, biking, or swimming, stimulates action in the brain and sort of clears out the fog!

The position of same arm and leg extended (#6) is a negative energy flow in the body. You will feel more of this charge in your energy field when you are tired, hungry, grumpy or afraid. Doing the Thymus Thump will rebalance your energy and bring a smile to your face!

I'm not saying that one of these energy flows is good and the other is bad. The human body has a certain charge to it when it is healthy and another charge to it when it is not! Every energy that you bring into your body just needs to fit within the range of health that you are emanating or moving towards!

Food Awareness Exercise

So, after mastering the bilateral awareness in your body, you can practice feeling the positive and negative charges of different foods:

1) Once you have a sense of the positive and negative flows, stand with your legs together and pick up a food. Just feel it.

2) Does it feel like the positive field?

3) Does it feel like a negative charge?

4) Does it have both feelings within it?

Trust your immediate reactions and thoughts, even if they don't totally make sense to your brain. Usually, all the sensations and information you are going to get come in the first five seconds! Thinking about what you're feeling much longer than that is a waste. When you just 'sit' with a feeling and feel it, evidently the brain will come to understand it and be able to give you words to describe it.

So, pick up a second food and compare the sensations, first, with the positive and negative stance feelings and, second, with the sensations from the food previously held.

Play with holding onto foods that you've had digestive problems with or one that I list as difficult-to-digest. Check out how they compare to foods that are easy-to-digest.

When you get good at this, you may even find that you can just look at a food and feel how your body energies react. When I eat out, I look over the menu and watch how my body reacts to the images of different foods. It's usually obvious what I should and shouldn't eat if I'm going to please my body!

SEASONAL EATING

Urban living tends to distract us from the natural flows of the planet, but bodies are strongly linked to these changes. As you heal your body, you may find that you become more aware of body changes and needs that are linked to seasonal changes.

As we go through annual changes, our bodies need different foods and different amounts of nutrients. It takes different vitamins and minerals to run our internal furnaces during the winter and our internal cooling systems during the summer.

One of the observations I have had concerning seasonal shifts occurred after I moved to New Mexico. It happened because the shifts are so obvious here.

About six weeks before a new season arrives, we will experience a week of that weather. So somewhere around mid-July there will be a hint of autumn in the air; the leaves will sound different in the wind, a tree or two will have a few yellowing leaves, the morning air will feel a fall chill, and the air will smell different. Then we go back to six weeks or so of summer. But six weeks later it will be Fall.

I have marked these changes on my calendar for fifteen years now and it is incredibly consistent. I mean, sometimes the new season will arrive in four or five weeks instead of six, but there is no doubt when we experience that week of change that the new season will be with us shortly.

Whether you are observing these six-week-before changes or not, your body will take note of them and start to respond to them. In midwinter it will start to crave fresh, raw greens. In midsummer it will start to crave heavier foods than you have been eating, like potatoes and rice.

The two most dramatic changes happen from winter into spring and summer into fall. The body needs to make some major changes during these times; it is literally either shutting off the heating system or stoking it up and/or revving up the cooling system or turning it off.

The needs for different vitamins and minerals can skyrocket during any of these seasonal shifts. Human bodies seem to be basically split on what nutrients they need, however. Some bodies require more vitamins in the winter and more minerals in the summer and some bodies are just the opposite; they need more minerals in the winter and more vitamins in the summer!

So, start watching for these six-weeks-before transitions and observe what changes your body goes through, what cravings come up, and what nutrients it might need. Start increasing your nutrient intake to compensate for the changes. When the new season arrives, feel out whether you need more vitamins or more minerals to stay balanced.

Also, be aware that you may feel a sense of vulnerability during these transitions. Try to take a little time each day to consciously tune your body into the transition and relax with it.

TEMPORAL TAP

Temporal Tap is the greatest quick little self-hypnosis trip I have ever seen! This technique is so powerful that you can 'tap in' so that you won't be able to respond to the GAG reflex, then stick your fingers down your throat and NOT gag!!!

The Temporal-Sphendiol Suture (see fig. 2 on the following page) is a fissure in the skull that has some remarkable techniques associated with it. The three major techniques I have used are:

1) There are spots all along it that correspond to all the muscles and organs in the body (see the table with fig. 2.) Properly manipulated, these points can dramatically affect the condition of the corresponding muscle or organ. Rub any of the points that are sore to the touch. With the index finger or thumb, make little circles on the tender spot just like you would rub any reflex point.

2) There are two specific points along the suture line that, within a moment or two, will relieve headaches. Read the section on Headaches in the Dis-ease and Dis-comfort chapter.

3) And there is a technique that will easily change and reprogram any habit, desire or pattern that you wish to change! This self-hypnosis technique can immediately erase the desire to smoke a cigarette,

wipe out the desire for sweets, change a negative emotional pattern or retrain your sleep patterns. It's uses are unlimited!!! Here's how to use it:

1) Look at the suture line in figure 2 and feel for the corresponding points on your head.

2) Decide what issue you want to work with and make up two statements about the change; the first statement must have a NOT in it and the second statement must be totally positive. You want the statements to counterbalance each other.

Figure 2, Temporal-Sphendiol Suture

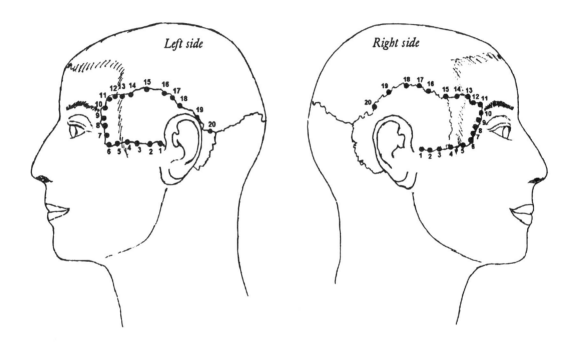

1) Kidneys	8) Reproductive Organs	15) Gall Bladder
2) Kidneys	9) Large Intestines	16) Stomach
3) Small Intestines	10) Circulation	17) Diaphragm
4) Adrenal Glands	11) Sinuses	18) Pancreas
5) Liver	12) Sinuses	19) Small Intestines
6) Small Intestines	13) Heart	20) Spleen
7) Large Intestines	14) Lungs	

For example, if you want to use the technique to stop smoking, you could use a statement like, *"I do NOT desire this cigarette."* and a corresponding positive statement like *"I am free of the desire for cigarettes."*

Or if you want to change an overeating pattern, you could use *"I will NOT eat any food today unless my body is truly hungry."* And *"I am free of the pattern of using food to stuff my emotions."*

Or, if you can't stop eating a sweet treat that is right in front of you, you could say *"I do NOT want any more of this treat."* and *"I am free of the desire for that sweet."*

3) Once you have decided on your statements, you are ready to 'tap them in.' And that is literally what you do!

Squeeze your index and middle finger together and place them on the suture line right in front of the ear on the right side of the head. Start lightly tapping these fingers on the suture line while you say your NOT statement.

Move your fingers forward along the suture line, then up around the temple, over the corner of the forehead, into the hairline, along the side of the head and around and down to the base of the ear. Keep repeating the NOT statement as you tap along, saying it as many times as it will 'fit in.'

4) Tap three complete circles along the right suture line, repeating the NOT statement.

5) Now move to the left side of the head and repeat the whole process but this time use the POSITIVE statement. 'Tap in' the positive statement again and again, making three complete circles along the suture line.

That's all it takes! I have used this technique for so many different things, I can't count them all!

There are two stories I like to tell, though. The first one has to do with food. A friend had made some decadent, chocolate dessert bars and I couldn't stop eating them. The hand to mouth reaction was on automatic.

So I 'tapped in' an *"I don't want any more of those"* message and put a plateful of the goodies in my lap. It stopped the desire for a half hour. I almost had taken another bite before I caught myself! So I tapped the messages in again and that was that!

The second story has to do with an emotional pattern change. I was at the end of a relationship and we were trying to talk things out. We started playing this game where he said something 'below the belt' like, *"You never really loved me!"* and I emotionally reacted. I saw the pattern but just couldn't stop myself from falling into it.

So, after an argument, when he started this game, I tapped in that I would not respond to his emotional goading and that I would stay cool, calm and collected. He tried to get the game rolling for three hours but couldn't break through and get me emotionally upset. I just responded with, *"Oh, you know that's not true!"*

After three hours, I could feel the hypnosis wearing off, so I tapped in the messages again and that was that!

Appendix

TABLE 1- FOOD AND MENU SUGGESTIONS

ABOUT USING HERBS: The only way to learn about herbs and spices is to use your nose! Smell what you are cooking and then sniff different herbs and spices and see which ones go well together. Keep sniffing the food as you add flavors to it and then go to the different seasonings.

ABOUT MICROWAVES: I don't suggest you use them. Radiation doesn't seem to be the problem. It seems they kill the life-force in the food, so it's truly like eating something dead.

The following suggestions are mainly for working with the three Basic Diets, but I eat much like this all the time. Recipes are listed here in all capital letters and appear in the back of this book.

SUGGESTIONS FOR THE SUPER CLEANSER DIET

BREAKFAST:

Quinoa:

As a hot cereal, with maple syrup or stevia and apricots, stewed with the quinoa and diluted, sweetened yogurt.

Pancakes: Finnish Pancakes, Pumpkin Pancakes, Quinoa Pancakes served with butter and maple syrup, APRICOT BUTTER PRESERVES, or MAPLE BLISS BUTTER GRANOLA

Eggs:

hard-boiled, soft-boiled, fried with ghee or butter, scrambled.

Omelette with veggies and yogurt cheese.

Serve cooked eggs on sprouted sourdough toast spread with MAYO SUBSTITUTE.

Serve cooked eggs with cooked spinach and toast.

Sprouted sourdough bread

Toasted and spread with dates and yogurt cheese.

Toasted and spread with homemade apricot jam.

French toast with apricot preserves, MAPLE BLISS BUTTER or maple syrup.

LUNCH:

With a glass of CREAM SODA.

A glass of DATE SMOOTHIE.

Sandwiches on sprouted sourdough:

Tuna or other cooked fish (moistened with MAYO SUBSTITUTE)

Grill the above sandwich in a little butter.

Grilled YOGURT CHEESE SPREAD sandwich.

Avocado with YOGURT CHEESE SPREAD and chiles.

EGG SALAD SANDWICH MIX

Steamed veggies.

DINNER:

> BASIC QUINOA with:
>> Curry, veggies and yogurt
>> Veggies and herbed WHITE SAUCE
>
> Quinoa Dishes: GENTLE SAVORY QUINOA, SPRINGTIME QUINOA, SPINACH TIMBALES
> Fresh cooked fish: CYNTH'S SMOKED TUNA PASTA 'ALFREDO,' DIANE'S SUSHI, GOURMET BROILED FISH, LOX and EGGS, POACHED SALMON WITH DILL, TIDEWATER CRABCAKES, YOGURT BAKED SWORDFISH STEAKS, YOGURT SALMON MOUSSE
> Steamed Veggies with AVOCADO DRESSING, GREEN GODDESS DRESSING, YOGURT HERB DRESSING
> Egg Dishes: EGG LASAGNE, SPINACH FRITTATA
> Salads: COLD QUINOA SALAD
> Soups: BASIC BORSCHT, CURRIED ZUCCHINI SOUP, PUMPKIN SOUP

SNACKS AND DESSERTS:

> Cheesecake: BAKED and LAYERED CHEESECAKE, CAROB CHEESECAKE, ORANGE CHEESECAKE
> Cookies: APRICOT BARS, CAROB FUDGE, MARSHA'S LACE COOKIES, QUINOA COOKIES
> Drinks: DATE SMOOTHIE, CREAM SODA
> Cakes: CAROB BROWNIES #1, CAROB BROWNIES #2, CARROT CAKE, DREAMY POPPY SEED CAKE, GINGERBREAD, ZUCCHINI SQUASH BREAD with APRICOT BUTTER PRESERVES, MAPLE BLISS BUTTER, MAPLE CARAMEL CRUNCH FROSTING, YOGURT CHEESE FROSTING or YOGURT CHEESE WHIPPING CREAM
> Crackers: CINNAMON MADNESS, FLAKY CRACKERS, SAVORY CRACKERS
> Ice Cream: FROZEN FRUIT YOGURT with APRICOT FOOL
> Pudding: ABBY'S BREAKFAST PUDDING, ABBY'S PUMPKIN PUDDING, QUINOA PUDDING, QUICK PUDDING
> Pies: PUMPKIN PIE with YOGURT WHIPPING CREAM

SUGGESTIONS FOR THE DEEP CLEANSER DIET

If you're following the Deep Cleanser Diet, you can eat anything on Super Cleanser Diet as well.

BREAKFAST:

> Sprouted Breads:
>> Sprouted Grain Toast with APRICOT PRESERVES.
>> Sprouted Grain French Toast.

Quinoa or quinoa flakes as hot cereal with:
>   diluted yogurt, maple syrup, pat of butter.
>   with SPROUTED SOY MILK.

GRANOLA with SPROUTED WHEAT FLAKES.

Eggs with:
>   Potatoes.
>   Sprouted grain toast.
>   Omelettes with kefir cheese, LOX and EGGS, veggies.

Chicken sausage.

Pancakes: FINNISH PANCAKES, POTATO PANCAKES, PUMPKIN PANCAKES, QUINOA PANCAKES with APRICOT BUTTER PRESERVES, FIG PRESERVES OR MAPLE BLISS BUTTER

LUNCH:

>   A glass of DATE SMOOTHIE.

>   Baked Potatoes with herbed YOGURT CHEESE.

>   Veggie Soup or Stew: SPROUTED PEA SOUP, SPROUTED PEA STEW, SHELLEY'S CHILI, SPROUTED BEAN CHILE, SPROUTED BEAN SOUP, BASIC BORSCHT, BORSCHT, CURRIED ZUCCHINI SOUP, PUMPKIN SOUP, TORTILLA SOUP, VEGETABLE CHOWDER.

>   Salads: COLD QUINOA SALAD, KIDNEY BEAN SALAD, raw veggies with AVOCADO DRESSING, GAZPACHO DRESSING, GREEN GODDESS DRESSING, YOGURT HERB DRESSING.

>   Crackers: CINNAMON MADNESS, FLAKY CRACKERS, GRAHAM CRACKERS, SAVORY CRACKERS, 'WHEAT THIN' CRACKERS.

>   Sprouted Bread Sandwiches made with:
>   >   Tuna, salmon, or other fish with MAYO SUBSTITUTE.
>   >   Avocado and kefir cheese or YOGURT CHEESE SPREAD.
>   >   EGG SALAD SANDWICH MIX.
>   >   SPROUTED SOYBURGERS
>   >   A glass of CREAM SODA/GINGER ALE, BANANA YOGURT SMOOTHIE or LASSI

>   Sprouted Bean: FRIJOLES, Burritos or tostados made with frijoles.

DINNER:

>   Salads: COLD QUINOA SALAD, KIDNEY BEAN SALAD, raw veggies with AVOCADO DRESSING, GAZPACHO DRESSING, GREEN GODDESS DRESSING, YOGURT HERB DRESSING.

>   Veggies: CYNTH'S FENNEL SAUTE W/CARAWAY, MARSHA'S GNOCCHI, T-BOO'S TURNIPS

Entrees of:

    Sprouted Bean Dishes: FRIJOLES, LENTIL KEDGEREE, OLD-FASHIONED BAKED BEANS.

    Quinoa dishes: ABBY'S QUINOA MEXICAN STYLE, BASIC QUINOA, GENTLE SAVORY QUINOA, SPINACH TIMBALES, SPRINGTIME QUINOA, STIR-FRY QUINOA, STUFFED GREEN PEPPERS WITH CHINESE BLACK MUSH-ROOMS.

    Egg dishes: CORN CUSTARD, EGG FOO YONG, EGG LASAGNE, EGG SALAD SANDWICH MIX, MUSHROOM CRUST QUICHE, SPINACH FRITTATA.

    Mixed dishes: ENCHILADAS, MUSHROOM CURRY, PIZZA, VEGGIES ENCHI-LADAS.

    Fish dishes: 'CRABMEAT' DIP, CYNTH'S SMOKED TUNA PASTA 'ALFREDO,' DELICATE SLEEPING FISH, DIANE'S SUSHI, FISH STEW, GOURMET BROILED FISH, POACHED SALMON WITH DILL, POTATO SALMON PANCAKES, TIDEWATER CRABCAKES, YOGURT BAKED SWORDFISH STEAKS, YOGURT SALMON MOUSSE.

    Quinoa with MOLE SAUCE, SPANISH and POTATO CHUTNEY, WHITE SAUCE.

SNACKS:

    Any cakes or cookies made with SPROUTED WHEAT FLOUR.

    Any cakes or cookies topped with YOGURT CHEESE FROSTING, YOGURT CHEESE WHIPPING CREAM.

    Breads: BANANA BREAD, ZUCCHINI SQUASH BREAD.

    Puddings: ABBY'S BREAKFAST PUDDING, ABBY'S PUMPKIN PUDDING, QUINOA PUDDING, QUICK PUDDING.

    Pies: MOCK PUMPKIN PIE, PUMPKIN PIE.

    Cakes: ABBY'S YUMMY CARROT-CORN BREAD, CARROT CAKE, DATE BREAD, DREAMY POPPY SEED CAKE, GINGERBREAD served with APRICOT BUTTER PRESERVES, FIG PRESERVES, MAPLE BLISS BUTTER OR MAPLE CARAMEL CRUNCH FROSTING.

    Cheesecakes: BAKED/LAYERED CHEESECAKE, CAROB or ORANGE CHEESECAKE.

    Cookies: ABBY'S CAROB COOKIES, APRICOT BARS, BASIC COOKIE RECIPE, CAROB BROWNIES #1, CAROB BROWNIES #2, FIG MOON COOKIES, MARSHA'S LACE COOKIES, QUINOA COOKIES.

    Candies: CAROB FUDGE.

    Frozen Goodies: ICE CREAM, SORBERT, FROZEN FRUIT YOGURT with APRICOT FOOL.

    Drinks: COCONUT CAROB DRINK.

SUGGESTIONS FOR THE BASIC BALANCER DIET

If you are following the Basic Balancer Diet, you can eat anything in the *Creating Heaven ON Your Plate* recipe section.

BREAKFAST:
>   Sprouted Breads:
>>   Sprouted Grain Toast with APRICOT PRESERVES, APRICOT BUTTER PRE-
>>   SERVES, or FIG PRESERVES.
>>   Sprouted Grain French Toast
>   Quinoa or quinoa flakes as hot cereal with:
>>   diluted yogurt, maple syrup, pat of butter
>>   with SPROUTED SOY MILK
>   GRANOLA with diluted, sweetened yogurt.
>   Eggs with:
>>   Potatoes
>>   Sprouted grain toast
>>   Omelettes with kefir cheese, LOX and EGGS, veggies.
>   'Toasted' corn tortilla spread with banana and yogurt.
>   Chicken sausage
>   Pancakes: BANANA FLATS, CORN CAKES, CORN FRITTERS, FINNISH PANCAKES,
>   POTATO PANCAKES, PUMPKIN PANCAKES, QUINOA PANCAKES.
>   ABBY'S BREAKFAST PUDDING

LUNCH:
>   APRICOT or DATE SMOOTHIE.
>   Baked Potatoes
>   Veggie Soup or Stew: SPROUTED PEA SOUP, SPROUTED PEA STEW, SHELLEY'S
>   CHILI, SPROUTED BEAN CHILE, SPROUTED BEAN SOUP, BASIC BORSCHT,
>   BORSCHT, CURRIED ZUCCHINI SOUP, PUMPKIN SOUP, TORTILLA SOUP,
>   VEGETABLE CHOWDER.
>   Salads: COLD QUINOA SALAD, KIDNEY BEAN SALAD, raw veggies with AVOCADO
>   DRESSING, GAZPACHO DRESSING, GREEN GODDESS DRESSING, YOGURT
>   HERB DRESSING, quinoa/corn pasta salad.
>   Crackers: CINNAMON MADNESS, FLAKY CRACKERS, GRAHAM CRACKERS, SA-
>   VORY CRACKERS, 'WHEAT THIN' CRACKERS served with YOGURT CHEESE,
>   APRICOT BUTTER PRESERVES OR MAPLE BLISS BUTTER.
>   Sprouted Bread Sandwiches made with:
>>   Tuna, salmon, or other fish with MAYO SUBSTITUTE.
>>   Avocado and kefir cheese or YOGURT CHEESE SPREAD.

EGG SALAD SANDWICH MIX.
SPROUTED SOYBURGERS
A glass of CREAM SODA/GINGER ALE, BANANA YOGURT SMOOTHIE, CO-CONUT MILK or LASSI.

Sprouted Bean: FRIJOLES, Burritos or tostados made with frijoles.

DINNER:

Salads: COLD QUINOA SALAD, KIDNEY BEAN SALAD, raw veggies with AVOCADO DRESSING, GAZPACHO DRESSING, GREEN GODDESS DRESSING, YOGURT HERB DRESSING.

Veggies: CYNTH'S FENNEL SAUTE WITH CARAWAY, MARSHA'S GNOCCHI, T-BOO'S TURNIPS.

Entrees of:

Sprouted Bean Dishes: FRIJOLES, LENTIL KEDGEREE, OLD-FASHIONED BAKED BEANS.

Quinoa dishes: ABBY'S QUINOA MEXICAN STYLE, BASIC QUINOA, GENTLE SAVORY QUINOA, SPINACH TIMBALES, SPRINGTIME QUINOA, STIR-FRY QUINOA, STUFFED GREEN PEPPERS WITH CHINESE BLACK MUSHROOMS, QUINOA NOODLE STOVE-TOP CASSEROLE.

Egg dishes: CORN CUSTARD, EGG FOO YONG, EGG LASAGNE, EGG SALAD SANDWICH MIX, MUSHROOM CRUST QUICHE, SPINACH FRITTATA, CHILE-CORN CASSEROLE, CORNBREAD CASSEROLE.

Mixed dishes: ENCHILADAS, KEFIR & VEGETABLE PASTA, MUSHROOM CURRY, PIZZA, VEGGIE ENCHILADAS.

Fish dishes: 'CRABMEAT' DIP, CYNTH'S SMOKED TUNA PASTA 'ALFREDO,' DELICATE SLEEPING FISH, DIANE'S SUSHI, FISH STEW, GOURMET BROILED FISH, POACHED SALMON WITH DILL, POTATO SALMON PANCAKES, TIDEWATER CRABCAKES, YOGURT BAKED SWORDFISH STEAKS, YOGURT SALMON MOUSSE, T-BOO'S SPINACH HAU PIA.

Serve fish with no-vinegar horseradish and yogurt sauce.

Chicken dishes: CHICKEN CACCIATORI, CYNTH'S SHISH-KA-BOB, DIANE'S OVEN 'FRIED' CHICKEN, MARSHA'S COCONUT-DIPPED CHICKEN, TORTILLA SOUP.

Make a stuffing with sprouted bread, eggs and herbs to stuff a chicken or turkey.

Quinoa with MOLE SAUCE, SPANISH and POTATO CHUTNEY, WHITE SAUCE.

Breads: ABBY'S CORN MUFFINS, ABBY'S CORNBREAD.

SNACKS:

APRICOT or DATE SMOOTHIE.
Yogurt and no-vinegar salsa dip with baked corn chips or veggies.
Any cakes or cookies made with SPROUTED WHEAT FLOUR.

Any cakes or cookies topped with YOGURT CHEESE FROSTING, YOGURT CHEESE
     WHIPPING CREAM.
Breads: BANANA BREAD, ZUCCHINI SQUASH BREAD.
Puddings: ABBY'S BREAKFAST PUDDING, ABBY'S PUMPKIN PUDDING, QUINOA
     PUDDING, QUICK PUDDING.
Pies: COCONUT CREAM PIE, COCONUT CUSTARD PIE, MOCK PUMPKIN PIE,
     PUMPKIN PIE with CORN FLAKE CRUST and YOGURT CHEESE WHIPPING
     CREAM.
Cakes: ABBY'S YUMMY CARROT-CORN BREAD, CARROT CAKE, DATE BREAD,
     DREAMY POPPY SEED CAKE, or GINGERBREAD served with APRICOT BUT-
     TER PRESERVES, FIG PRESERVES, MAPLE BLISS BUTTER OR MAPLE CARA-
     MEL CRUNCH FROSTING.
Cheesecakes: BAKED and LAYERED CHEESECAKE, CAROB CHEESECAKE, ORANGE
     CHEESECAKE.
Cookies: ABBY'S CAROB COOKIES, APRICOT BARS, BASIC COOKIE RECIPE,
     CAROB BROWNIES #1, CAROB BROWNIES #2, FIG MOON COOKIES,
     MARSHA'S LACE COOKIES, QUINOA COOKIES.
Candies: CAROB FUDGE
Frozen Goodies: ICE CREAM, SORBERT, FROZEN FRUIT YOGURT, VANILLA CUS-
     TARD ICE CREAM with APRICOT FOOL.
Drinks: COCONUT CAROB DRINK, CREAM SODA and GINGER ALE, BANANA
     YOGURT SMOOTHIE, LASSI.

SUGGESTIONS FOR ONCE A WEEK COOKING

Set aside a two to three hour period once a week (making it the same day and time each week, working it into your life's schedule, makes following the whole diet routine easier) and cook a bunch of different foods. Then, when you get ready to leave the house, it's easy to grab up some stuff to take with you. And, when you get home from a long day, it's easy to throw some stuff together, warm it up and be sitting down to eat with 15-20 minutes!

Of course, if you have the time and like to cook, the recipe section and the separate volume of recipes, *Creating Heaven ON Your Plate*, have lots of goodies to play with!

As you are planning your week's eating ideas, keep in mind a wide range of choices and taste treats. As you go through the program and can add new foods, like nuts and regular grains, you can add new variety and recipes.

Here's one week's suggestion:

**Buy a loaf of sprouted bread, potatoes, veggies, butter, yogurt, some fresh salmon, fruit, carob powder, maple syrup, quinoa.

**Cook a pan of BASIC QUINOA. Steam a number of different veggies, either separately or mixed together, depending upon your future plans. Make a double pan of cornbread. Make a pan of CAROB BROWNIES. Bake ten potatoes. Make a recipe of APRICOT PRESERVES.

From these prepared items you could make all the following meals:

Breakfasts: Potatoes and eggs. Sliced and 'fried' cornbread served with maple syrup like pancakes. Veggie omelettes. Hot quinoa 'cereal' with butter and maple syrup. Sprouted toast with apricot preserves. 'Refried' potatoes.

Lunches: Avocado or tuna sandwich on sprouted bread. Cornbread with apricot preserves. Mix veggies and potatoes or quinoa into veggie or chicken broth for a quick soup. Mash a cooked potato or two and fry like a pancake. Reheat veggies. Have a carob brownie.

Dinners: Reheated quinoa as a bed for curried veggies or Mexican spiced veggies or tomato sauce with veggies. Add some tamari and sprouted mung beans to veggies and serve over quinoa. Make Egg Foo Yong. Mash potatoes, mix in veggies and reheat like a Shepherd's Pie.

Snacks: Make a QUINOA PUDDING. Eat Carob Brownies. Make some YOGURT CHEESE WHIPPING CREAM.

Here's another week's ideas:

**Bake some QUINOA COOKIES. Make some Zucchini Bread. Cook a big pot of VEGGIE CHOWDER. Cook a bunch of chicken. Steam a bunch of veggies. Make a pan of quinoa. Bake a couple of winter squashes or pumpkin. Make some frozen yogurt and yogurt cheese. Make a batch of FRIJOLES. From these foods you could make or eat the following:

Breakfasts: Hot quinoa cereal. Pumpkin pancakes. Sprouted French toast. Toasted sprouted essene bread with yogurt/kefir cheese. Omelette with yogurt cheese and veggies. Polenta or corn grits. Toast a tortilla, then spread with banana and yogurt cheese.

Lunches: Veggies and quinoa. Veggie Chowder. Frijoles in warmed corn tortillas. Veggies in corn tortillas with yogurt cheese. Chicken sandwich with baked corn chips.

Dinners: Chicken soup with veggies and quinoa. Chicken curry over quinoa. Pumpkin Soup. Veggie enchiladas.

Snacks: Quinoa cookies with yogurt cheese icing. Zucchini bread with yogurt cheese whipping cream. Pumpkin pie. Any of the cheesecakes. No-vinegar salsa and baked corn chips.

The following recipes are great reheated or eaten cold:

KIDNEY BEAN SALAD	COLD QUINOA SALAD	EGG FOO YONG
GENTLE SAVORY QUINOA	SPROUTED SOYBURGER	FISH STEW
OLD-FASHIONED BAKED BEANS	FRIJOLES	EGG LASAGNE
STIR-FRY QUINOA	SPRINGTIME QUINOA	PIZZA
CHILE-CORN CASSEROLE	TORTILLA SOUP	VEGETABLE CHOWDER
MUSHROOM-CRUST QUICHE	PUMPKIN SOUP	SPINACH FRITTATA
SPROUTED PEA SOUP	SPROUTED PEA STEW	SHELLEY'S CHILI
SPROUTED BEAN CHILE	SPROUTED BEAN SOUP	BASIC BORSCHT
BORSCHT	CURRIED ZUCCHINI SOUP	

I tend to eat simply on a regular basis and eat the same things over and over, changing more with the seasons than with any other influence. Then occasionally, I go all out and make a 'real' meal, with leftovers in mind. The most important thing you want to do with your food and diet is to try alot of different ideas and find new, fun foods to eat. Don't make it difficult unless you want to do that.

TABLE 2 - FOOD CATEGORIES

Foods fall into different digestive categories. The following lists show how different foods digest.

PROTEINS

These foods need hydrochloric acid in the stomach to properly digest.

MEATS:
- bear
- beef
- buffalo
- chicken
- duck
- elk
- goat (chevon)
- goose
- lamb
- moose
- organ meats
- pork
- rabbit
- turkey
- veal (beef)
- venison (deer)

FISH:
- cod
- halibut
- orange roughi
- maui-maui
- salmon
- sole
- trout
- tuna

DAIRY:
- buttermilk
- cheeses:
  - hard
  - soft
  - cottage cheese
  - cream cheese

DAIRY cont'd:
- eggs
- goat cheeses
- kefir
- kefir cheese
- milk:
  - cow or goat
- sour cream
- yogurt
- yogurt cheese

NUTS & SEEDS:
- almonds
- black walnuts
- Brazil nuts
- cashews
- chestnuts

- filberts
- hazelnuts
- hickory
- macadamia nuts
- peanuts
- pecans
- pine nuts
- pistachios
- pumpkin seeds
- sesame seeds
- sunflower seeds
- walnuts

MISC.:
- brewers yeast
- carob powder
- nutritional yeast

STARCHES

These foods need pancreatic enzymes to properly digest. You may have noticed that I talk about starches instead of carbohydrates. Carbohydrates are foods the quickly turn into digestible sugars, so they include fruits, veggies and starches. Because of the 'don't combine starches with proteins' rule, it is important to differentiate between carbohydrates and starches.

amaranth	millet	soy powders	textured vegetable products
barley	oats	spelt	triticale
buckwheat	rice	teff	unsprouted beans & legumes
couscous	rye	tempeh	wheat
kamut	soy cheeses	tofu	

SWEETENERS

Natural sweeteners are the only sugars I suggest using.

blackstrap molasses
cane syrups:
  granulated cane juice
  Sucanat
date sugar
fructose
sorghum molasses
maple syrup or granulated
malt syrup
barley malt syrup
honey
rice syrup
rice bran syrup
stevia (an herb)

OILS

Oils and fats take bile, a soap-like substance, from the liver and gallbladder to digest properly.

almond oil
butter
canola/rapeseed oil
corn oil
grape seed oil
mayonnaise
olive oil
peanut oil
safflower oil
sesame oil
soy/soya oils
soy margarine
sunflower oil

FRUITS

Fruits can be fresh, dried, cooked, canned or juiced. They digest by fermenting in the intestines; this process is accelerated by enzymes that speed up the fermenting.

apples
apricots
avocado
bananas
berries:
  blackberries
  blueberries
  gooseberries
  raspberries
  strawberries
  cherries
citrus:
  grapefruit
  lemons
  limes
  oranges
  pineapple
  tangelos
  tangerines
coconut
cold-processed
  coffee extract
currants
dates
figs
grapes
guava
kiwi
mangoes
nectarines
papaya
peaches
pears
melons:
  cantaloupe
  crenshaw
  honeydew
  muskmelon
  watermelons
plums
quinoa
rhubarb
persimmons

VEGGIES

Like fruits, veggies basically ferment in the intestines, a process accelerated by additional enzymes.

agar-agar	endive	parsnip	sprouted:
arrowroot	fennel	peas:	beans
artichokes	garlic	green	grains
asparagus	greens:	snap	legumes
beans:	arugula	sugar	squash, summer:
green	beet greens	peppers:	crookneck
limas	chicory	chili	patty pan
sprouted	corn salad	green/red/yellow	zucchini
beets	dandelion	jalapeno	squash, winter:
broccoli	escarole	poppy seeds	acorn
brussels sprouts	radicchio	potatoes:	banana
bok choy	turnip greens	white	butternut
cabbage	watercress	colored	delicata
capers	horseradish	sweet	hubbard
carrots	Jerusalem artichoke	pumpkins	spaghetti
cauliflower	jicama	radishes	Swiss chard
celeriac	kale	rutabaga	tapioca
celery	kohlrabi	salisfy	tomatillo
chives	leeks	scallions	tomatoes
collards	lettuce	seaweeds	turnips
corn	mushrooms	shallots	wild rice
cornmeal	mustard greens	sorrel	yams
cranberries	okra	spinach	eggplant
cucumbers	olives	onions	

HERBS & SPICES

It would be impossible to list all available medicinal herbs, so I am listing the most common ones along with cooking herbs and spices. In their various forms, herbs and spices digest like veggies.

COOKING HERBS:

anise	chili powder	marjoram	rosemary
basil	chives	mustards:	sage
bay leaves	cilantro	powder	savory
caraway	cumin	seed	sorrel
cardamom	curry powder	oregano	tarragon
cayenne	dill	paprika	thyme
celery seed	fennel	parsley	tumeric
chervil	lovage	pepper	

SPICES:

allspice	cloves	ginger	nutmeg
cinnamon	coriander	mace	saffron

TEAS:

black teas	chamomile	lavender	peppermint
catnip	green teas	lemon balm	spearmint

COMMON MEDICINAL HERBS:

alfalfa	eyebright	mullein	saw palmetto
aloe vera	fennel	myrrh	scullcap
barberry	fenugreek	nettle	shepherd purse
bayberry	garlic	oat straw	slippery elm
black cohosh	ginger	parsley	squaw vine
black walnut	ginseng	passion flower	St. Johnswort
blessed thistle	golden seal	pennyroyal	strawberry
blue cohosh	gotu kola	peppermint	thyme
burdock	hawthorn	plantain	uva ursi
cascara sagrada	hops	pleurisy root	valerian root
catnip	horseradish	poke root	vervain
cayenne	horsetail	psyllium	white oak bark
chamomile	hyssop	queen of the meadow	wild yam
chaparral	juniper	raspberry	willow
chickweed	kelp	red clover	wintergreen
comfrey	licorice	rose hips	witch hazel
damiana	lobelia	rue	wood betony
dandelion	mandrake	saffron/safflowers	wormwood
echinacea	marshmallow	sage	yarrow
eucalyptus	mistletoe	sarsaparilla	yellow dock
			yerba santa

SPECIALTY FOODS

VINEGAR AND ITEMS WITH IT:

catsup	mayonnaise	salsa
chutneys	mustard	worcestershire sauce
horseradish	pickles	

TABLE 3 - WHERE CAN I GET......?

The following section lists companies making products you can eat on Basic Diets 1-3. As you move into Phase 2 and on, you will find products listed in the second section. Many of the companies listed in the first section also make products you can only add from Phase 2 and on.

For a free catalog of health foods, grains, flours, and additional products which meet the diet needs outlined in this book, call 800-235-6570 and request *The Summers Approach Products Catalog.*

CORN PRODUCTS

ARROWHEAD MILLS, Box 2059, Hereford, TX 79045, (806) 364-0730 -- FAX (806) 364-8242
Products: Corn Flakes, Puffed Corn, white & yellow Corn Grits, cornmeal (blue, Hi-Lysine, yellow, white.)

BARBARA'S BAKERY, INC, 3900 Cypress Dr, Petaluma, CA 94954
Products: Barbara's Amazing Bakes (corn/quinoa baked corn chips): Lightly Salted, Blue Corn, Quinoa, and Pesto.

GARDEN OF EATIN', 5300 Santa Monica Blvd, Los Angeles, CA 90029
Products: California Bakes (baked corn chips) and blue and yellow tortillas.

PACIFIC GRAIN PRODUCTS, PO Box 2060, Woodland, CA 95776
Products: Nutty Corn cereal (corn and honey.)

SANTA CRUZ CHIPS COMPANY, P.O. Box 1153, Boulder Creek, CA 95006
Products: Baked Blue Corn Chips

WEETABIX COMPANY, 20 Cameron St, Clinton, MA 01510
Products: GRAINFIELD brand name — the very best CornFlakes!!! They're made with corn and malt syrup only. (And for later in the diet, try their Rasin Bran and Crispy Rice.)

MAPLE SUGAR PRODUCTS

MAPLE GROVE FARMS OF VERMONT, 167 Portland St, St. Johnsbury, VT 05819
Products: maple syrup and maple candies.

VERMONT COUNTRY MAPLE, INC, PO Box 53, Jericho Center, VT 05465
Products: maple syrup, maple candies and maple sprinkles.

THE VERMONT COUNTRY STORE, PO Box 3000, Manchester Center, VT 05255-3000
for credit card orders: (802)362-2400
Products: maple syrup, powder and candies.

WOOD HOMESTEAD, RD 1 Box 107, Stamford, NY 12167
Products: maple syrup candies.

QUINOA PRODUCTS

If you are using alot of quinoa grain and flour, I suggest that you look into buying it bulk and grinding it yourself. Or, find a friend with a flour mill.

ARROWHEAD MILLS, Box 2059, Hereford, TX 79045, (806) 364-0730 -- FAX (806) 364-8242
Products: whole grain quinoa.

EDEN FOODS, 701 Tecumseh Road, Clenton, Michigan 49236, (517) 456-7424, FAX (517) 456-6075
Products: Eden Foods is a great source for quinoa grain. It is clean and needs little or no rinsing.

QUINOA CORPORATION, PO Box 1039, Torrance, CA, (800)237-2304FAX (310) 530-8764
Brand name: ANCIENT HARVEST. Products: Pastas: *Elbows, Shells, Rotelle and Garden Pagoda*: Corn flour, Quinoa flour, (Garden Pagoda also contains red bell pepper, dried spinach.) Quinoa Grain, Quinoa Flakes (like rolled oats.)

SPROUTED GRAIN PRODUCTS

When I first started looking for sprouted grain products, I found one bread. It was delicious, but it used cashews as a binder, so many people couldn't digest it for months. Now there are so many sprouted grain products on the market I can't keep track of them all. But a word of WARNING. Some of the labeling done by bakery companies is misleading, to say the least! Even if it says '100% sprouted' on the front of the package, read the ingredient list to make sure ALL grains in it are sprouted.

ALSO, Gluten Flour is the protein of wheat flour and so, is NOT a problem for most people. Remember, sweeteners are added to breads for the yeast to grown on, so basically, no sugars are left.

All these products are baked, frozen and shipped that way. I try to buy them still frozen; sometimes the stores put them out on the shelves where they can either dry out or get moldy. I'd rather thaw them out myself and keep them in the fridge.

THE SUMMERS APPROACH PASTA CO., P.O. Box 216, Torreon, NM 87061
100% Sprouted SPELT PASTA, approved for all diet phases; mild, lighter-than-whole-wheat taste; numerous styles. Write for more information.

ALVARADO STREET BAKERY, Rohnert Park, CA, (707) 585-3293
These products are great; they make the best sourdough on the market. But read their labels carefully; there's some confusion there. It seems that when they say *"organically grown ...... kernels"* that they mean sprouted and when they say *"100% sprouted"* across the front of the label, it doesn't mean

the whole bread IS sprouted. The following three breads are safe bets: *Sprouted Sourdough, Sprouted Whole Wheat, Sprouted Rye Bread.*

BERLIN BAKERY, PO Box 311, Berlin, OH 44610, (216) 893-2734--FAX (216) 893-2157

As far as I know, this is the only bakery making their own sprouted <u>flours</u> and making breads with them. All the other sprouted bread companies that I am aware of are using sprouted *grains* in their breads, not sprouted flour. They also sell both the sprouted flours they make, that is, sprouted spelt flour and sprouted wheat flour (panocha flour.) Ask your health food store to carry the flours or deal with the bakery directly. From my contacts with these people, I'd have to say, they are wonderful! And their products match that wonderfulness!

Sprouted Spelt Bread: Sprouted whole spelt flour, water, honey, canola oil, yeast, sea salt.

Sprouted Seed Bread: Sprouted seed flour (wheat, barley, soy beans, lentils, millet, oats,) water, honey, yeast, sea salt.

CASADOS FARMS / Juanita Casados, Box 852, San Juan Pueblo, NM 87566, (505)852-2433 or 753-8180

These wonderful people make sprouted wheat flour (panocha flour) and sell it by the pound. They will direct ship from 1# up at the cost of $1 per pound plus shipping.

Panocha Flour has lost all its gluten, so some must be added if you want to make light-textured goodies. Check out the recipes that use it.

FOOD FOR LIFE, PO Box 1434, Corona, CA 91719, (909)279-5090

I love this company and I love their products. Their labeling is clear, their product line is extensive, they keep adding new products and their foods are yummy!

**Seven-Grain Sprouted Bread*: sprouted wheat, water, pure honey, molasses, sprouted rye, sprouted barley, sprouted oats, sprouted millet, sprouted corn, sprouted brown rice, fresh yeast, lecithin, malted barley, sea salt.

**Cinnamon Raisin Bread*: sprouted wheat, raisins, malted barley, water, raisin juice, sprouted rye, sprouted barley, sprouted oats, sprouted millet, sprouted corn, sprouted brown rice, yeast, lecithin, malt, sea salt, cinnamon.

**Bran Plus -- High Fiber Bread*: Sprouted wheat, water, wheat bran, malted barley syrup, raisin juice concentrate, fresh yeast, sea salt.

**Ezekiel 4:9*: sprouted wheat, malted barley, sprouted millet, sprouted barley, sprouted lentils, sprouted soybeans, sprouted whole oats, fresh yeast, water, sea salt.

**Sprouted Whole Grains*: sprouted wheat, water, honey, molasses, fresh yeast, lecithin, malted barley, sea salt.

**California Raisin*: Sprouted wheat, California raisins, malted barley, water, raisin juice, sprouted rye, sprouted barley, sprouted oats, sprouted millet, sprouted corn, sprouted brown rice, fresh yeast, lecithin, malt, sea slat, cinnamon.

**Organic Ezekiel 4:9 Cinnamon Raisin*: organic sprouted wheat, organic raisins, organic sprouted barley, organic sprouted millet, malted barley, organic sprouted lentils, organic sprouted soybeans, organic sprouted spelt, fresh yeast, water, sea salt, cinnamon.

**Sprouted Whole Wheat*: sprouted wheat, water, honey, molasses, fresh yeast, lecithin, malt, sea salt.

**All Natural Whole Grain, Sprouted Grain Bread* (Low Sodium): sprouted wheat, water, fresh yeast, lecithin, carob pod meal.

**7 Sprouted Grains, Low Sodium Bread*: sprouted Wheat, water, honey, molasses, sprouted rye, sprouted barley, sprouted oats, sprouted millet, sprouted corn, sprouted brown rice, fresh yeast, lecithin, malt.

**Organic Ezekiel 4:9 Bread Rolled in Sesame Seeds*: organic sprouted wheat, water, organic sprouted barley, organic sprouted millet, malted barley, organic sprouted lentils, organic sprouted soybeans, organic sprouted spelt, fresh yeast, sea salt. Rolled in organic unhulled sesame seeds.

GARDEN OF EATIN, 5300 Santa Monica Blvd., Los Angeles, CA. 90029, (213) 462-5406

Products: Onderful essene bread.

NATURES PATH AND MANNA, 7453 Progress Way, Delta, B.C. V4G 1E8 CANADA,
(604) 940-0505, (FAX) (604)940-0522

These are great products, though the labeling is odd. They definitely state on the label that all the grains are sprouted, but the ingredient lists don't quite state it clearly. Nature's Path does make sure that their grains are all certified organic and their ingredients are top-notch.

The Manna Breads they make are wonderful and there are quite a few selections. Their information says: No Yeast, No Salt, No Sugar, No Oil, No Preservatives, No Flour, Simply Sprouts!

Nature's Path also makes a number of cereals, though none of them, at this writing, are made with sprouted grains. Their Corn Flakes cereal is made with mixed fruit juices, which can definitely cause some problems with hypoglycemics, especially early on in the diet. You might want to try them after you are through the final phase; these particular flakes are very crisp and crunchy.

**Sprouted 9-Grain Bread*: Sprouted whole wheat kernels, vital wheat gluten, millet, brown rice, barley, sunflower oil, malt, yeast, soybeans, rye, flax, oats, oat bran, cornmeal, raisin syrup, sesame seeds, soya lecithin, sea salt.

**Sprouted 9-Grain Sesame Bread*: Sprouted whole wheat kernels, vital wheat gluten, millet, brown rice, barley, sunflower oil, malt, soybeans, rye, flax, oats, oat bran, sea salt, yeast, cornmeal, raisin syrup, sesame seeds, soya lecithin.

Manna Bread Varieties: *Carrot Raisin, Sunseed, Carrot Raisin Rye, Whole Rye, Fruit and Nut, Whole Wheat, Millet Rice, Sun-Spelt, Multigrain Oatbran*

OASIS BREADS, 440 Venture St. , Escondido, CA , (619) 747-7390

These breads are the best. The taste, texture, and flavors are like good homemade breads. They are also sold under the Trader Joe label, a gourmet chain-store in California. Here's a quote from some of the literature they send me:

"We started making sprouted whole grain breads because we were excited by the high nutrition claims made about sprouts. The nourishing properties of sprouts are amazing. Sprouts have the most nutrients per unit of any food known to man. We also discovered that sprouts are more easily digestible than whole grains or flour.

Sprouting creates enzymes and develops amino acids which aid digestion, makes dissolvable compounds out of insoluble oils and turns whole grains into a complete protein food."

Sprouted 7 Grain: Ground wheat, rye, corn, barley, millet, oats and rice sprouts with water, honey, yeast and salt.

Sprouted Wheat: Ground wheat sprouts with water, honey, yeast and salt.

Flourless Pumpernickel Bread: Ground wheat and rye sprouts with water, honey, molasses, caraway seed, yeast and salt.

Flourless Sprouted Rye Bread: Ground wheat and rye sprouts with water, honey, yeast, ground caraway seed and salt.

Sunflower Seed: Ground wheat sprouts with water, sunflower seeds, honey, yeast and salt.

California Fruit Loaf: Ground wheat sprouts with water, raisins, honey, sunflower seeds, dates, yeast and salt.

Oat Bran: Ground wheat sprouts, oat bran, honey, yeast, salt and topped with oat flakes.

Raisin Oat Bran: Ground wheat sprouts, raisins, oat bran, honey, water, yeast, salt and oat flakes.

Salt Free 7 Grain: Same ingredients as the Sprouted 7 Grain without the salt. Ground wheat, rye, corn, barley, millet, oats and rice sprouts with water, honey and yeast.

Sprouted Kashi: Wheat sprouts, Kashi sprouts (a blend of whole oats, long grain brown rice, rye, hard red winter wheat, triticale, raw buckwheat, barley and sesame seeds,) honey, yeast, oat bran, wheat gluten, and salt.

(*Special Sprouted* and *Sprouted Kamut Bread* are not all sprouted.)

TRADER JOE'S (Main Office), 538 Mission St, South Pasadena, CA 91031

Products: Most of the Trader Joe's stores carry sprouted Oasis Breads under their own label.

DISTRIBUTORS FOR SPROUTED BREADS

Before you directly call a company listed above, you might let your health food store look at the following list. If they deal with one of these distributors, they will be able to get sprouted breads for you.

FOOD FOR HEALTH, 3655 W. Washington St, Phoenix, AZ 85009, (602) 269-2371

Regions: Arizona, California, Colorado, Idaho, Montana, Nebraska, Nevada, New Mexico, Oklahoma, South Dakota, Texas, Utah, Wyoming, and the panhandle of Kansas.

RAINBOW NATURAL FOODS , 4850 Moline St, Denver, CO 80239, (303) 373-1144

Regions: Colorado, Illinois, Iowa, Kansas, Missouri, Nebraska, New Mexico, S. Dakota, and Wyoming.

NATURES BEST, PO Box 2248, Brea, CA 92622, (714) 441-2378

Regions: California, Hawaii, Nevada (Reno and Las Vegas only)

TREE OF LIFE WEST, 9501 El Dorado Ave., Sun Valley, CA 91352, (818) 768-2330
   Region: Southern California

TREE OF LIFE HAYWARD, 3371 Arden Rd, Hayward, CA 94545, (415) 783-1996
   Region: Northern California

CEDARLINE NATURAL FOODS, 131 S. Maple #4, So. San Francisco, CA 94080, (415) 742-0444
   Region: Northern California

TREE OF LIFE MIDWEST, 225 Daniels Way, Bloomington, IN 47402, (812) 333-1511
   Regions: Alabama, Georgia, Illinois, Indiana, Iowa, Michigan, Minnesota, Missouri, Mississippi, North Carolina, Ohio, Pennsylvania, Virginia, Wisconsin, and parts of North and South Dakota

SOURCES FOR VITAMINS AND MINERALS

BERNARD JENSEN PRODUCTS, Box 8, Solana Beach, CA 92075, (619) 755-4027, FAX (619) 55-2026
   Products: Alfalfa tablets; Dulse powder, tablets and liquid; chlorophyll tablets, concentrate and liquid; bee pollen tablets; spirulina tablets and powder; Cell Salts; Sun Chlorella; Vitalfa.

CELL TECH, 1300 Main, Klamath Falls, OR 97601, (800)800-1300, (503)882-5406, FAX (503)884-1869
   Products: blue-green algae tablets and powder. This is a networking company, so call and ask who your local distributor is.

FIRST NATURE, PO Box 1656, Capitola, CA 95010, (408) 475-6986
   Products: SIX TASTES NURTURING POWER

FUTUREBIOTICS, 72 Cotton Mill Hill, Brattleboro, VT 05301, (802) 257-5691
   Products: Alfalfa Juice Concentrate, Barley Juice Concentrate, Vital Green, Alfalfa-Barley Chlorella, Aqua Greens, Echinacea, Propolis and Vitamin C combination, a line of regular vitamins, minerals and herbs and extracts.

GREENS + ORANGE PEEL ENTERPRISES, 2183 Ponce de Leon Cr, Vero Beach, FL 32960, (800) 643-1210, (407) 562-2766, FAX (407) 562-9848
   Products: Greens+ tablets contain: chlorella, extracts of milk thistle, echinacea, bilberry, green tea, grape seed, licorice root, ginseng, and ginkgo, wheat sprouts, spirulina, juice powders of acerola berries, alfalfa, red beet and wheat, bee pollen, dulse, dunaliella salina, ultra lecithin, astragalus, natural Vit. E, 4 bowel cleansers, and probiotic culture. (These are not listed in order of quantity.)

GREEN FOODS CORPORATION, 620 Maple Ave, Torrance, CA 90503, (800)777-4430, (310) 618-0678, FAX (310) 618-9246
   Products: Green Magma (retail) tablets and powder, Barley Green (distributors) tablets and powder, Beta Carrot, Green Essence, and Wheat Germ Extract.

THE HERITAGE STORE, PO Box 444-V, Virginia Beach, VA 23458-0444, (800)TO-CAYCE
   Products: They carry all the Edgar Cayce remedies as well as Diodes, liquid sea lettuce seaweed, blue-green algae, a liquid Vit. B with iron, and tinctures of myrrh, valerian, slippery elm and eyebright.

KAL , PO Box 4023, Woodland Hills, CA 91365-4023, (818) 340-3035
   Products: Alfalfa and alfalfa seed tablets, chlorophyll, Chlorella, Kelp tablets, and a wide variety of vitamin and mineral supplements.

MEZOTRACE COMPANY, 5184 E. Winnamucca Blvd, Winnamucca, NV 89445 (800)843-9989, (702) 623-1151
   Products: Mezotrace mineral tablets.

MIRACLE EXCLUSIVES, INC., 3 Elm St./PO Box 347, Locust Valley, NY 11560
   Products: Flora-dix (liquid vitamins)

NATURE'S SOURCE INTERNATIONAL, Corona, CA, (800)995-6607
   Products: LIQUID LIFE, Body Booster (see Table 6 for analysis.)

NATURE'S WAY PRODUCTS, 10 Mountain Springs Pkwy, Springville, UT 84663, (800)926-8883
   Products: Alfalfa leaves, alfalfa concentrate, Barley Grass, Chlorella, Kelp, Nettle Herb, Parsley Herb, Spirulina, Black Walnut Hulls, Dong Quai, Echinacea, Valerian Root, Bee Pollen, Aloe Vera, Uva Ursi, Red Clover, Licorice Root, Damiana, Blessed Thistle and many more.

NEW MOON EXTRACTS, INC, PO Box 1947, Brattleboro, VT 05302, (802) 257-0018
   Products: Ocean Herbs, ginger products, vitamins & herbs.

PINES INTERNATIONAL, Box 1107, Lawrence, KS 66044 (800)MY-PINES, FAX (913)841-1252
   Products: Wheat Grass tablets/powder, Barley Grass Tablets, Alfalfa Tables, Green Energy (wheat/barley grass powder,) herbs, and Rhubarb juice powder.

REACH FOR LIFE, 6846 S. Canton, St. 100, Tulsa, OK 74136 (800)258-5028, FAX (918)492-9546
   Products: Body Booster (liquid mineral supplement,) Liquid Life (liquid vitamin and mineral,) assorted other vitamin and mineral products, enzymes and oils.

SOLGAR VITAMIN AND HERB CO., 500 Willow Tree Rd., Lenora, NJ 07605
   Products: Earth Source Greens and More (powdered greens mix.)

THE SYNERGY COMPANY, PO Box 2901 CVSR, Moab, UT 84532, (800)723-0277

Products: *Algae Powder:* spirulina, Klamath Lake blue green, open-celled chlorella, Australian dunaliella salina, red dumontiaceae, wild-crafted kelp, blad-derwrack, Irish Moss, dulse and alaria. *Green Juice Powder:* green kamut grass juice, barley grass juice, oat grass juice, wheat grass juice, spelt grass juice, alfalfa grass juice, spinach octocosanol.

THE VITAMIN SHOP, (800)223-1216

Mail order source for many vitamin and mineral supplements I suggest as well as a number of food products like quinoa.

WORLD ORGANICS CORP., 5242 Bolsa Ave #3, Huntington Beach, CA 92649, (714) 892-0017

Products: Liquid Kelp, Alfalfa juice powder, Kelp and Iron tabs., liquid Vit. B, bee pollen wafers, liquid vitamins, chlorella, Chloro-Greens (5 concentrated green foods.)

SOURCES FOR READING INFORMATION

RECIPE BOOKS:

Creating Heaven Through Your Plate, (see recipe section, back of book) by Shelley Summers, (Warm Snow Publishers, (800) 235-6570)

Creating Heaven ON Your Plate, Volume II, (more recipes for diet programs outlined in above book) by Shelley Summers, (Warm Snow Publishers, (800) 235-6570)

Sugarfree Cooking, by Nicole Walker, 3116 W Nebraska St, Tucson, AZ 85746. (send $4.50)

BOOKS ON NUTRITION:

Let's Eat Right to Keep Fit, by Adelle Davis, (Harcourt Brace Janovitz)

Fit for Life, by Harvey Diamond, (Warner Books)

Nutrition Almanac, by Nutrition Search, Inc., John D. Kirschmann, (McGraw-Hill)

ON PHYSIOLOGY:

The Human Body, by Iaasc Asimov, (New American Library)

The 12 Stages of Healing, by Donald M. Epstein, (Amber-Allen Publishing)

ON HEALTH & WELLNESS:

To receive a complete catalog of books at discount prices on wellness, holistic health and alternative medicine, call **800-235-6570** and request a free copy of *"The Whole Health Book Catalog."*

SOURCE FOR 'ALCOHOL HERBS'

DELIGHTS THROUGH ALCHEMY, P.O. Box 2248, Tijeras, NM 87059

Products: Imbibers Sanity and energetic vitamin/mineral supplements.

SOURCE FOR DIODES

L.I.F.E., PO Box 144, Pullman, WV 26421, (304) 659-3193
    Products: Wayne & Wanda Cook diodes, retreat center, and assorted other goodies.

SOURCES FOR FLOWER ESSENCES

FLOWER ESSENCE CONNECTION, Bert Norgorden, PO Box, Torreon, NM 87061
    Products: Emergency Mix, 60 other combination SW essences, Chaco Canyon essences, essences to give your veggie and fruit plants.

BACH FLOWER ESSENCES, Available at most herb or health food stores.
    Products: Rescue Remedy in liquid and cream, 37 other flower essences.

CATHERINE RICH, 201 Hawthorne Ave, Larkspur, CA 94939
    Products: Liquid 911, other flower essences, skin creams.

PACIFIC ESSENCES, Box 8317, Victoria, B.C. V8W 3R9 Canada, (684)384-5568, FAX (684)382-4488
    Products: Sea essences, Goddess remedies, flower essences.

PERELANDRA, PO Box 3603, Warrenton, VA 22186, (703) 937-2153
    Products: numerous flower essences.

RUNNING FOX FARMS, 74 Thrasher Hill Road, Worthington, MA 01098, (413) 238-4291
    Products: flower essences of many herbs, childbearing kit and special kits.

SOURCES FOR ICE CREAMS AND ICE CREAM MAKERS

GARDEN OF EATIN,' INC., 5300 Santa Monica Blvd, Los Angeles, CA 90020, (213) 462-5406, FAX (213) 462-0517
    Products: (Go light on these and try them AFTER you've mostly completed the program, because they contain mixed fruits,) FROZEN JOY (in Lemon-Lime, Watermelon, Cantaloupe, Strawberry, Mango, Pina Colada) and FRUIT GLACE (in Mango, Lemon, Pineapple, Passion Fruit, Raspberry, Pina Colada.)

GLACIERWARE INC., 1 Ferry St, Easthampton, MA 01027, (413) 527-7141
    Products: freezer/paddle style ice cream makers.

DONVIER ICE CREAM MAKER
    This is the brand name of my ice cream maker and I love it. For a free catalog of ice cream makers, yogurt makers, and additional health products, call (800)235-6570.

SOURCE FOR OTHER NATURAL CANDIES

SOKENSHA CO. LTD, PO Box 883033, San Francisco, CA 94188-3033
Products: Soken Candies (made with rice syrup.)

SOURCE FOR NATURAL CHOCOLATE

MERCANTILE FOOD CO., PO Box SS, Philmont, NY 12565, (518) 672-0190
Products: Organic chocolate candies made with granulated cane juice!

SOURCES FOR NATURAL GRAIN PRODUCTS

HEALTH VALLEY FOODS, INC., 16100 Foothhill Blvd., Irwindale, CA 91706-7611
Products: Once you've gone through the whole diet program, you will want to occasionally 'embellish' yourself with some of this company's cereals. They all contain some mixed fruit juices and other sweeteners.

PACIFIC GRAIN PRODUCTS, PO Box 2060, Woodland, CA 95776
Products: As well as their Nutty Corn cereal, they make a variety of crackers and 'puffs' made mostly with potato flour called NO FRIES. They taste great, but unfortunately they contain rice flour, so they can't be eaten with proteins and some of their products contain sour cream making a starch and protein combination. But when you can eat rice, enjoy the following NO FRIES varieties: Puffs: Potato Snacks, BBQ Potato Snacks, Cheese Puff Snacks and Crackers: Plain Potato Snacks, BBQ, Au Gratin and Tortilla Crackers: Plain.

PURITY FOODS INC., 2871 W Jolly Rd, Okemos, MI 48864, (517) 351-9231, FAX (517) 351-9391
Products: They specialize in Spelt flour products, some of their noodles are made without eggs, they sell Delta Fiber flakes (a sugarbeet fiber flake,) and sell 'white' and whole spelt flours.

SHAFFER, CLARKE AND CO., 3 Parkland Dr, Damien, CT 06820-3639, (203) 655-3555
Products: RyVita crackers: two all rye flour crackers, Tasty Dark Rye and Tasty Light Rye.

SOURCES FOR NATURAL SWEETENERS

SUCANAT NO. AMERICAN CORP., 58 Meadowbrook Parkway, Milford, NH 03055
Products: Sucanat granulated cane juice.

SUNRIDER INTERNATIONAL, 1625 Abalone Ave, Torrance, CA 90501, (310) 781-3808
Products: Stevia extract--this product can NOT be sold as a sweetener, but is part of their facial products. That won't stop you from using it as a sweetener if you wish. Call their L.A. number and ask for your local Sunrider distributor.

T AND A GOURMET, (800)762-2135
Products: rice syrup, fruit jams and syrups (THE BEST!!!)

BODY-ECOLOGY CO. , Donna Gates, 327 Buckhead Ave, Atlanta, GA 30305 (800)896-7838.
Products: white stevia powder

SOURCE FOR NATURAL TOBACCO

SANTA FE NATURAL TOBACCO CO., PO Box 25140, Santa Fe, NM 87504-5140, (800)332-5595,
(505) 982-4257, FAX 1-(505) 982-0156
Products: They sell natural tobacco (Natural American Spirit brand) in filtered cigarettes,
non-filtered cigarettes, menthol filter cigarettes, pouch tobacco, a pow-wow mix, natural tobacco leaves
and all kinds of accessories. All their tobacco's are chemical-free.

SOURCES FOR NO-VINEGAR SALSA

GARDEN OF EATIN,' INC, 5300 Santa Monica Blvd., Los Angeles, CA 90029, (213) 462-5406,
FAX (213) 462-3268
Products: Great Garlic Salsa and Hot Habanero Salsa

GARDEN VALLEY NATURALS, 1333 Marsten Rd, Burlingame, CA 94010, (415) 579-5565
Products: no-vinegar salsa

UNCLE GRANTS FOODS, PO Box 210638, San Francisco, CA 94121
Products: no-vinegar salsa

TABLE 4 - ASSOCIATION OF VITAMINS/MINERALS & DEFICIENCIES

Listing of Vitamins and Minerals and their typical deficiency symptoms. For more information,
I suggest you read *The Nutrition Almanac* by Nutrition Search, Inc. for a concise overview of how the
vitamins and minerals work in your body, and Adelle Davis's *Let's Eat Right to Keep Fit* for a more
in-depth study.

Vitamins are either fat-soluble or water-soluble. That is, fat-soluble vitamins must have fats
present to be properly utilized and can be easily stored in the body. Water-soluble vitamins are easily
flushed from the body with little or no storage abilities.

VITAMIN A -- A fat-soluble vitamin.
NEEDED FOR: maintaining good vision, resisting infections, development of bones and tooth
enamel, good appetite, good digestion, reproductions, lactation, the formation of red and white blood
corpuscles, the promotion of longevity and resistance to senility!

NATURAL SOURCES: apricots, butter, cream, egg yolks, fish-liver oils, green veggies like spinach, yellow veggies like carrots and winter squashes, green pasture crops like alfalfa, liver, seaweeds, yams and sweet potatoes.

DEFICIENCIES CAUSE:

eyes:	eye strain	mucus membranes:	infections:
bad night vision	eyeball pain	develop poorly	boils
burning	hair:	aids bacteria production	carbuncles
inflamed	dandruff	skin:	impetigo
itching	dry, lackluster	acne, blackheads	warts
light sensitive	fingernails:	dry	whiteheads
sties	ridged, peel easily	'goose pimples'	

VITAMIN B COMPLEX -- A water-soluble vitamin.

There are quite a few different substances that make up the Vitamin B's. They are: Biotin, Choline, Folic Acid, Inositol, PABA (Para-aminobenzoic Acid,) Thiamine (B1,) Riboflavin (B2,) Niacin (B3,) Pyridoxine (B6,) Cyanocobalatin (B12,) Orotic Acid (B13,) Pangamic acid (B15,) and Laetrile (B17.) Since they must all be available to make any one of them usable, I am going to list their functions, sources and deficiencies all together. If you want more information on the specific B's, check out the suggested reading material.

NEEDED FOR: needed for almost every function in the body in some way and provides the body with energy, needed for fat and protein metabolism, balances the nervous system by keeping the nerves healthy, keeps the intestines strong, keeps the eyes, hair, liver, mouth and skin healthy.

NATURAL SOURCES: acidophilus, brewer's yeast, green veggies, kefir, liver, whole grains, yogurt

VITAMIN B DEFICIENCIES CAUSE:

bad breath	hair:	mouth:	skin cont'd:
blood:	baldness	canker sores	psoriasis
anemia	graying	corner cracks	scaly
high blood pressure	thinning	lip sores	tingling
high cholesterol	headaches	tender gums	tongue:
constipation	hormone imbalances	nails:	bacteria-coated
dizziness	hypoglycemia	brittle	enlarged or
eyes:	insomnia	moons	swollen
burning	loss of memory	ridged	grooved
cornea changes	moods:	splitting	red-tipped
dilation	confusion	poor appetite	shiny
fatigue	depression	skin:	ulcers
gritty	irritability	acne	
poor vision	nervousness	burning feet	
heart::	stressed	eczema	
disease	suicidal	edema	
irregularities	tiredness	oily	

VITAMIN C -- A water-soluble vitamin.

NEEDED FOR: maintains health of skin, ligament and bone connective tissue, heals wounds and burns, helps form red blood cells, prevents hemorrhaging, fights off infections and allergens, works with amino acids, calcium, folic acid, riboflavin, pantothenic acid, thiamine, Vitamin A and Vitamin E.

NATURAL SOURCES: fresh fruits and veggies.

DEFICIENCIES CAUSE:

blood:	heart attacks	joint problems	shortness of breath
anemia	nosebleeds	low resistance	skin:
bleeding gums	strokes	poor digestion	flexibility
capillary health	bones:	poor lactation	overall health
clotting	slow healing	teeth - cavities	

VITAMIN D -- A fat-soluble vitamin.

NEEDED FOR: need for bone formation, absorption of calcium, normal childhood growth, normal blood clotting, and heart action, for maintaining a healthy nervous system, and for breaking down and using phosphorus.

NATURAL SOURCES: Our bodies make Vitamin D by first interacting with sunlight and surface skin oils. Fish and fish oils are the only natural source.

DEFICIENCIES CAUSE:

bones:	muscles:	poor calcium absorption
enlarged joints	numbness	poor metabolism
rickets	spasms	poor teeth
weak formation	tingling	hormone imbalances
nearsightedness		

VITAMIN E -- A fat-soluble vitamin.

NEEDED FOR: stops oxidizing of oxygen in the blood so aids the use of Vit. A, B, C and E by increasing muscle action, increasing endurance and stamina, dilating blood vessels, carrying nutrients, strengthening blood walls, and protecting red blood cells. It helps eyesight, hormone balance, the flushing of toxins and is needed in every cell.

NATURAL SOURCES: veggie oils, nuts, seeds, and soybeans.

DEFICIENCIES CAUSE:

blood problems:	phlebitis	hormone imbalances	sterility
anemia	strokes	enlarge prostate	old age spots
clots	varicose veins	infertility	
heart attacks	internal fatty deposits	premature birth w/deficits	

VITAMIN F -- A fat-soluble vitamin consisting of unsaturated fatty acids.

NEEDED FOR: regulates rate of blood clotting, breaks up cholesterol, keeps adrenals and thyroid functioning properly, keeps skin, nerves and mucus membranes cells healthy, helps calcium, phosphorus and Vitamin A absorption.

NATURAL SOURCES: veggie oils

DEFICIENCIES CAUSE:

allergies	hair:	heart disease	skin:
diarrhea	brittle	kidney problems	acne
gallstones	dandruff	nail problems	dry
poor teeth	dull	weight loss	eczema

VITAMIN K -- A fat-soluble vitamin.

NEEDED FOR: blood clotting, glucose storage, liver functions, vitality and longevity.

NATURAL SOURCES: green veggies and plants, seaweeds, milk, yogurt, eggs, molasses, oils and intestinal bacteria.

DEFICIENCIES CAUSE:

nosebleeds	diarrhea
hemorrhaging	malabsorption
slow clotting	miscarriages

VITAMIN P OR BIOFLAVONOIDS-- A water-soluble vitamin.

NEEDED FOR: proper use of Vit. C and together for: healthy collagen, capillary strength and permeability, to prevent hemorrhages and infections.

NATURAL SOURCES: all fruits and veggies, especially apricots, blackberries, cherries, currants, grapefruits, grapes, lemons, plums, and rosehips.

DEFICIENCIES CAUSE:

blood:	heart attacks	bones:	shortness of breath
anemia	intense bruising	slow healing	skin:
bleeding gums	nosebleeds	joint problems	flexibility
capillary health	strokes	low resistance	overall health
clotting	poor lactation	poor digestion	teeth/cavities

VITAMIN T -- A fat-soluble vitamin.

NEEDED FOR: keeping the blood healthy by promoting blood platelet formation.

NATURAL SOURCES: egg yolks and sesame seeds.

DEFICIENCIES CAUSE:

anemia	hemophilia	memory loss

VITAMIN U -- A water-soluble vitamin.

NEEDED FOR: the health of the intestinal tract

NATURAL SOURCES: fresh, raw cabbage and homemade sauerkraut.
DEFICIENCIES CAUSE:

colitis	stomach ulcers	intestinal lesions

ALUMINUM

NEEDED FOR: No one is sure what aluminum is good for in the body, though it appears naturally in animal and plant foods. Negative affects are known. Ranges of 10-100 mg. is normal in a daily diet, but higher levels move into poisoning levels.
ALUMINUM OVERDOSES CAUSE:

digestion:	diarrhea	low energy	skin:
colic	loss of appetite	muscle twitches	excessive sweat
colitis	nausea		numbness
constipation			outbreaks

CALCIUM

Like many nutrients, calcium needs other vitamins and minerals present to properly function. Actually, calcium needs alot of help; it needs magnesium, phosphorus, and vitamins A, C and D. Calcium is the most abundant mineral in the body.

NEEDED FOR: builds and maintains bones and teeth, builds healthy blood, regulates heartbeat, balances blood clotting and ph levels, works with nerve health to maintain muscle balance, helps the passage of nutrients and toxins in and out of the cells, gets some enzymes going, and aids the use of iron.

NATURAL SOURCES: dairy products and green veggies
DEFICIENCIES CAUSE:

bones:	heart:	muscles:
brittle	palpitation	cramps
deformities	slowed pulse	irritability
rickets	tooth decay	joint pains
slow growth	nervousness	numbness
insomnia		tingling

CHLORINE

Chlorine is found in the body formed with potassium or sodium, as in table salt, sodium chloride.

NEEDED FOR: regulates the body ph, balances the nutrient/toxin flow in and out of the cells, increases HCL, helps the liver filter the blood of toxins, keeps flexibility in the tendons and joints, and helps hormones get around in the body.

NATURAL SOURCES: sea greens and seaweeds, olives and rye
DEFICIENCIES CAUSE:

intestinal distress	muscle weakness	teeth/gum problems	thinning hair

COBALT
NEEDED FOR: making of Vit. B12, maintains proper functioning of all the cells, especially the blood cells, and kicks enzymes into action.

NATURAL SOURCES: meats, especially liver, milk products, seaweeds

DEFICIENCIES CAUSE:

nerve disorders	pernicious anemia	stunted growth

COPPER
NEEDED FOR: proper formation of hemoglobin and red blood cells, skin and hair colorations, health of nerve endings, helps utilized Vit. C, helps enzyme production, builds elastin, bones and RNA.

NATURAL SOURCES: almonds, green leafy veggies, sprouted legumes, liver and whole grains.

DEFICIENCIES CAUSE: It's not clear what copper deficiencies cause except that it's linked to iron deficiency problems like acne, anemia, edema, kwashiorkor, labored breathing, and low energy.

FLUORINE
Fluorine is present in every cell in the body.

NEEDED FOR: strengthening the bones and protecting against tooth decay.

NATURAL SOURCES: seafood and greens and gelatin.

DEFICIENCIES CAUSE: tooth decay

OVERDOSES CAUSE: a malfunction in the use of vitamins by the body, inhibits enzyme production and attacks brain cells.

IODINE
NEEDED FOR: maintaining the general healthy of the thyroid gland by aiding body energy, growth and development, metabolism rate, fat burning and the general health of hair, skin, teeth and nails; speech, mental alertness and cholesterol balance are all maintained.

NATURAL SOURCES: all sea plants and animals, mushrooms and the herb, Irish Moss.

DEFICIENCIES CAUSE:

dry hair	heart:	slow digestion	nervous
goiters	rapid beat	thyroid problems	weight problems
irritable	palpitations		

IRON
NEEDED FOR: making hemoglobin with proteins and copper, giving the red color to blood, and transporting oxygen in the body; needed for the making of enzymes to break down proteins.

NATURAL SOURCES: organ meats, lean meats and leafy green veggies.

DEFICIENCIES CAUSE:

anemia	labored breathing	constipation
bad nails	low energy	pale skin coloring

MAGNESIUM

NEEDED FOR: helps the absorption of other minerals and Vit. B, C, and E, helps building of bones, maintains nerves and muscles, balances ph levels, gets starch enzymes going, helps the amino acids, stabilizes body temperatures, and balances blood sugar levels.

NATURAL SOURCES: chlorophyll and green veggies, nuts (especially almonds,) seeds, corn, figs, soybeans, apples.

DEFICIENCIES CAUSE:

moods:	related to:	alcoholism	blood clots
confused	calcium deposits	hypoglycemia	heart disease
disoriented	diarrhea	kidney problems	high-starch diet
tentative	diabetes	vomiting	

MANGANESE

NEEDED FOR: activating several enzymes that utilize Vit. B and C, works with fatty acids and cholesterol, is part of the makeup of proteins, carbohydrates, and fats, helps bone development, helps form blood and urea, helps produce milk, balances sex hormones and balances the nervous system.

NATURAL SOURCES: green veggies, egg yolks and whole grains

DEFICIENCIES CAUSE:

dizziness	in infants:	deafness
hearing problems	blindness	paralysis
hypoglycemia	convulsions	lack of muscle coordination

MOLYBDENUM

Molybdenum is found in practically all foods we eat and no known deficiency effects are known.

NEEDED FOR: major part of 2 important enzymes in the use of iron and fats.

NATURAL SOURCES: dark leafy greens, sprouted legumes, whole grains

OVERDOSES CAUSE: anemia, depressed growth, diarrhea.

PHOSPHORUS

This is the second most common mineral in the body, is in all the cells and plays a part in most body actions.

NEEDED FOR: growth, repair, reproduction and maintenance of the cells, maintains body energy, needed for absorption of several Vit. B's, needed for bone and tooth growth, nerve health and kidney functions, help ph balance, sex hormone balance and pull substances through the cell walls.

NATURAL SOURCES: all meats and fish, eggs, nuts, seeds and whole grains.

DEFICIENCIES CAUSE:

bones:	rickets	confusion	weight:
arthritis	stunted growth	irregular breathing	overweight
disorders	tooth decay	low energy	underweight
pyorrhea	nervousness		

POTASSIUM

High salt and low fruit and veggie intake can throw out the balance of potassium.

NEEDED FOR: regulates flow of nutrients/toxins into the cells, needed for healthy nerves, normal growth, and a balance of ph, keeps the skin, heartbeat and muscle system healthy, functions with calcium, helps change glucose to glycogen, stimulates the kidneys, helps the liver, metabolism enzymes, and amino acid levels.

NATURAL SOURCES: all veggies, especially leafy greens, potatoes, bananas, oranges, sunflower seeds, mint family and whole grains.

DEFICIENCIES CAUSE:

acne	dry skin	muscle disorders	diarrhea
constipation	heart irregularity	nerve disorders	insomnia
diabetes	hormone imbalances	poor reflexes	sodium increases

SELENIUM

NEEDED FOR: promotes fertility, general growth, tissue elasticity, and works with Vit. E.

NATURAL SOURCES: veggies, especially broccoli, onions, and tomatoes, whole grain brans and germs, and in tuna.

DEFICIENCIES CAUSE: loss of skin elasticity and early aging.

SODIUM

NEEDED FOR: pulls nutrients/toxins out of the cells, balances ph levels, helps muscle contraction and nerve stimulation, keeps minerals in the blood soluble, keeps the lymph system healthy, aids protein digestion and other enzyme production.

NATURAL SOURCES: fish and meats, seaweeds, carrots and beets

DEFICIENCIES CAUSE:

arthritis	nerve pains	vomiting	joint problems
gas	small muscle development	weight loss	

SULFUR

NEEDED FOR: keeps the hair and skin healthy through collagen production, helps maintain nails, regulates insulin, works with Vit. B's and lipoic acid for healthy nerves, releases energy through proper use of oxygen, helps with overall body health.

NATURAL SOURCES: meats, fish, sprouted legumes, nuts, cabbage family, and eggs.

DEFICIENCIES CAUSE: There are no known symptoms.

ZINC

NEEDED FOR: needed for absorption of most vitamins and minerals, especially B's, is a part of most digestive enzymes, insulin, and DNA, promotes healthy growth, reproduction, hormone balance, starch and phosphorus metabolism, helps heal wounds and burns, and is needed for alcohol breakdown.

NATURAL SOURCES: most proteins, brewer's yeast, pumpkin seeds, whole grains.
ZINC DEFICIENCIES CAUSE:

atherosclerosis	infections	poor healing	heart problems
confusion	liver problems	prostate problems	poor appetite
dwarfism	loss of taste	sterility	ulcers
fatigue	retarded growth		

TABLE 5 - HERBS AS SOURCES FOR VITAMINS AND MINERALS

The following is a list of herbs that are known to be good sources of their corresponding vitamins and minerals; these herbs can all be ingested on a regular basis as food supplements. This list is reprinted from *Herbally Yours*, by Penny C. Royal.

There are other herbs that are also high in individual vitamins and minerals, but since they also work on specific areas in the body, it is not wise to take large amounts of them for long periods of time. I have listed them in parenthesis.

VITAMIN A	Alfalfa, Burdock, Cayenne, (Dandelion,) Garlic, Kelp, (Marshmallow,) Papaya, Parsley, (Pokeweed,) Raspberry, Red Clover, (Saffron,) Watercress, (Yellow Dock.)
VITAMIN B-1	Cayenne, (Dandelion,) (Fenugreek,) Kelp, (Thiamine) Parsley, Raspberry.
VITAMIN B-2	Alfalfa, Burdock, (Dandelion,) (Fenugreek,) (Riboflavin) Kelp, Parsley, (Saffron,) Watercress.
VITAMIN B-3	Alfalfa, Burdock, (Dandelion,) (Fenugreek,) (Niacin) Kelp, Parsley, (Sage.)
VITAMIN B-6 (Pyridoxine)	Alfalfa.
VITAMIN B-12 (Cyanocobalamin; Cobalt)	Alfalfa, Kelp.
VITAMIN C	Alfalfa, Burdock, (Boneset,) Catnip, Cayenne, Chickweed, Comfrey, (Dandelion) Garlic, (Hawthorn,) (Horseradish,) Kelp, (Lobelia,) Parsley, Plantain, (Pokeweed,) Papaya, Raspberry, Rose Hips, Shepherd's Purse, Strawberry, Watercress, (Yellow Dock.)

VITAMIN D	Alfalfa, Watercress.
VITAMIN E	Alfalfa, (Dandelion,) Kelp, Raspberry, Rose Hips, Watercress.
VITAMIN G	Alfalfa, Cayenne, (Dandelion,) (Gota Kola,) Kelp.
VITAMIN K	Alfalfa, Plantain, Shepherd's Purse.
VITAMIN P (Rutin)	(Dandelion,) Rose Hips, (Rue.)
VITAMIN T	Plantain.
VITAMIN U	Alfalfa.
ALUMINUM	Alfalfa.
CALCIUM	Alfalfa, (Blue Cohosh,) (Camomile,) Cayenne, (Dandelion,) (Horsetail,) (Irish Moss,) Kelp, (Mistletoe,) Nettle, Parsley, Plantain, (Pokeweed,) Raspberry, Rose Hips, Shepherd's Purse, (Yellow Dock.)
CHLOROPHYLL	Alfalfa.
CHLORINE	Alfalfa, (Dandelion,) Kelp, Parsley, Raspberry.
COPPER	Kelp, Parsley.
FLUORINE	Garlic.
IODINE	Dulse, Garlic, (Irish Moss,) Kelp, (Sarsaparilla.)
IRON	Alfalfa, Burdock, (Blue Cohosh,) Cayenne, (Dandelion,) Dulse, Kelp, Mullein, Nettle, Parsley, (Pokeweed,) (Rhubarb,) Rose Hips, (Yellow Dock.)
LITHIUM	Kelp.
MAGNESIUM	Alfalfa, (Blue Cohosh,) Cayenne, (Dandelion,) Kelp, (Mistletoe,) Mullein, Peppermint, (Primrose,) Raspberry, (Willow,) (Wintergreen.)

MANGANESE   Kelp.

PHOSPHORUS   Alfalfa, (Blue Cohosh,) (Caraway,) Cayenne, Chickweed,(Dandelion,)
                           Garlic, (Irish Moss,) Kelp, (Licorice,) Parsley, Purslane, (Pokeweed,)
                           Raspberry, Rose Hips, Watercress, (Yellow Dock.)

POTASSIUM   Alfalfa, (Blue Cohosh,) (Birch,) Borage, (Camomile,) Clotsfoot,
                           Comfrey, (Centaury,) (Dandelion,) Dulse, Eyebright, (Fennel,) (Irish
                           Moss,) Kelp, (Mistletoe,) Mullein, Nettle, Papaya, Parsley, Peppermint,
                           Plantain, (Primrose,) Raspberry, Shepherd's Purse, (White Oak Bark,)
                           (Wintergreen,) (Yarrow.)

SELENIUM   Kelp.

SILICON   Alfalfa, (Blue Cohosh,) (Burdock,) (Horsetail,) Kelp, Nettle.

SODIUM   Alfalfa, (Dandelion,) Dulse, (Fennel,) (Irish Moss,) Kelp, (Mistletoe,)
                           Parsley, Shepherd's Purse, (Willow.)

SULFUR   Alfalfa, (Burdock,) Cayenne, Coltsfoot, Eyebright, (Fennel,)
                           Garlic, (Irish Moss,) Kelp, Mullein, Nettle, Parsley, Plantain,
                           Raspberry, (Sage,) Shepherd's Purse, (Thyme.)

ZINC   Kelp, (Marshmallow.)

TRACE MINERALS   Kelp.
(Boron, Bromine, Nickel,
Strontium, Vanadium)

TABLE 6 - CHEMICAL ANALYSIS

VITALFA, ALFALFA CONCENTRATE POWDERS, A-30 AND A-100

NUTRITIONAL INFORMATION: On the average* a 100 gram portion of Alfalfa Concentrate
Powder contains the following:

Calories	289 (approx)		
Crude protein (nx6.25)	23 g	or	23.00%
Crude Fat (either extract)	4.20 g.	or	4.20%
Carbohydrates (Nitrogen fee extract)	39.80 g.	or	39.80%
Crude Fiber	15.00 g.	or	15.00%
Ash (Mineral Matter)	12.00 g.	or	12.00%
Moisture	6.00 g.	or	6.00%

VITAMIN and MINERAL PROXIMATE* ANALYSIS (per 100/grams):

Vitamin A (as Beta Carotene)	15,000.00 I.U.	Para-Amino Benzoic Acid	1.00 ppm.
Vitamin E	20.90 I.U.	Calcium	1,750.00 mg.
Vitamin K	8.00 mg.	Phosphorus	500.00 mg.
Ascorbic Acid (Vit. C)	50.00 mg.	Iron	300.00 mg.
Thiamin (Vit B1)	.55 mg.	Iodine	.90 mg.
Riboflavin (Vit B2)	1.50 mg.	Zinc	12.00 mg.
Niacin or Niacinamide	9.00 mg	Magnesium	900.00 mg.
Pyridoxine (Vit B6)	1.20 mg.	Copper	.50 mg.
Folacin (Folic Acid)	1.00 mg.	Potassium	3,800.00 mg.
Biotin	100.00 mcg.	Sodium	350.00 mg
Inositol	680.00 mg.	Selenium	.78 ppm.
Choline	2.50 mg.	Manganese	8.10 mg.
Pantothenic Acid	6.00 mg.	Nickel	2.00 mg.

A Test Laboratories Company

BEE POLLEN CHEMICAL ANALYSIS

In general, one ounce or two tablespoons of Bee Pollen contain:

28 Calories   7 grams of Carbohydrates
15% Lecithin   25% Protein

VITAMINS

	%		%
Provitamin A	5-9 mg.	Folic Acid	5 mcg.
Vitamin B-1	9.2 mcg.	Inositol	5 mcg.
Vitamin B-2	5 mcg.	Pantothenic Acid	20-50 mcg.
Vitamin B-3	5 mcg.	Rutin	13-16 mg.
Vitamin B-5	5 mcg.	Vitamin C	5 mcg.
Vitamin B-6	5 mcg.	Vitamin D	5 mcg.
Biotin	5 mcg.	Vitamin K	5 mcg.
Choline	5 mcg.		

MINERALS

Boron	trace	Molydbenum	trace
Calcium	1-15% of ash	Phosphorus	1-20% of ash
Chlorine	trace	Potassium	20-45% of ash
Copper	.05-.08% of ash	Silica	2-10% of ash
Iodine	trace	Sodium	trace
Iron	1-12% of ash	Sulphur	1% of ash
Magnesium	1-12% of ash	Titanium	trace
Manganese	1.4% of ash	Zinc	trace

MICRO-NUTRIENTS -- trace amounts

Alpha-Amino-Butyric Acid	Kinins
Auxins	Lycopene
Brassins	Monoglycerides
Crocetin	Nucleosides
Diglycerides	Peutosaus
Gibberellins	Triglycerides
Guanine	Vernine
Hexodecanol	Xanthine
Hypoxalthine	Zeaxanthin

ENZYMES and COENZYMES

Amylase	Lactic dehydrogenase
Catalase	Pectase
Cozymase	Phosphatase
Cytochrome systems	Saccharase
Diaphorase	Succinic dehydrogenase
Disstase	

FATS and OILS

Alpha-amino butyric acid	
Fatty acid 5%	Hexadecanol .14%

FATTY ACIDS from Conifer Pollen

Arachidic -- C-20	Limolenic -- C-18
Benemic -- C-22	Linoleic -- C-18**
Brucic -- C-22	Myristic -- C-14
Capric -- C-10	Oleic -- C-18**
Caproic -- C-6	Palmitic -- C-16**
Caprylic -- C-8	Palmitoleic -- C-15
Eicosanoic -- C-20	Stearic -- C-18**
Lauric -- C-12	Uncowa -- C-18
	**Major fatty acids

PIGMENTS

Ammpcyamin--in hand-collect only	Lycopene
Carotates--Alpha and Beta Carotenes	Xannmepayll
Chlorophyin hand-collected only	Zaaxanmin
Crocetin	

PROTEINS, GLOBULINS, PEPTONES, AMINO ACIDS

Alanine	trace	Leucine	5.6 %
Arginine	4.7 %	Lysine	5.7 %
Aspartic Acid	trace	Methionine	1.7 %
Butyric Acid	trace	Phenylalanine	3.5 %

Cystine	0.6 %	Proline	trace
Glutamic Acid	9.1 %	Serine	trace
Glycine	trace	Thresonine	4.6 %
Histidine	1.5 %	Tryptophan	1.6 %
Hydroxyproline	trace	Tyrosine	trace
Isoleucine	4.7 %		

CARBOHYDRATES

Gums, Pentosans, Cellulose	Total Sugars
Sporonine	Sucrose
Starch	Levulose or fructose
	Glucose

MISCELLANEOUS

Amines	Nuclein
Flavonoids	Phenolic Acids
Glucoside of Isorhanetin	Resins
Glycosides of Quercetir	Selenium
Growth Factors	Steroids
Growth Inhibitors	Tarpenes
Lecithin	Waxes
Nucleic Acids	

Reprinted from: TSI--Total Success Inc., 7975 N. Hayden Rd. Ste #A-201, Scottsdale, AZ 85258 (800)824-7888 Operator 552 or for California (800)852-7777 Operator 552.

BARLEY GREEN ANALYSIS
By Volume

Fiber	0.1 to 1.0%	Carbohydrates	23.0 to 40.0%	
Chlorophyll	0.9 to 1.5%	Protein	25.0 to 48.0%	Fats (lipids)
1.5 to 4.5%				

Minerals	15.0 to 25.0%	**Vitamins**	
(per 100 grams)		Carotene	52,000 IU.
Calcium	1,108 mg.	B1	1.29 mg.
Copper	1.36 mg.	B2	2.75 mg.
Iron	15.8 mg.	B6	0.03 mg.
Magnesium	224.7 mg.	Biotin	48.0 mg.
Phosphorus	594 mg.	Choline	260 mg.
Potassium	8,880 mg.	Folic Acid	640 mg.
Sodium	775 mg.	Pantothenic	2.48 mg.
Zinc	7.33 mg.	Nicotinic Acid	10.6 mg.
		C	238 mg.
		E	51 mg.
		Chlorophyll	1,490 mg.

Reprinted from *GREEN BARLEY ESSENCE, the Ideal "Fast Food"* by Yoshihide Hagiwara, M.D.

LIQUID LIFE ANALYSIS and BODY BOOSTER
BODY BOOSTER contains only trace minerals listed below. Reprinted from label panel:

Potassium	500 mg.	Vitamin B1	87 mg.
Magnesium	100 mg.	B2	9 mg.
Calcium	25 mg.	B3	1 mg.
Zinc	10 mg.	B5	1 mg.
Selenium	50 mcg.	B12	60 mcg.
Chromium	50 mcg.	Folic Acid	12 mg.
Vitamin C	60 mg.	Biotin	16 mg.
Vitamin A	500 IU	Pantothenic Acid	625 mg.
Vitamin D3	40 mg.	Iron	965 mg.
Vitamin E	3 IU	Copper	0.78 mg.

Trace Amounts of the following:

Calcium	Cerium	Lanthanum	Samarium
Chloride	Cesium	Lead	Scandium
Magnesium	Chromium	Lithium	Selenium
Phosphorus	Cobalt	Lutelium	Silicon
Potassium	Copper	Manganese	Silver
Sodium	Dysprosium	Mercury	Strontium
Sulfur	Erbium	Molybdenum	Tartalum
Arsenic	Europium	Neodymium	Terbium
Aluminum	Fluorine	Nickel	Thulium
Barium	Gadolinum	Niobium	Tin
Beryllium	Gallium	Nitrogen	Titanium
Boron	Holmium	Oxygen	Vanadium
Bromine	Hydrogen	Praseodymium	Yterbium
Cadmium	Iodine	Rubidium	Yttrium
Carbon	Iron	Ruthenium	Zinc
			Zirconium

MEZOTRACE ANALYSIS
Each FOUR TABLETS contains an average of the following amounts:

		%R.D.A.*
Calcium	1,300 mg.	163%
Magnesium	800 mg.	229%
Phosphorus	3.0 mg.	.39%
Iron	2.5 mg.	25%
Copper	41 mcg.	2.5%
Zinc	81.0 mcg.	.54%
Iodine	6.5 mcg.	4.3%

Sodium	1.2 mg.	**
Potassium	2.5 mg.	**
Sulphur	350 mcg.	**
Molybdenum	52.0 mcg.	**
Manganese	240 mcg.	**
Chromium	27.0 mcg.	**
Selenium	71.0 mcg.	**

Trace Elements:

Bismuth	Gallium	Silver
Boron*	Germanium	Strontium
Bromine*	Gold	Tin
Chlorine	Hydrogen	Tungsten
Cobalt	Lithium	Vanadium
Fluorine	Nitrogen	Zirconium

QUINOA ANALYSIS:

Reprinted from Eden Foods, Inc. and pertains to Eden Quinoa only.

Information on Cholesterol content provided for individuals who, on the advice of a physician, are modifying their total dietary intake of cholesterol.

NUTRITIONAL INFORMATION: Serving size 2 oz.

Calories 200	Protein 8 g	Carbohydrates 38 g
Fat 4 g	Cholesterol 0 mg/100 g	Sodium less than 30 mg
Potassium 270 mg		

PERCENTAGE OF U.S. RDA

Protein	10 %	Iron	15 %
Vitamin A	*	Vitamin D	*
Vitamin C	*	Vitamin E	6 %
Thiamine, B-1	25 %	Vitamin B-6	15
Riboflavin, B-2	10 %	Vitamin B-12	*
Niacin--B-3	2 %	Phosphorus	25 %
Calcium	2 %	Zinc	8 %

* Contains less that 2% of the U.S. RDA.

TOTAL AMINO ACID PROFILE-MG/G

Alanine	6.21	Lysine	8.43
Arginine	11.10	Methionine	1.68
Aspartic Acid	12.50	Phenylalanine	5.74
Cycstine	1.39	Proline	6.19
Glycine	8.27	Serine	6.37
Glutamic Acid	20.60	Threonine	5.24
Histidine	4.96	Tryptophan	1.69
Isoleucine	5.13	Tyrosine	3.82
Leucine	9.03	Valine	6.29

PINES WHEAT GRASS and GREEN BARLEY ANALYSIS

Nutrient	Total	% US RDA
Calories	29	**
Protein	2,630 mg.	4.63
Carbohydrates	4 g.	**
Sodium	3 mg.	**

Antioxidants

	Total	% US RDA
Beta-carotene		
(in Vit. A units)	5005 I/U	91.00
Vitamin C	32 mg.	53.00
Vitamin E	3 mg.	33.80

Vitamins

	Total	% US RDA
Vitamin K	46 mcg.	1100.00
Thiamine	29 mcg.	2.25
Choline	3 mg.	150.00
Riboflavin	203 mcg.	13.00
Pyridoxine	129 mcg.	7.26
Vitamin B12	3 mcg.	150.00
Niacin	752 mcg.	4.50
Pantothenic Acid	240 mcg.	**
Biotin	11 mcg.	**
Folic Acid	109 mcg.	57.50

Minerals

	Total	% US RDA
Calcium	52 mg.	6.50
Phosphorus	52 mg.	6.50
Potassium	320 mg.	**
Magnesium	10 mg.	3.20
Iron	6 mg.	50.00
Selenium	10 mcg.	16.00
Zinc	50 mcg.	***
Iodine	20 mcg.	13.00
Copper	.06 mg.	**
Cobalt	5 mcg.	**
Sulphur	20 mg.	**
Other Trace minerals	369 mg.	**

Amino Acids

Lysine	83 mg.	Histidine	46 mg.
Arginine	112 mg.	Aspartic Acid	223 mg.
Threonin	106 mg.	Glutamic Acid	243 mg.
Proline	94 mg.	Glycine	117 mg.
Alanine	137 mg.	Valine	126 mg.
Isoleucine	89 mg.	Leucine	163 mg.
Tyrosine	52 mg.	Phenylalanine	109 mg.
Methionine	43 mg.	Cystine	23 mg.
Tryptophan	11 mg.	Arnide	29 mg.
Purines	6 mg.	Serine	243 mg.

Superoxide Dismutase (SOD)   31,450 I/U

Chlorophyll   53 mg.

Crude Fiber   1,620 mg.

(Based on 21 tabs. or 3 tsp. powder)

** No Recommended Daily Allowance has been established.

*** Contains less than 2% of RDA.

TABLE 7 - COMMUNITY SUPPORTED AGRICULTURE
FARMS AROUND THE U.S.

For more information write or call: BIO-DYNAMIC Farming & Gardening Assn.
PO Box 550, Kimberton, PA 19442, (610) 935-7797

ALABAMA
CSA, Rt. 1 Box 306-D, Coker, AL 35452

ARKANSAS
DRIPPING SPRINGS GARDEN, Rt. 4 Box 158, Huntsville, AR 72740

CALIFORNIA
HOMELESS GARDEN PROJECT, 219 Pearl St., Santa Cruz, CA 95060
MARKLEY FARM, 17148 Old Bambetta Rd., Mokalumme Hill CA 93245
MOORE RANCH CSA, 5844 Castina Pass Rd., Carpinteria, CA 93013

COLORADO
COMMUNITY SERVICE AGRICULTURE, 1090 Rock Creek Canyon Rd., Colorado Springs CO 80926
HAPPY HEART FARM CSA, 2820 W. Elizabeth, Ft. Collins, CO 80521

CONNECTICUT
MILL RIVER VALLEY GARDENS, 3600 Ridge Rd, North Haven, CT 06473
NW CONNECTICUT CSA, Town Street, Cornwall, CT 06796

GEORGIA
CSA, Box 163, Talking Rock, GA 30175
UNION AGRICULTURAL INSTITUTE, Rt. 4 Box 4635, Blairsville, GA 30512

ILLINOIS
WHITE OAK FARM CSA, Bear Creek Rd. Rt. 4, Pana, IL 62557

INDIANA
EARTHWORKS, 9805 Union Rd., Plymouth, IN 46563

KENTUCKY
RENAISSANCE FARM, Rt. 3, Bedford, KY 40006

MAINE
BEECH HILL FARM, HCR 62 Box 307, Mt. Desert, ME 04660
CSA, RR 1 Box 471, Anon, ME 04911

CSA, RR 1 Box 2151, Morrill, ME 04952
THE TURKEY FARM, RFD 1, Box 2445, Rt. 27, New Sharon, ME 04955
WILLOW POND FARM, RR 2 Box 4105, Rt. 9, Sabettus, ME 04735
WOOD PRAIRIE FARM, RFD 1 Box 164, Bridgewater, ME 04735

MARYLAND
CHESAPEAKE CSA, 11904 Old Marlboro Pike, Upper Marlboro, MD 20772
CSA, 4621 S. Chelsea Ln., Bethesda, MD 20814
CSA, 5760 Brookswoods Rd., Lothian, MD 20711
CSA EHRHARDT ORGANIC FARM, 1032 Hoffmaster Rd., Knoxville, MD 21758
EARTH PATH, 16820 York Rd., Hereford, MD 2111

MASSACHUSETTS
BROOKFIELD FARM, 4 Hulst Road, Amherst, MA 01002
CARETAKER FARM, Hancock Rd., Williamstown, MA 01267
CSA at NEW ALCHEMY INSTITUTE, 237 Hatchville Rd, E. Falmouth, MA 02536
INDIAN LINE FARM, RR 3 Box 85, Jug End Road, Great Barrington, MA 01230
MAHAIWE HARVEST CSA, RD 2, East Rd., W. Stockbridge, MA 01266
MARLBOROUGH COMMUNITY FARM, Box 705, Marlborough, MA 01701
STEARNS ORGANIC FARM, 859 Edmonds Rd, Framingham, MA 01701

MICHIGAN
COMMUNITY FARM OF ANN ARBOR, 1283 W. Huron River Dr, Dexter, MI 48130
COMMUNITY HARVEST PROGRAM, 7831 E. Main St, Kalamazoo, MI 49001

MINNESOTA
CAMPHILL VILLAGE MN, Rt 3 Box 249, Sauk Centre, MN 56378
COMMON HARVEST COMMUNITY FARM, 2406 31st Ave S., Minneapolis, MN 56406
CSA, Rt. 1 Box 405, Park Rapids, MN 65470
THE SECRET GARDEN, Rt. 1 Box 404, Park Rapids, MN 56470

MISSOURI
CSA, PO Box 110, Dutzow, MO 63342
NELSON and SON FAMILY FARMS, Rt. 2 Box 79, Lincoln, MO 65338

MONTANA
DIXON PARTNERSHIP FARM, PO Box 26, Dixon, MT 59831

NEW HAMPSHIRE
EARLE FAMILY FARM, RFD Box 27, Ctr. Conway, NH 03813

HOLLYHOCK GARDENS, 674 Old Walpole Rd, Surry, NH 03431
TEMPLE-WILTON COMMUNITY FARM, RR 1, W. Wilton, NH 03086

NEW JERSEY
CSA AT GENESIS FARM, Silver Lake Rd, RD 3 Box290A, Blaintown, NJ 07825
WATERSHED ORGANIC FARM, 260 Wargo Rd, Pennington, NJ 08534

NEW MEXICO
BENEFICIAL FARMS CSA, 366 Ojo de la Vaca, Santa Fe, NM 87505
FARMS FOR FAMILIES CSA, 26 Sile Road, Pena Blanca, NM 87041
TIERRA MADRE ORGANIC CSA, PO Box 142, Ojo Calliente, NM 87549

NEW YORK
BEAN POLE FARM CSA, PO Box 14063, Fredonia, NY 14063
CRESSET-RICHVIEW CSA, RD 1, Britt Rd, Aurora, NY 13026
CSA GARDEN, 34 Park St., Buffalo, NY 14201
CSA OF KINGSTON, Box 1399, Manor Lake Farm, Kingston, NY 12401
DAMASCUS RD. COMMUNITY GARDEN, PO Box 1603, East Quogue, NY 11942
FULL CIRCLE FARM, Box 2078, Sag Harbor, NY 11963
PROMISED LAND FARM, PO Box 1728, Amagansett L.I., NY 11930
ROSE VALLEY FARM, Rose Valley Farm, Rose, NY 14542
ROXBURY ORGANIC FARM, RD 1 Box 186-D, Hudson, NY 12534
SEEDS, 5954 Rt. 41, Homer, NY 13077

NORTH CAROLINA
UWHARRIE FARM, Rt. 5 Box 256, Ashboro, NC 27203
WALK SOFTLY CSA, Rt. 2 Box 201, Born Creek, NC 27207

OHIO
LAKE-GRAUGA CSA, 1345 Brakeman Rd., Leroy Township, OH 44077
RIVERBEND FARM, 30500 Ferguson Rd., Tippacanoe, OH 44699

PENNSYLVANIA
C.H. VILLAGE/KIMBERTON HILLS, PO Box 155, Kimberton, PA 19442
CSA, 929 Georgetown Rd, Paradise, PA 17562
CSA OF THE POCONOS, RD 1 Box 332A, Effort, PA 18330
FELLOWSHIP FARM, 107 Kathleen Drive, Coatesville, PA 19320
FLICKERVILLE MT. FARM, Rt. 1 Box 765, Warfordaburg, PA 17267
KIMBERTON CSA, PO box 192, Kimberton, PA 19442
MOURNING CLOAK FARM, RD 4, Box 5738, Newport, PA 17074
SYCAMORE GARDEN, RR 1, Box 421, Juilian, PA 16844

RHODE ISLAND
EARTHLY DELIGHTS CSA, 27 Princeton Ave, Providence, RI 02906
PHOENIX GARDENS, 358 South Rd, Wakefield, RI 02879

TENNESSEE
CSA, Box 163, Red Boiling Sprgs, TN 27150

TEXAS
CONSUMER SUPPORTED AGRICULTURE, 207 S Elanon Rd., DeSoto, TX 75115
MUSTARD SEED FARMS, 8619 FM 359, Richmond, TX 77469

VERMONT
BLUE FLAG FARM, Box 1040, Marshfield, VT 05658
CSA AT SNOW/BAKER FARM, RR 1 Box 880, Plainfield, VT 05667
INTERVALE COMMUNITY FARM, 128 Intervale Rd, Burlington, VT 05401
PEACE/CARROTS ORGANIC FARM, RD 1 Box 5380, Worcester, VT 05682
WORKING LAND FUND, Box 190, S. Stafford, VT 05070

VIRGINIA
BRAMBLE BUSH FARMS CSA, 2205 Link Road, Lynchburg, VA 24503
CIRCLE HARVEST PARTNERSHIP, PO Box 1721, Charltonville, VA 22902
JORDAN RIVER FARM, Miriam Harris, Huntly, VA 22640
SEVEN SPRINGS FARM, Rt 1. Box 229C, Check, VA 24072

WEST VIRGINIA
SLEEPY CREEK SEED CO, Box 42, Berkeley Springs, WV 25411

WISCONSIN
AQUA GAIA FARMS, 402 Water St., Cambridge, WI 53523
CSA, N3823 W. Cedar, Cambridge, WI 53523
CSA, Rt. 4 Box 460F, Elkhorn, WI
CSA, 2409 N Wahl Ave., Milwaukee, WI 53211
CSA, RR 1 Box 180, Osceola, WI 54220
CSA, 1109 Vernon St., Stoughton, WI 53569
CSA, W759 Hwy. 19, Waterloo, WI 53594
GENESSEE COMMUNITY FARM, 513 Grove St., Waulimba, WI 53186
SPRINGDALE FARM, N4544 Silver Spring Lane, Plymouth, WI 53073
SUNNYFIELD FARM, 38 Maria Drive, Elkhorn, WI 53121
WELLSPRING, 4382 Hickory Rd., West Bend, WI 53095
ZEPHYR FARM, 2625 Oaklawn Rd., Stoughton, WI 53589

Creating Heaven
ON Your Plate

A Collection of Shelley and Friends' Recipes

Featuring Recipes from
Ruty Magidish
author of
Creating Heaven ON Your Plate, Volume II

Recipes Contents

BASIC BALANCER DIET RECIPE LIST

HOW TO MAKE SECTION
- COCONUT MILK
- GHEE
- SPROUTED BEANS & LEGUMES
- SPROUTED SOY MILK
- SPROUTED WHEAT FLAKES
- SPROUTED WHEAT FLOUR
- YOGURT CHEESE

BEVERAGES
- COCONUT CAROB DRINK
- CREAM SODA & GINGER ALE
- BANANA YOGURT SMOOTHIE
- DATE SMOOTHIE
- LASSI

BREADS
- ABBY'S CORN MUFFINS
- ABBY'S CORNBREAD
- DATE BREAD
- ZUCCHINI SQUASH BREAD

CEREALS
- GRANOLA

CRACKERS
- CINNAMON MADNESS
- FLAKY CRACKERS
- GRAHAM CRACKERS
- SAVORY CRACKERS
- 'WHEAT THIN' CRACKERS

PANCAKES
- BANANA FLATS
- CORN CAKES
- CORN FRITTERS
- FINNISH PANCAKES
- POTATO PANCAKES
- PUMPKIN PANCAKES
- QUINOA PANCAKES

CRUSTS & TOPPINGS
- CORN FLAKE CRUST
- MAPLE BLISS
- MAPLE CARAMEL CRUNCH
- YOGURT CHEESE FROSTING
- YOGURT CHEESE WHIPPING CREAM

DESSERTS
- ABBY'S CAROB COOKIES
- ABBY'S YUMMY CARROT-CORN BREAD
- APRICOT BARS
- BAKED & LAYERED CHEESECAKE
- BANANA BREAD
- BASIC COOKIE RECIPE
- CAROB BROWNIES #1, #2, and #3
- CAROB CHEESECAKE
- CAROB FUDGE
- CARROT CAKE
- DREAMY POPPY SEED CAKE
- FIG MOON COOKIES
- GINGERBREAD
- MARSHA'S LACE COOKIES
- ORANGE CHEESECAKE
- QUINOA COOKIES

FROZEN GOODS
- ICE CREAM
- SORBET
- FROZEN FRUIT YOGURT
- VANILLA CUSTARD ICE CREAM

PIES
- COCONUT CREAM PIE
- COCONUT CUSTARD PIE
- MOCK PUMPKIN PIE
- PUMPKIN PIE

PUDDINGS
ABBY'S BREAKFAST PUDDING
ABBY'S PUMPKIN PUDDING
CAROB MOUSSE
QUINOA PUDDING
QUICK PUDDING

DRESSINGS
MAYO SUBSTITUTE
AVOCADO DRESSING
GAZPACHO DRESSING
GREEN GODDESS DRESSING
YOGURT HERB DRESSING

ENTREES
ABBY'S QUINOA MEXICAN STYLE
BASIC QUINOA
CHILI-CORN CASSEROLE
CORN CUSTARD
CORNBREAD CASSEROLE
EGG FOO YONG
EGG LASAGNE
EGG SALAD SANDWICH MIX
ENCHILADAS
GENTLE SAVORY QUINOA
KEFIR AND VEGETABLE PASTA
MUSHROOM CURRY
MUSHROOM-CRUST QUICHE
PIZZA
SPINACH FRITTATA
SPINACH TIMBALES
SPRINGTIME QUINOA
STIR FRY QUINOA
STUFFED GREEN PEPPERS WITH
    CHINESE BLACK MUSHROOMS
T-BOO'S SPINACH HAU PIA
VEGGIES ENCHILADAS

CHICKEN CACCIATORI
'CRABMEAT' DIP
CYNTH'S SHISH-KA-BOB
CYNTH'S SMOKED TUNA PASTA
    'ALFREDO'
DELICATE SLEEPING FISH
DIANE'S OVEN 'FRIED' CHICKEN
DIANE'S SUSHI
FISH STEW
GOURMET BROILED FISH
LOX & EGGS
MARSHA'S COCONUT-DIPPED
    CHICKEN
POACHED SALMON WITH DILL
POTATO SALMON PANCAKES
TIDEWATER CRABCAKES
YOGURT BAKED SWORDFISH STEAKS
YOGURT SALMON MOUSSE

SALADS AND SPREADS
COLD QUINOA SALAD
YOGURT CHEESE SPREAD

SAUCES
APRICOT BUTTER PRESERVES
APRICOT FOOL
APRICOT PRESERVES
FIG PRESERVES
MOLE SAUCE
SPANISH & POTATO CHUTNEY
WHITE SAUCE

SOUPS
BASIC BORSCHT
BORSCHT
CURRIED ZUCCHINI SOUP
PUMPKIN SOUP
TORTILLA SOUP
VEGETABLE CHOWDER

SPROUTED BEANS & LEGUMES
FRIJOLES
KIDNEY BEAN SALAD
LENTIL KEDGEREE
SHELLEY'S CHILI
SPROUTED BEAN CHILE
SPROUTED BEAN SOUP
SPROUTED SOYBURGERS

SPROUTED PEA SOUP
SPROUTED PEA STEW

VEGGIES
CYNTH'S FENNEL SAUTE W/CARAWAY
MARSHA'S GNOCCHI
T-BOO'S TURNIPS

DEEP CLEANSER DIET RECIPE LIST

HOW TO MAKE SECTION
GHEE
SPROUTED BEANS
SPROUTED SOY MILK
SPROUTED WHEAT FLAKES
SPROUTED WHEAT FLOUR
YOGURT CHEESE

BEVERAGES
CREAM SODA/GINGER ALE
BANANA YOGURT SMOOTHIE
DATE SMOOTHIE
LASSI

BREADS
DATE BREAD
ZUCCHINI SQUASH BREAD

CEREALS
GRANOLA

CRACKERS
CINNAMON MADNESS
FLAKY CRACKERS
GRAHAM CRACKERS
SAVORY CRACKERS
'WHEAT THIN' CRACKERS

PANCAKES
FINNISH PANCAKES
POTATO PANCAKES
PUMPKIN PANCAKES
QUINOA PANCAKES

CRUSTS & TOPPINGS
MAPLE BLISS
MAPLE CARAMEL CRUNCH
YOGURT CHEESE FROSTING
YOGURT CHEESE WHIPPING CREAM

DESSERTS
ABBY'S CAROB COOKIES
ABBY'S YUMMY CARROT-CORN BREAD
APRICOT BARS
BAKED & LAYERED CHEESECAKE
BANANA BREAD
BASIC COOKIE RECIPE
CAROB BROWNIES #1, #2 and #3
CAROB CHEESECAKE
CAROB FUDGE
CARROT CAKE
DREAMY POPPY SEED CAKE
FIG MOON COOKIES
GINGERBREAD
MARSHA'S LACE COOKIES
ORANGE CHEESECAKE
QUINOA COOKIES

FROZEN GOODS
ICE CREAM, SORBERT
FROZEN FRUIT YOGURT

PIES
MOCK PUMPKIN PIE
PUMPKIN PIE

PUDDINGS
ABBY'S BREAKFAST PUDDING
ABBY'S PUMPKIN PUDDING
CAROB MOUSSE
QUINOA PUDDING
QUICK PUDDING

DRESSINGS
MAYO SUBSTITUTE
AVOCADO DRESSING
GAZPACHO DRESSING
GREEN GODDESS DRESSING
YOGURT HERB DRESSING

ENTREES
ABBY'S QUINOA MEXICAN STYLE
BASIC QUINOA
CORN CUSTARD
EGG FOO YONG
EGG LASAGNE
EGG SALAD SANDWICH MIX
ENCHILADAS
GENTLE SAVORY QUINOA
MUSHROOM CURRY
MUSHROOM-CRUST QUICHE
PIZZA
SPINACH FRITTATA
SPINACH TIMBALES
SPRINGTIME QUINOA
STIR FRY QUINOA
STUFFED GREEN PEPPERS W/CHINESE
    BLACK MUSHROOMS
VEGGIES ENCHILADAS

ENTREES WITH FISH & CHICKEN
'CRABMEAT' DIP
CYNTH'S SMOKED TUNA PASTA
    'ALFREDO'
DELICATE SLEEPING FISH
DIANE'S SUSHI
FISH STEW
GOURMET BROILED FISH
LOX & EGGS
POACHED SALMON WITH DILL
POTATO SALMON PANCAKES
TIDEWATER CRABCAKES
YOGURT BAKED SWORDFISH STEAKS
YOGURT SALMON MOUSSE
SALADS AND SPREADS
COLD QUINOA SALAD
YOGURT CHEESE SPREAD

SAUCES
APRICOT BUTTER PRESERVE
APRICOT FOOL
APRICOT PRESERVES
FIG PRESERVES
MOLE SAUCE
SPANISH & POTATO CHUTNEY
WHITE SAUCE

SOUPS
BASIC BORSCHT
BORSCHT
CURRIED ZUCCHINI SOUP
PUMPKIN SOUP
TORTILLA SOUP
VEGETABLE CHOWDER

SPROUTED BEANS & LEGUMES
FRIJOLES
KIDNEY BEAN SALAD
LENTIL KEDGEREE
OLD-FASHIONED BAKED BEANS

SHELLEY'S CHILI
SPROUTED BEAN CHILE
SPROUTED BEAN SOUP
SPROUTED SOYBURGERS
SPROUTED SOYBURGERS
SPROUTED SPLIT PEA SOUP
SPROUTED SPLIT PEA STEW

VEGGIES
CYNTH'S FENNEL SAUTE W/CARAWAY
MARSHA'S GNOCCHI
T-BOO'S TURNIPS

SUPER CLEANSER DIET RECIPE LIST

HOW TO MAKE SECTION
GHEE
YOGURT CHEESE

BEVERAGES
CREAM SODA
DATE SMOOTHIE

BREADS
ZUCCHINI SQUASH BREAD

CEREALS
GRANOLA

CRACKERS
CINNAMON MADNESS
FLAKY CRACKERS
SAVORY CRACKERS

PANCAKES
FINNISH PANCAKES
PUMPKIN PANCAKES
QUINOA PANCAKES

CRUSTS & TOPPINGS
MAPLE BLISS
MAPLE CARAMEL CRUNCH
YOGURT CHEESE FROSTING
YOGURT CHEESE WHIPPING CREAM

DESSERTS
BAKED & LAYERED CHEESECAKE
APRICOT BARS
CAROB BROWNIES #1, #2, and #3
CAROB CHEESECAKE
CAROB FUDGE
CARROT CAKE
DREAMY POPPY SEED CAKE
GINGERBREAD
MARSHA'S LACE COOKIES
ORANGE CHEESECAKE
QUINOA COOKIES

FROZEN GOODS
ICE CREAM
FROZEN FRUIT YOGURT

PIES
PUMPKIN PIE

PUDDING
ABBY'S BREAKFAST PUDDING
ABBY'S PUMPKIN PUDDING
CAROB MOUSSE
QUINOA PUDDING
QUICK PUDDING

DRESSINGS
    MAYO SUBSTITUTE
    AVOCADO DRESSING
    GREEN GODDESS DRESSING
    YOGURT HERB DRESSING

ENTREES
    BASIC QUINOA
    EGG LASAGNE
    EGG SALAD SANDWICH MIX
    GENTLE SAVORY QUINOA
    SPINACH FRITTATA
    SPINACH TIMBALES
    SPRINGTIME QUINOA

ENTREES WITH FISH & CHICKEN
    CYNTH'S SMOKED TUNA PASTA
        'ALFREDO'
    DIANE'S SUSHI
    GOURMET BROILED FISH
    LOX & EGGS

    POACHED SALMON WITH DILL
    POTATO SALMON PANCAKES
    TIDEWATER CRABCAKES
    YOGURT BAKED SWORDFISH STEAKS
    YOGURT SALMON MOUSSE

SALADS AND SPREADS
    COLD QUINOA SALAD
    YOGURT CHEESE SPREAD

SAUCES
    APRICOT BUTTER PRESERVE
    APRICOT FOOL
    APRICOT PRESERVES
    WHITE SAUCE

SOUPS
    BASIC BORSCHT
    CURRIED ZUCCHINI SOUP
    PUMPKIN SOUP

A companion book of recipes, *"Creating Heaven ON Your Plate, Volume II"* includes scores of additional recipes organized by diet programs outlined in this book. Available Spring, 1996. To order, write or call Warm Snow Publishers, Box 75, Torreon, NM 87061, 800-235-6570.

RECIPES - GENERAL COOKING SUGGESTIONS

⇨   All diets can use extracts, like vanilla, in cooking.

⇨   Baking sodas and powders are fine for all diets.

⇨   Salt is always an optional ingredient.

⇨   Experiment and have fun!!!

⇨   If you are following Basic Diet #3, remember to keep foods in your life simple.

⇨   Quinoa and Panocha flours can be used in any recipe you convert, but be aware neither will hold as much oils as regular flour. Try cutting fat needed in half and adding an extra egg for more moisture.

⇨   When you convert a baked goods recipe, decrease overall liquid amounts because of liquid sweeteners.

⇨   ABOUT USING HERBS: The only way to learn about herbs and spices is to use your nose! Smell what you are cooking and then sniff different herbs and spices and see which ones go well together. Keep sniffing the food as you add flavors to it and then go to the different seasonings.

⇨   ABOUT MICROWAVES: I don't suggest you use them. Radiation doesn't seem to be the problem. It seems they kill the life-force in the food, so it's truly like eating something dead.

⇨   Spray-on PAM and other lecithin-based butter and oil alternatives are fine to use.

⇨   Please note: I don't use the food category called 'carbohydrates.' This group of foods is made of fruits, veggies, beans, legumes and starches, like grains and soy products. It's important to divide this group into individual sections because of different ways they digest and because of future digestive rules.

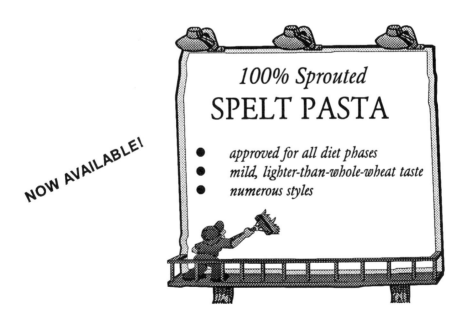

NOW AVAILABLE!

100% Sprouted
SPELT PASTA

- *approved for all diet phases*
- *mild, lighter-than-whole-wheat taste*
- *numerous styles*

For more information, write:
The Summers Approach PASTA Co.,
P.O. Box 216, Torreon, NM 87061

HOW TO MAKE COCONUT MILK
For Basic Diet #1

A rich milk for sauces, puddings, or a super-rich drink. Blend for 3 minutes:

1 c. shredded dried coconut	3 c. water
1 tsp sweetener	a pinch of salt

Strain. Makes 2+ c.

MAKING COLD-PROCESSED COFFEE EXTRACT
For Diets From Phase 4 Diet and Beyond

Mix in a large bowl:

1 lb. coffee, regular grind	12 c. cold water

Let this sit on the counter for 36 hours. Filter the grounds and liquid extract. **Refrigerate the extract. For 1 cup of coffee (taking cup size, extract strength, and personal taste into account):

1-4 tbsp. extract	boiling hot water

*Note: *'The Toddy'* coffee maker is a commercial product for making cold-processed coffee. My proportions are different and come with alot of experimenting to get the most for your money!

I use a 3-qt. strainer lined with moist coffee filters. Scoop most of the grounds onto the filters to hold them in place. Run all the rest of the liquid through the grounds, saving it in jars. I usually run 1-2 cups of plain cold water over the grounds and mix this slightly diluted extract equally through the stronger mix. And remember this coffee digests as a fruit!!!

HOW TO MAKE GHEE
All Basic Diets

Ghee is clarified butter, that is, butter with the excess water and few protein molecules skimmed off or cooked out of the oil. One of the advantages of ghee is that it can be heated to high temperatures without burning, since the excess water and proteins are what makes butter burn easily.

HOW TO SPROUT BEANS AND LEGUMES

Sprouting beans and legumes (that is, peas and lentils) changes them from a starch product which is indigestible (hence all that gas) to a vegetable that is a pure delight!

Sprouted beans and legumes can be used in any of the recipes that regular beans and legumes are called for. I've noticed one slight taste change, and that is, some beans take on a slight sweet taste. It's never hurt anything I've ever made with them.

I suggest making enough sprouts to cook and freeze for later use, so you don't have to be sprouting them all the time. They come out of the freeze in great condition, so there's no problem there.

THE SPROUTING PROCESS

1) After rinsing the beans to remove any dust or dirt, put them in a bowl and cover them with several inches of water.

2) Let them soak up the water for 24 hours.

3) Dump them into a colander you can leave them in.

4) Cover them with a damp towel so they don't dry out.

5) Rinse them morning and evening to remove any bacteria, mold or fungus buildup.

6) Sprouted tails need to be 3/4" to 1" long. For most beans this will take 3-4 days in the colander.

BEAN SPROUTING PROBLEMS

**Always try to purchase beans and legumes that were last year's crop. As beans age they lose the ability to germinate and grow. When you are trying to sprout them, then, they only rot and get moldy.

**Only do one kind of bean in any one colander. Mixing different varieties of beans can be a problem because some of them sprout faster or slower than others.

**Beans sprout and grow in the ground only when the ground temperature gets to 70 degrees. Except for fava beans, beans are considered a hot weather crop. So, if your kitchen drops much below 70, you may have a rotting problem.

**Split peas can be sprouted, but they are very tricky. Half of them will sprout tails and the other half will start to convert its starches into sugars. But there is a time when that other half will just start to rot. You have to catch them just before that time and cook them all.

I suggest you try sprouting other beans before you try peas. Also, some health food stores now carry WHOLE dried peas. You might have better luck sprouting them.

HOW TO MAKE SPROUTED SOY MILK
For Basic Diets #1 and #2

This is a 'hot water method' of making soy milk developed by Cornell University. It produces a nutritious and good tasting milk. Using boiling water inactivates the enzyme lipoxidase which tends to make soy milk bitter tasting.

If sprouted soybeans are used, the resulting product will be digested as a vegetable by the body.

1 c sprouted soybeans	8-10 c boiling water
1 tbsp melted butter	1/4 tsp salt
2 tbsp honey	

Check soybeans over, discarding broken beans. Soak in 3 c. water for 12 hours. Rinse and Drain. Bring all the water to a rolling boil and keep it boiling. Preheat blender by using 2 c. boiling water and run blender for 2 minutes. Wrap Blender top with a towel to protect yourself from getting burned. Empty blender. Now blend 1/3 of the soaked beans with 1 1/3 c. BOILING water for 3 minutes. Strain through cheesecloth. Repeat process. Add the butter, honey and salt to the strained milk and add extra water to make 1 quart of milk. Heat strained milk in DOUBLE BOILER for 30 minutes. Refrigerate.

HOW TO MAKE SPROUTED WHEAT FLAKES
For Basic Diets #1 and #2

Soak wheat berries in water for at least 36 hours. You should just see a small tip emerging at the pointed end of the grain. You may need to change the water once or twice. Spread the soaked berries out on a hard, flat surface. Smash them flat with a rolling pin. Or cover them with a cotton cloth and smash them with a piece of 2x4. Scrap them off the surface and spread them on a screen to dry. Use wheat flakes just like rolled oats for cooking as a hot cereal, for granola, in cookies or meat loaf!

HOW TO MAKE SPROUTED WHEAT FLOUR (PANOCHA FLOUR)
For Basic Diets #1 and #2

Soak wheat berries in water for at least 36 hours. You should just see a small tip emerging at the pointed end of the grain. You may need to change the water once or twice. Spread the berries out on screens to dry, use a cool dehydrator, or dry in a 100 degree oven. When thoroughly dry, grind the berries is a regular flour mill.

HOW TO MAKE YOGURT CHEESE
For All Basic Diets

In a cheese cloth bag or a yogurt cheese funnel, pour 1 c. yogurt. Place in fridge over a container and let the excess whey drip out. Takes 12-24 hours.

RECIPES

BEVERAGES

COCONUT CAROB DRINK
For Basic Diet #1

Blend all ingredients:

1 qt. coconut milk	3 tbsp. melted butter
4 tbsp. sweetener	1 1/2 tsp. vanilla
4 tsp. carob powder	a pinch salt

CREAM SODA AND GINGER ALE
For All Basic Diets

Mix in a glass:

1 tbsp. maple syrup	3+ drops of vanilla

Pour in plain bubbly water.
For Ginger Ale, add slices of fresh ginger.

BANANA YOGURT SMOOTHIE
For Basic Diets #1 and #2

Blend until smooth.

2 c. plain yogurt	3/4 tsp cinnamon
2 overripe bananas	2 pinches nutmeg
4 tsp sweetener (or more)	1/4 tsp vanilla

Variation: add 8 tbsp peanut butter!

DATE SMOOTHIE
(Thanks to Ruty Magidish)
For All Basic Diets

Pit and slice a handful of dates. Blend with a few tbsp. of water until it is a paste.
Add into blender:

1 c. yogurt	1 c. crushed ice

(Put ice cubes in plastic bag and hammer into small pieces first.) Blend until
foamy. Add and blend optional ingredients of:

1 egg	1 tsp. carob powder

LASSI
For All Basic Diets

Blend until smooth:

1 c. yogurt	3/4 c. water
6 tbsp sweetener (or to taste)	1/4 c. ground cardamom
8 drops rose water	

BREADS

ABBY'S CORN MUFFINS
(Thanks to Abby Remer, NY)
For Basic Diet #1

Mix together:

1 c. cornmeal	3 tsp. baking powder
1 c. quinoa flour	1 1/2 tsp. baking soda

Separately cream together:

1 egg	1/4 c. butter
1/4 c. maple syrup	

Add to creamed mix:

1 c. yogurt or kefir

Mix dry and wet ingredients. Pour into greased muffin tin. Bake at 375° for 20
minutes.

Variations:

Add 1 c. corn kernels.

Add grated zucchini, mashed bananas and another tbsp. maple syrup.

ABBY'S CORNBREAD
(Thanks to Abby Remer)
For Basic Diet #1

In mixing bowl, combine:

1 1/2 c. cornmeal	1 1/2 tsp. baking soda
1/2 quinoa flour	1 tsp. salt (opt.)
3 tsp. baking powder	

In a separate bowl, beat together:

1 egg	1/4 c. soft butter
1 c. yogurt or kefir	

Add flour mixture into liquids. Pour into greased 9" skillet that has been heated for 3 minutes. Bake at 375° for 20 minutes or until center is done.

Variations:

Add 3+ tsp. poppy seeds and few drops lemon extract.

Cut a piece in half, through cornbread, and fry for a quick pancake.

DATE BREAD
(Thanks to Ruty Magidish)
For Basic Diets #1 and #2

Preheat oven on lowest setting, then turn off. In a bowl, combine and rub into breadcrumbs:

1 c. quinoa flour	3 tbsp. butter

Soften 1 cube/envelope/tbsp. baking yeast in 3 tbsp. warm water. Make a well in the center of the flour mix and pour in yeast. Add and mix into a soft yet manageable dough:

1 egg	1/4 tsp. salt

Flour your table with quinoa flour. Roll out dough. Make into a rectangle 1/8" thick. Pit and blend into a paste:

a handful of dates	water or yogurt to blend

Spread paste over dough with a rubber spatula. Roll the dough up into a sausage, from the long side of the rectangle and across it. Gently place on a buttered cookie sheet and let rise in the pre-warmed (and turned off) oven for 30-60 minutes. Remove bread and heat oven up to 350*. Bake for 30 minutes. Serve with Maple Bliss or plain with tea.

ZUCCHINI SQUASH BREAD
For All Basic Diets

Mix together:

    1 1/2 c. each quinoa & corn flour or 3 c. quinoa flour

    1 tsp. baking soda   1/2 tsp. salt

    2 tsp. cinnamon   1/2 tsp. baking powder

Cream together:

    1 c. maple syrup   1/2-1 c. melted butter

    3 eggs

Add 1 c. grated or 3 c. sliced zucchini. Mix dry and wet ingredients. Bake in 2 greased pans at 350° for 1 hour or longer.

CEREALS

GRANOLA
For All Basic Diets

Mix together:

    3 c. sprouted wheat flakes   or quinoa flakes

    or air-popped popcorn (broken or blended into small pieces)

    Delta Fiber flakes   or any combination of them

Mix together:

    1/3-1/2 c. liquid sweetener   1 tsp. vanilla or almond extract

    1/4-1/3 c. melted butter   pinch of cinnamon

Coat all dry ingredients with liquid mix. Spread out on a greased cookie sheet. Bake at 250° for about 1 hour stirring occasionally. When toasted mix is cool add any ONE of the following:

    coconut, shredded (can be stirred into toasting mix also)

    dates, chopped

    dried bananas or apricots, chopped

CRACKERS

CINNAMON MADNESS
(Thanks to Ruty Magidish)
For All Basic Diets

Following the Flaky Cracker Recipe directions below, combine:

    1/2 stick butter   1 pinch baking powder

    1 c. quinoa flour   1 pinch baking soda

    1 1/2 tsp. cinnamon   1 egg, slightly beaten

    4 tbsp. maple syrup

Before baking, brush top with a thin film of maple syrup and cinnamon. Serve with fresh fruit as dessert.

FLAKY CRACKERS
(Thanks to Ruty Magidish)
For All Basic Diets

Cut into chunks 1 stick butter.
Add:

> 1 1/3 c. quinoa flour   1 tbsp. maple syrup
> 1 pinch baking powder

Rub between fingers until it resembles bread crumbs. Then press together to form dough. Shape into 1 1/2" roll or use a cookie press. Spread butter on a cookie sheet. Sprinkle quinoa flour over butter. Slice crackers off roll. Bake at 350° for 10 minutes. Remove carefully with a spatula.

Suggestions:

For freshly cooked crackers, for a special treat, keep the cracker roll in the fridge, slice off and bake in the toaster oven! Use of a cookie press (a basic $10 item) makes the crackers into cute shapes. So does flattening the roll on two sides and making a dent on one end for a heart shape.

GRAHAM CRACKERS
For All Basic Diets

Mix:

> 2 c. panocha flour (sprouted wheat flour*)
> 1 1/2 c. quinoa flour   1/2 tsp baking powder

Add and mix:

> 3/4 c. maple syrup
> (or later, 1/4 c. molasses and 1/2 c. other liquid sweetener)
> 1/4 c. water

Let this dough stand for 30 minutes. Roll out on cookie sheet to about 1/8 inch thickness. With a long knife or spatula, make indented lines on the crust for graham cracker pieces. Bake at 350° for 25-30 minutes, until the crackers are golden. Immediately remove from cookie sheet and cool.

SAVORY CRACKERS
(Thanks to Ruty Magidish)
For All Basic Diets

Following the Flaky Cracker Recipe directions above, combine:

> 1 pinch salt   1 tsp. onion powder
> 1 egg   1 pinch baking powder
> 3 Tbsp. maple syrup   1/3 tsp. paprika
> 1 stick butter, in chunks   1/2 tsp. finely minced garlic
> 1 1/2 c. corn or quinoa flour

Serve with fish stew or as hors d'oeurves, topped with yogurt or kefir cheese or veggies.

"WHEAT THIN" CRACKERS
For All Basic Diets

Mix:

    2 c. panocha flour (sprouted wheat flour*)
    1 1/2 c. quinoa flour
    3/4 tsp. baking powder
    herbs and spices to taste (I usually use cayenne, onion and garlic powders
    and green chili flakes)

Add and mix 1 1/2 c. water. Let the dough stand for 30 minutes. Roll out very thinly on cookie sheets and cut into 1" x 1" squares. Bake at 350° for 20-25 minutes. Remove immediately from the cookie sheet with a spatula.

PANCAKES

BANANA FLATS
For Basic Diet #1

Mix:

    1 c. corn flour   3/8 tsp. baking soda
    a pinch of salt

In a separate bowl mix together:

    2 eggs   1/2 c. yogurt
    1/2 c. water

Mix flour and liquid together until smooth. Peel 3 bananas, cut in 1/2, then in 1/3's, lengthwise. Dip banana lengths in batter and fry on hot griddle.

CORN CAKES
For Basic Diet #1

Mix:

    1/2 c. yellow corn flour   1/2 c. white corn flour
    1/2 tsp. baking soda

In a separate bowl, beat together:

    1/2 c. yogurt   1 egg
    1/2 water   1 tbsp. maple syrup

Mix corn and liquids together. Cook on hot griddle.

CORN FRITTERS
For Basic Diet #1

Grate off ears 2 cups of fresh corn. Mix into corn:

    2 egg yolks   1 tsp. sweetener
    1/2 tsp. salt

Beat until stiff and then fold into corn mixture:

2 egg whites   2 pinches cream of tartar

Fry over medium heat by dropping spoonfuls into hot butter.

Serving suggestions: For Breakfast: serve with maple syrup. To eat with soup or salad: add 4 tbsp. chopped parsley and a pinch onion powder to batter.

FINNISH PANCAKE
For All Basic Diets

Melt 4 Tbsp. butter in deep dish pan. Mix together:

2 c. yogurt with 2 Tbsp. cornstarch mixed in 1 c. quinoa flour

4 Tbsp. maple syrup   4 eggs

1/4 tsp. salt

Pour into baking dish. Bake at 350° till golden. Serve with butter and maple syrup.

POTATO PANCAKES
For Basic Diets #1 and #2

Grate on finest blade and squeeze all liquid out, leaving 2 heaping c. peeled, raw potatoes. Add:

2 beaten eggs   2 tbsp. onion, finely chopped

1 tsp. salt

Drop by spoonfuls into hot butter and fry until golden brown on both sides. These are great served with sour cream and apple sauce.

PUMPKIN PANCAKES
For All Basic Diets

For Diets 1 & 2: Combine following, let stand for 5 minutes (omit for Diet #3):

1/2 c. cornmeal   1 c. boiling water

Mix together (and with above, if appropriate)

1 c. yogurt   1 Tbsp. soft butter

1 egg, slightly beaten   1 Tbsp. maple syrup

1/2 c. pumpkin puree

Add in:

1 c. quinoa flour   1 tsp. allspice

(1 1/2 c. for diet #3)   3/4 tsp. salt (opt)

2 1/2 tsp. baking powder

Fry in ghee or butter with 1/4 c. portions. Cook 1-2 minutes on each side. Top with butter and maple syrup.

QUINOA PANCAKES:
For All Basic Diets

In bowl #1, Mix together:

1 c. quinoa flour	1 3/4 tsp baking powder
1 tsp salt	1/2-1 tsp nutmeg

In bowl #2 blend together until smooth:

2 egg YOLKS	2 tbsp oil
2 tbsp melted butter	2-3 tbsp sweetener
2 ripe bananas	2 tsp vanilla (2 tsp optional)

1 c. yogurt, sour cream, or kefir
(Omit bananas for Basic Diet 3--use dates blended with yogurt)
In bowl #3 beat until stiff:

3 egg whites

Gently combine first 2 mixtures until batter is barely moist. Fold in the egg whites. The more gently you do this, the lighter the pancakes will be. Fry over moderate heat. Makes about 50 3 inches pancakes.

ZUCCHINI PANCAKES
For All Basic Diets

Combine:

3 c. grated zucchini	1 tsp. baking powder
1/2 c. quinoa flour	salt and pepper to taste

Add and mix:

1 egg, beaten

Drop mixture by large tablespoonfuls onto hot buttered griddle. Cook until brown.

CRUSTS and TOPPINGS

CORNFLAKE CRUST
For Basic Diet #1

Crush enough cornflakes to make 1 1/2 to 2 c. crumbs. Mix with:

2 Tbsp. maple syrup	2 Tbsp. soft butter

Press into pie pan for baking dish.

MAPLE BLISS BUTTER
(Thanks to Ruty Magidish)
For All Basic Diets

Make 1/2 recipe of MAPLE CARAMEL CRUNCH. While it is still warm, add:

1 stick butter

Melt together on low heat and stir in:

a dash of cinnamon

Stir until butter is completely incorporated. Pour into jar or porcelain bowl. Refrigerate and use when cool. Use as frosting/spread on DREAMY POPPY SEED CAKE or other cakes and baked goods.

MAPLE CARAMEL CRUNCH FROSTING
(Thanks to Ruty Magidish)
For All Basic Diets

In a heavy frying pan, on medium heat, slowly pour maple syrup in until it just covers the bottom. When it feels warm to the touch, add 4 heaping tbsp. plain yogurt. Stir constantly until it thickens. Immediately smear it on top of the cake. Do not attempt to cover the cake completely. Maple Crunch is best used as a quick glaze. Ideas: It is sticky enough to hold small flowers for decorations. Use half the recipe for frosting and make Maple Bliss with the rest, to spread over the cake slices!

YOGURT CHEESE FROSTING
For All Basic Diets

Mix until smooth:

1 c. YOGURT cheese	1/3 c. melted butter
3-6 tbsp. liquid sweetener	1 1/2 tsp. vanilla
drops of lemon or orange extracts to taste	

Variations: Carob Frosting: add 1/4 c. carob powder; omit rinds. Fruit Frosting: add 1/2 c. additional yogurt cheese, then add pureed dates or apricots or other fruits to taste.

YOGURT CHEESE WHIPPING CREAM
For All Basic Diets

With a hand whip, beat until fluffy:

1 c. thinned yogurt cheese (the consistency of sour cream)	
2+ tbsp. sweetener	drops of vanilla

DESSERTS: CAKES, CANDIES and COOKIES

ABBY'S CAROB COOKIES
(Thanks to Abby Remer)
For Basic Diets #1

Cream together:

    1/2 c. melted butter   1/2+ c. maple syrup

    3 eggs   2 tsp. vanilla

Separately, mix together:

    2 c. corn flour   2 c. quinoa flour

    1/2 c. carob powder

Mix together wet and dry ingredients. Add yogurt or kefir to moisten, if needed.

    Variations:

    Add unsweetened coconut.

    Change extract to 1 tsp. vanilla and 1 tsp. almond extract.

ABBY'S YUMMY CARROT-CORN BREAD
(Thanks to Abby Remmer)
For Basic Diet #1

In a saucepan, bring to a boil, stirring frequently:

    1 lb. carrots, grated   1 1/4 c. thinned yogurt or plain kefir

Simmer for 5 minutes. Stir. Remove and cool. Cream together:

    2 beaten eggs   1/2 c. maple syrup

    2 tbsp. melted butter

Add:

    2 1/2 c. corn flour   2 tsp. baking powder

    2 tsp. baking soda

Mix into carrot mix. Pour into greased loaf pan. Bake at 375° for 60-70 minutes or until knife comes out clean.

APRICOT BARS
(Thanks to Ruty Magidish)
For All Basic Diets

Mix and form a dough:

    1 1/2 c. quinoa flour   1/2 c. butter

    2 tbsp. maple syrup

Pat it into the bottom of a 9x13 pan. Bake at 350° for 15 minutes. Cool. Spread on top of dough:

    5-7 fresh apricots sliced or

    1 c. cut-up dried apricots soaked in 1 c. boiling water

Beat together and pour over apricots:

  3 eggs   2 tbsp. maple syrup

  a dash of salt

Bake at 350° for 20 minutes or until eggs are set. Cool slightly and cut into bars.

  Variations:

  Use dates or figs instead of apricots.

BAKED & LAYERED CHEESECAKE
For All Basic Diets

With the following ingredients at room temperature, cream together:

  8 oz. cream-, kefir- or yogurt cheese

  1/2 c. liquid sweetener (or to taste)

Beat and add to cheese mix:

  2 eggs   1/2 tsp. vanilla

Pour into Nut crust or Sprouted Grain crust or no crust (pour into greased pie pan)

Bake at 325° for 20 minutes or until firm.

Mix:

  2 c. sour cream or thinned yogurt cheese

  1/4 c. liquid sweetener (or to taste)

  1/2 tsp. vanilla

  1/8 tsp. cinnamon

Spread over baked cheese mix. Bake for 5 minutes at 325. Cool, then chill.

BANANA BREAD
(Thanks Cynthia Mayer)
For Basic Diets #1 and #2

Cream together:

  1/2 c. melted butter   1/2 c. maple syrup

Add in:

  (2 eggs, slightly beaten--eggs are totally optional!!)

  3 ripe, mashed bananas   juice of one lemon, or to taste

Mix in:

  1 c. quinoa flour   1/2 tsp. baking powder

  1. c. cornmeal   1/2 tsp. salt

  1/2 tsp. baking soda

Pour into greased loaf pan. Bake at 375° for 45 minutes.

BASIC COOKIE RECIPE
(Thanks to Toby Tarnow)
For All Basic Diets

Dissolve:

    1/2 tsp. baking soda   1/4 c. boiling water

Cream together:

    1 c. butter   1 c. maple syrup

Add:

    soda water   1 tsp. vanilla

Add in a little at a time:

    3 3/4 c. panocha flour

Variations:

    Add chopped dates, apricots or coconut.

    Add quinoa flakes.

Drop from spoon onto greased cookie sheet, flatten with fork. Bake at 350° for 15-20 minutes. Cool on cookie sheet.

CAROB BROWNIES #1
For All Basic Diets

Beat together:

    1/2 c. melted butter   1+ c. maple syrup (to taste)

    2 eggs   1 tsp. vanilla

Add in:

    1/2 c. carob powder

Add in:

    1 c. quinoa or panocha flour   1 tsp baking powder

Pour into 8x8 pan. Bake at 350° for 40 minutes or until toothpick comes out clean.

CAROB BROWNIES #2
For All Basic Diets

Cream together:

    1/4 c. melted butter   1/4 c. yogurt

    1/2 c. maple syrup   2 eggs

    1 tsp. vanilla

Add:

    1/2 c. carob powder   1 c. quinoa flour

    1 tsp. baking powder

Pour into 8x8 greased pan. Bake at 350° for 40 minutes or until knife comes out clean. Serve with yogurt and toasted coconut.

CAROB BROWNIES #3
(Thanks to Nancy Kintisch)
For All Basic Diets

Mix or blend:

       1 c. carob powder   2/3 c. melted butter
       1/2+ c. maple syrup

In another bowl, beat until light:

       4 eggs

Beat in carob mix. Stir in:

       5 tbsp. quinoa flour   2 tsp. vanilla

Spread evenly in a greased 9x9 pan. Bake at 325° for 30 minutes or until surface is firm.

CAROB CHEESECAKE
For All Basic Diets

Blend until velvety:

       1 c. plus 2 tbsp. sour cream (or some combo of yogurt/yogurt cheese, kefir cheese, or kefir to match the consistency of sour cream)
       4 eggs   2 c. or more of maple syrup
       1/4 c. soft butter

While blending, drop in bits of:

       1 1/2 lbs. kefir cheese or yogurt cheese

Add in:

       1-3 tsp. rum extract   8 tbsp. carob powder
       1 tsp. almond extract   1 tsp each cinnamon

Line a 9" x 13" pan with a nut crust or Sprouted Grain crust or grease pie pan directly. Pour filling into crust or pan. Bake at 350° for 35-40 minutes or until a toothpick comes out clean. Cool and spread with 1 c. sweetened sour cream or yogurt. Great decorated with fruit on top!

CAROB FUDGE
For All Basic Diets

Mix into a smooth, stiff dough:

       1 tbsp. soft butter   1/2 c. carob powder
       1/2 tsp. vanilla   1/4 c. + 1 tbsp. sweetener

Add toasted quinoa flakes for a crunch. Spread in a pan or roll in balls. Chill.

CARROT CAKE
For All Basic Diets

Cream together:

       1 1/2 c. soft butter   2 c. maple syrup

Beat in 4 eggs.

Sift into creamed mixture and mix well:

       2 c. quinoa flour   2 tsp. baking powder

       2 tsp cinnamon

Let dough stand for 10 minutes. Stir in:

       2 c. grated carrots

Turn into greased and floured pans. Bake at 350° (35-40 minutes for two 9" pans) (55 minutes for 9x13.) Cool for 10 minutes and turn onto cake rakes. Frost with Yogurt Cheese Frosting.

DREAMY POPPY SEED CAKE
(Thanks to Ruty Magidish)
For All Basic Diets

Preheat oven to 350°. Separate 4 eggs. Beat whites until stiff. Cream together:

       1 stick butter   1/4 c. maple syrup

When smooth, add the egg yolks. Mix in:

       4 heaping tbsp. quinoa flour

Rub butter into a shallow baking dish and, using 1 c. poppy seeds, cover it with seeds. (Any pan shape will do, but a ring shape is great.) Add remaining poppy seeds to batter and mix well. Gently fold in egg whites. Pour batter into baking dish and bake for 30 minutes until a toothpick comes out clean. Frost sparingly with Maple Caramel Crunch and spread with Maple Bliss and tea..

FIG MOON COOKIES
(Thanks to Ruty Madidish)
For Basic Diets #1 and #2

Mix the following to form a dough:

       a handful of fresh or dried figs, rinsed and finely minced

       (if hard and dry, soak in a cup of boiling water until soft)

       1 1/4 c. quinoa flour   1/2 c. soft butter

       2 tbsp. maple syrup   1 tsp. baking powder

       a dash each cinnamon, nutmeg and cloves

With a tbsp. of dough, shape into circles. Place on a greased cookie sheet. Refrigerate until firm. Bake at 350° for 15 minutes, until dry but NOT brown. When cool, pack into a plastic bag and keep in an airtight container. Serve with tea.

GINGERBREAD
For All Basic Diets

Cream together:

> 1/2 c. honey
> 1/2 c. maple syrup
> 1 tbsp. butter

Beat and cream into above until smooth:

> 2 eggs

Add and mix well:

> 2 1/2 c. panocha or quinoa flour
> 2 tbsp. ground ginger
> 1 tsp. baking powder
> 1 tsp. cinnamon
> 1/2 tsp. nutmeg

Spread in 8x8" greased and floured pan. Bake at 350° for 25-30 minutes.

MARSHA'S LACE COOKIES
(Thanks to Marsha Porcell)
For All Basic Diets

Bring to a boil and froth:

> 1/2 c. maple syrup   1/2 c. butter

Turn off heat and add:

> 1/3 quinoa flour

Spoon onto cookie sheet. They will spread alot. Bake at 350° for 8 minutes or until lightly brown around edges — time will vary based on size of cookie. Spatula carefully onto a plate. They will be very soft when removed and will harden within seconds after removal from the cookie sheet. They can be rolled immediately and filled with preserves, frosting, or whatever when cool. Store in closed container.

ORANGE CHEESECAKE
For All Basic Diets

Blend:

> 2 c. Yogurt or kefir cheese   1+ tsp. orange extract
> 2 eggs   1/8 tsp. almond extract

In a small saucepan, heat until dissolved:

> 6 tbsp. flaked Agar-Agar   1/2 c. maple syrup

Slowly beat agar-agar into cheese mixture. Pour into a prepared Quinoa Pie Crust or a greased pan. Chill for at least 4 hours.

QUINOA COOKIES
For All Basic Diets

For the Basic Recipe, cream together:

  1/4 c. soft butter   1 c. maple syrup

Add in and beat until smooth:

  1 egg   1 tsp vanilla

Add:

  2 c. quinoa flour

Put small spoonfuls on oiled cookie sheet. Flatten with a fork. Bake at 325° for 18-20 minutes.

 Variations:

  <u>Anise Cookies</u>: Add 1/2 tsp Anise Extract INSTEAD of the vanilla. Crushed Anise seeds can also be added.

  <u>Ginger Snaps</u>: Add 1 tbsp ginger powder or more to taste.

  <u>Lemon Drops</u>: Omit vanilla and add 1 tsp lemon extract

  <u>Date Cookies</u>: Add 1/2-1 cup chopped dates.

FROZEN GOODIES

There are a number of brand name ice cream makers out there, that are simple and easy to use. The one I own, a Donvier, has a small metal tub that you freeze. Then you make the 'ice cream' mixture in the blender and pour it into the center of the frozen tub. A paddle goes into the mix and the lid and turn-handle go on top.

As the mixture freezes against the side of the tub, the paddle scrapes it off. With a few turns of the paddle and 20 minutes, you have a great frozen treat! For information on ordering the Donvier Ice Cream Maker, call (800)235-6570 for a catalog.

Several of the following recipes can also be done in ice trays. They are the ones with Slippery Elm added to them. For some reason Slippery Elm powder keeps the ice crystals from forming for a day or two. It also gives a slight malt taste to the mixture.

REMEMBER: If it tastes good in the blender, it will taste good frozen!!!

ICE CREAM
For All Basic Diets
For 5 c. ice cream makers

Blend:

  3-4 eggs   1 c. sour cream or thinned yogurt

cheese

  1 c. yogurt or kefir cheese 1/2-1 c. sweetener (to taste)

  1 tsp.+ vanilla

Taste as you go along. Pour into ice cream maker and follow their directions.

Ice Cream Variations:
  French Vanilla: Add more vanilla extract to taste
  Add your favorite jam as flavoring.
  Use any of the flavored extracts.

SORBERTS
Blend:

  1/2-1 c. sour cream or thinned yogurt cheese
  3-4 eggs   3-4 c. fresh/canned/reconstituted fruit
  1/2+ c. sweetener   1 tsp. vanilla extract (optional)
Taste as you go along. Obviously, different fruits will need different amounts of sweeteners and extracts. Pour into ice cream maker and follow their directions.
Variations: Add chunks of fruit after blending is complete.

FROZEN FRUIT YOGURT
For All Basic Diets
In a mixing bowl, beat together:
  2-3 c. yogurt cheese   1 c. sweetener
  1 1/2 tsp. slippery elm powder
Add desired fruit. Spread in ice trays and freeze.

VANILLA CUSTARD ICE CREAM
For Basic Diet #1
Blend until smooth:
  1 1/2 c. grated fresh coconut   2 1/4 c. water
Strain and and enough water to make 2 1/4 c. coconut milk. Blend:
  2 c. coconut milk   3/4 c. plus 2 tbsp. melted butter
  1 tbsp honey
Refrigerate until cold and slightly thickened. Beat:
  5 egg yolks   1/2 c. sweetener
  1/4 c. coconut milk
Cook in double boiler, stirring constantly, until thick. Chill, then add 2 tsp. vanilla. Whip until stiff, but not dry:
  2 egg whites
Mix the coconut cream and egg yolk mixture together. Fold in the stiff egg whites. Pour into ice cube trays or shallow pans and freeze.

PIES

COCONUT CREAM PIE
(Thanks to Ruty Magidish)
For Basic Diet #1

Mix together:

      3/4 c. corn flour   1/4 c. butter

      2 tbsp. maple syrup

Press into a greased, floured pie pan.

Beat together:

      3 eggs   2 tbsp. maple syrup

      1 can coconut milk (or 1 2/3 c. coconut milk from recipe in *Beverages*)

Pour into crust. Bake at 350° for 45 minutes or until set. Serve warmish with dollop of yogurt.

COCONUT CUSTARD PIE
For Basic Diet #1

Blend until smooth:

      2 2/3 c. sour cream   7 tbsp. soft butter

      4 tsp. vanilla   1 1/3 c. coconut shreds

      2/3 c. sweetener   dash of salt

      6 eggs

Oil pie pan and dust with quinoa flour or arrowroot. Bake at 325° for approximately one hour. Sprinkle with toasted coconut 5 minutes before pie is done.

MOCK PUMPKIN PIE
Everyone will think it's pumpkin!!!
For Basic Diets #1 and #2

Blend until smooth:

      1 1/2 c. sprouted, cooked soybeans

      1 1/2 c. yogurt/sour cream/kefir

      3/4 c. sweetener   8 tsp. arrowroot

      1 tsp. ground ginger   1 tsp. cinnamon

      1/4 tsp. EACH: A few drops lemon extract to taste

         nutmeg, mace, allspice

Cook in double boiler until mixture thickens. Cool slightly.

Beat together:

      2 eggs   2 tbsp. melted butter

While constantly stirring, drizzle soybean mix into eggs. Return to double boiler and cook until thick. Pour into a prepared Walnut Crust. Bake at 350° for 25 minutes or until knife comes out clean.

PUMPKIN PIE
For All Basic Diets

Mix well:

1 1/2 c. pumpkin puree	1 tsp. cinnamon
1 egg yolk, slightly beaten	1/2 tsp. ginger
1 1/2 c. yogurt	1/4 tsp. salt
(+1 tsp corn starch)	1/4 tsp. nutmeg
1/2 c. maple syrup	1/4 tsp. cloves
2 Tbsp. melted butter	

Beat stiff 3 egg whites. Fold them carefully into rest of mix. Place in pie crust or greased pan. Bake at 450° for 10 minutes, then reduce heat to 350° for 20-25 minutes or until knife comes out clean.

PUDDINGS

ABBY'S BREAKFAST PUMPKIN PUDDING
For All Basic Diets

Mix together:

1 c. pumpkin	1-2 tsp. cinnamon
1 c. yogurt	1 tsp. vanilla
1 egg	

Pour into greased muffin tins. Bake at 400° for 40-45 minutes. Serve with yogurt and/or mashed banana.

ABBY'S PUMPKIN PUDDING
(Thanks to Abby Remer)
For All Basic Diets

Mix together:

1 c. yogurt	2 Tbsp. cinnamon
2 eggs	1 Tbsp. maple syrup
1/2-3/4 c. pumpkin puree	1 tsp. vanilla or maple extract

Pour into baking dish. Bake at 400° for 40-45 minutes.
  Variations: Add mashed banana.

A companion book of recipes, *"Creating Heaven ON Your Plate, Volume II"* includes scores of additional recipes organized by diet programs outlined in this book. To be published Spring, 1996. To order, write or call Warm Snow Publishers, Box 75, Torreon, NM 87061 USA, 800-235-6570.

CAROB MOUSSE
(Thanks to Nancy Kintisch)
For All Basic Diets

Combine in a small saucepan:

        1/4 c. water   1/4 c. carob powder

        1/4 maple syrup

Bring to a boil and simmer for 5 minutes, stirring constantly. Remove from heat and cool for 2 minutes. Mix into carob mix, gradually:

        2 egg <u>yolks</u>   2 tbsp. butter

Stir briskly over low heat until mixture thickens. Stir in 1 tsp. vanilla. Separately, beat 2 egg whites until stiff but not dry. Stir a spoonful of whites into carob mix, then fold in remainder. Combine thoroughly. Pour into 4 serving dishes and freeze for 15-20 minutes.

QUINOA PUDDING
For All Basic Diets

Beat together:

        1 c. yogurt, kefir or sour cream   3 eggs

        1/2 c. maple syrup (to taste)   1 tsp. vanilla

        1-2 drops lemon extract

Add in:

        1 1/2 c. cooked quinoa

Place in greased 8x8 pan (or 6x9 or something equivalent) and place that pan in another pan with water in it. Bake at 350° for 40 plus minutes or until a toothpick comes out clean.

  Variations:

        Add 1/2 c. of any dried or fresh fruit.

        Add carob powder to taste.

        Pour on top of a crushed corn flake crust or a sprouted grain crust.

        Mash bananas into the bottom of the pan.

QUICK 'PUDDING'
For All Basic Diets

In a cup, put:

        1/4 c. sour cream or thinned yogurt cheese

        1-2 tbsp. maple syrup

        1 tsp. carob powder (to taste)

        drops of extract (vanilla, orange, or strawberry)

Whip until smooth and frothy. Enjoy!

DRESSINGS

MAYO SUBSTITUTE
For All Basic Diets

Mix:

1 c. sour cream or yogurt/kefir cheese blend the consistency of sour cream
1/4 tsp. powdered mustard   garlic powder to taste
onion powder to taste   a dash or two of cayenne

AVOCADO DRESSING
For All Basic Diets

Blend:

2 c. yogurt (sour cream or plain kefir)
1/2 tsp. tamari (omit for Basic Diet #3)
2 lg. avocados   2 green onions
a dash garlic powder   a dash chili powder

Thin with water if needed.

GAZPACHO DRESSING
For Basic Diets #1 and #2

Blend until smooth:

1/2 c. water   2 tbsp. chopped parsley
5 tbsp. catsup   1/2 tsp. dill weed
1/4 tsp. tamari   1/2 tsp. basil
3 small tomatoes   4 thick slices cucumber
2 green onions   1/4 tsp. garlic powder
1/2 green pepper

GREEN GODDESS DRESSING
For All Basic Diets

Blend until smooth:

1/2 c. sour cream or thinned yogurt cheese
1/2 c. yogurt or kefir cheese   3 tbsp. chives, chopped
3 tbsp. chopped parsley   1 clove garlic
green onion to taste

Thin with yogurt or water if needed.

YOGURT HERB DRESSING
For All Basic Diets

Blend until smooth:

1 c. plain yogurt	1 tsp. sweetener
1/4 c. celery leaves, chopped	a few drops tamari-omit for #3
1/4 c, parsley, chopped	a pinch each: dill weed, thyme, sweet basil
1 green onion	1 clove garlic

ENTREES

ABBY'S QUINOA MEXICAN STYLE
(Thanks to Abby Remer)
For Basic Diet #1

In 1/4 c. veggie broth, braise:

1/2 c. onions, chopped	1/2 c. corn kernels
1/2 c. chopped zucchini	1 tsp. garlic, minced

Add:

3/4 c. veggie stock	1 c. juice from tomatoes
1 c. quinoa, well rinsed	1/2-1 jalapeno pepper, chopped
1 can tomatoes, drained	1/2 tsp. cumin or to taste

Reduce heat and cover. Cook for 20 minutes or until tender. Sprinkle with 2 Tbsp. chopped cilantro.

BASIC QUINOA
For All Basic Diets

Add one part quinoa to two parts boiling water. Add a tsp. of butter or oil. Cover and simmer at lowest heat for 20-30 minutes until all water is absorbed.

CHILE-CORN CASSEROLE
For Basic Diet #1

Beat well:

3/4 c. diluted sour cream or yogurt
1/3 c. olive oil
2 eggs

Stir in:

1 sm. can creamed corn or corn cut off two ears

Add and mix well:

1 c. cornmeal	2 tsp. baking powder
1/2 tsp. salt	

Pour 1/2 mixture into 9x9" casserole dish.

Spread over top:
> 3/4 c. chopped chili peppers
> 8 oz. kefir cheese, dropped onto layer in chunks

Pour on the rest of the corn mixture.

Spread over top:
> 1/4 c. chopped chili peppers
> 8 oz. kefir cheese, dropped onto layer in chunks

Bake at 350° for 50-60 minutes. or until knife comes out clean.

CORN CUSTARD
For Basic Diet #1

Beat 3 egg WHITES till they are stiff.

Beat together:

3 egg yolks	1 Tbsp. maple syrup
1 can cream corn	1 Tbsp. cornstarch
1 c. yogurt or kefir	1/2 tsp. salt
2 Tbsp. melted butter	pepper to taste

Carefully fold in stiff egg whites. Bake at 350° for 1/2 hour.

CORNBREAD CASSEROLE
For Basic Diet #1

Mix in a lg. bowl:

1 c. tomato juice or broth	3 eggs 3/4 c. water
1/4 tsp. cayenne	1/4 c. melted butter
1/4 tsp. rosemary	3/4 tsp. each: sage, thyme, savory, marjoram

Add and mix well:

5 c. dry cornbread crumbs	3 c. sprouted bread crumb
(For Basic Diet #3 use 8 c. sprouted sourdough crumbs)	
1/3 c. grated carrots	1 1/2 c. chopped chives
1/4 c. chopped parsley	1 c. celery, finely chopped
1 clove garlic, minced	
1 c. chopped mushrooms (omit for Basic Diet #3)	

Spread in a 9x13" oiled pan. Bake at 375° for 45 minutes.

Variation: Bake in 2 loaf pans for 1 1/2 hours.

EGG FOO YONG
For Basic Diets #1 and #2
Mix in a large bowl any of the following (and/or anything else,) making 3-4 cups:

Grated carrots	Chopped onions or green onions
Sprouted Mung beans	Chopped summer squashes
Chopped celery	Chopped green pepper
1-2 c. cooked quinoa	

Beat 3 eggs in a separate bowl. Add 1-2 tbsp tamari. Add eggs to veggie mix and mix thoroughly. Fry large spoonfuls of the mix (flattened out like 4-5 inch pancakes) in a pan with butter, turning them just like pancakes.

EGG LASAGNE
For All Basic Diets
Beat and fry in a 10-15" buttered pan like an flat omelette:

3 eggs	3 tbsp. water

Slide the flat omelette out onto a large, rimmed cookie sheet.
Mix together for filling:

1/2-1 c. chopped spinach	1/2 c. sliced black olives
2 8 oz. cans of tomato sauce (save 1/2 c. for topping)	

Spread filling on the half of the omelette. Drop small chunks of yogurt or kefir cheese on the filling (appx. 1/2 c.) and roll the omelette over. Cover the 'egg roll' with the remaining Tomato Sauce. Bake at 375° for 20 minutes.

EGG SALAD SANDWICH MIX
For All Basic Diets
Mix together:

> 6 hard-boiled eggs, peeled and chopped
> 1 stalk celery, chopped
> 3 green onions, chopped
> 1/2 green or red pepper, minced (omit for Diet #3)
> any of the following herbs to taste: marjoram, sweet basil, cayenne, garlic powder, pepper, oregano, dill weed, chili powder

Add and mix well: 1/4-1/2 c. Mayo Substitute.
Spread on Sprouted Bread, Sprouted Wheat Thins or salad greens.

ENCHILADAS
For Basic Diet #1

Blend until smooth:

3-4 ripe avocados	3/4 tsp. tamari
1 tsp. chili powder	1/4 tsp. cumin powder
3/4 tsp garlic powder	cayenne to taste
1 c. sour cream or yogurt	1/2 tsp. onion powder

In a large saucepan, heat this mix slightly, adding water if needed. Dip 12 corn tortillas in avocado mix and fill with any of the following:

Frijoles	olives
onions	green chiles
cooked chicken	green onions
sauteed veggies	yogurt or kefir cheese
chopped spinach	

Place rolled enchiladas in a baking dish. Pour leftover avocado mix over top. Bake for 20-30 minutes until thoroughly hot.

GENTLE SAVORY QUINOA
(Thanks to Ruty Magidish)
For All Basic Diets. An excellent bed for other dishes of veggies, fish or chicken.

Saute:

1 onion or 3 shallots or a bunch of chives

Add and mix:

1 sprig fresh tarragon	2 tbsp. butter
2 carrots, shredded	

Add and continue stirring:

1 c. quinoa

Add and bring to boil:

2 c. water

Simmer for 20 minutes.

KEFIR AND VEGETABLE PASTA
(Thanks to Corinne Smith, NY)
For Basic Diet #1

1 lb. quinoa pasta, thin spaghetti	2 med. carrots, julienned
2 med. squash sliced	4 scallions, chopped
2 tblspns. olive oil or butter	2 sliced leeks
2 tblspns. spiced mustard, opt'l.	2 stalks julienned celery
8 oz. kefir cheese or yogurt	3/4 kefir or diluted yogurt

Heat olive oil or butter and saute carrots, clery over medium heat for 5 minutes.
Add squash and scallions and leeks for 2 or 3 more minutes. Cook pasta, until al dente.

MUSHROOM CURRY
For Basic Diets #1 and #2

Saute:

2 lg. onion, chopped   1 carrot, chopped
2 cloves garlic

Add, cover and simmer for 10 minutes:

1 lb. mushrooms, sliced   1 tsp. cumin powder
4 tomatoes, chopped   1/2 tsp. cardamom powder
1 tbsp. grated ginger root   1/2 tsp. paprika
a dash cayenne   tamari to taste

Remove from heat. Stir in:

1 c. plain yogurt

Serve over sprouted wheat noodles, cooked quinoa, or sprouted bread toast.

MUSHROOM-CRUSTED QUICHE
For Basic Diets #1 and #2

CRUST:

Saute: 3/4 lb. mushrooms, finely chopped
          3 tbsp. butter

Remove from heat and add:

1/2 c. sprouted bread crumbs

Press into a 9" pie pan, evenly on sides and bottom.

FILLING:

Saute and spread on crust:

1 med. onion, chopped

Spread on top of onion:

8 oz. tub of kefir cheese, pieces dropped on layer

Blend and pour over onion-cheese layers:

3 eggs   8 oz. kefir or yogurt
dash of cayenne

Bake at 325° for 35+ minutes or until knife comes out clean.

PIZZA
For Basic Diets #1 and #2

CRUST #1:

Mix together flours of quinoa, corn and/or panocha (sprouted wheat flour) to make about 3 cups. In a jar shake together 3/4 c. water and 1/4 c. oil or melted butter. Mix the flours and liquid together and spread by hand or with a rolling pin on a 12 x 15 inch cookie sheet. (I usually pinch the sides up 1/2 inch or more to help keep all the ingredients I pile on top on the crust.)

CRUST #2:

Mix together:

    1 c. quinoa flour   1 c. panocha flour (sprouted wheat flour)

    1 c. cornmeal

Mix in 1 c. water. Knead for 10-15 minutes. The stiffer the dough, the crunchier the crust. Roll out crust to 1/4". Place in oiled cast iron pan. Oil crust.

CRUST #3:

Make a simple pancake batter with: quinoa or panocha flour, water, oil and baking powder. Pour into hot cast iron pan and let bake in oven for 5-10 minutes at 450°.

TOPPINGS:

I've listed the usual toppings I use for a 12 x 15 inch pizza but you can use anything! I tend to spice everything alot because it all mellows out as it's cooked.

    1 1/2 c. tomato sauce (I spice this up with garlic, onion powder, pepper, green chili pieces, cayenne, basil, marjoram.)

    1 lb. spiced, cooked ground turkey or chicken (again, I spice this up heavily with all the things in the sauce. If I want an Italian assuage taste I add alot of sage and thyme as well.)

    1 med. onion, chopped   1 bell pepper, chopped

    sliced mushrooms   1 can ripe olive pieces

    green chili pieces   2 med. carrots, grated

    2-3 med. tomatoes, sliced

CHEESE:

Cook the pizza for 15 minutes, pull it out and drop small pieces of yogurt/kefir cheese over the pizza, and put it back in the oven for 5 more minutes.) BAKE at 450° for 20 minutes.

QUINOA NOODLE STOVE-TOP CASSEROLE
For Basic Diet #1

In a pan with a small amount of boiling water, add:

    quinoa/corn pasta

    small pat of butter

    raw chopped veggies or dried veggies

    spices of: garlic/onion powder, cayenne, basil/marjoram/oregano, if you are adding tomato sauce, curry powder, dill if you are adding fish.

Simmer for 10+ minutes or until noodles and veggies are cooked. OR: Cook noodles with butter and spices only. When noodles are done, add already cooked veggies. For all versions, add any of the following:

    tuna or other cooked fish   tomato sauce

    spoonful of dairy: sour cream, kefir cheese or yogurt

Gently reheat and serve.

SPINACH FRITATTA
For All Basic Diets

Mix together:

1 c. chopped chives or 2 med. onions, chopped

10 eggs, beaten   2 bunches spinach, finely chopped

3 cloves garlic, minced   2 c. sprouted bread crumbs

1 c. kefir cheese in bits   1 c. chopped parsley

2 tsp. tamari (omit for Diet 3) 1/3 c. melted butter

1/2 tsp each: oregano, basil, marjoram

Spread in 9x13" oiled pan. Bake at 325° for 45 minutes.

SPINACH TIMBALES
For All Basic Diets

Steam:

1 lb. cleaned, chopped spinach

Blend with:

2 eggs, beaten   1/2 c. yogurt

1/4 tsp. nutmeg   salt and pepper to taste

1 head garlic, roasted with veggie or chicken broth

Pour into timbales molds. Bake at 375° for 45 minutes in large pan of water.

SPRINGTIME QUINOA
(Thanks to Ruty Magidish)
For All Basic Diets

Simmer and cook:

Steam (carrots will be done first) and cool:

2 c. boiling water   1 c. quinoa

2 beets   2 carrots

4 asparagus

Remove beet skins and cut into small cubes. Slice carrots. Slice asparagus into thin slices. In a small sauce pan, saute:

2 cloves garlic, finely minced

2 tbsp. butter

Add to saute:

4 stalks cilantro, very finely chopped

Pour herbs over quinoa and mix. Add and mix veggies. Serve.

STIR-FRY QUINOA
(Thanks to Ruty Magidish)
For Basic Diet #1

Stir fry:

    1 onion, chopped fine   1 tbsp. butter

    a dash salt

Add and continue to stir fry until slightly cooked:

    1/4 red cabbage, fine shredded

Pour into a bowl.

Saute for 1 minute:

    3 cloves garlic, minced   1/2" thick fresh ginger slice, minced

    1 tbsp. butter

Add and saute until wilted:

    5 mushrooms, thinly sliced

Add 2 tbsp. tamari. Remove from heat, add to the mushroom/garlic mix and toss:

    1 c. cooked quinoa

    1 c. well chopped mild greens (spinach, lettuce, chard)

    onion/cabbage mix

Beat 3 eggs and fry in butter. Cut into small rectangles. Add veggie/quinoa mix with eggs in a large bowl. Toss. Serve with chopped green onion as garnish.

STUFFED GREEN PEPPERS WITH QUINOA
& CHINESE BLACK MUSHROOMS
For Basic Diets #1 and #2

Steam 4-6 green peppers till soft but not limp. Cool.

Cook at a simmer:

    1 c. quinoa   2 c. boiling water

    1 tsp. butter

Saute in ghee or butter:

    chopped onions   chopped zucchini

    chopped parsley   chopped garlic

    chopped mushrooms   chopped softened black Chinese
                               mushrooms

Mix cooked veggies with cooked quinoa. Stuff peppers and place in greased baking dish. Bake at 350° until top is dry.

T-BOO'S SPINACH HAU PIA
(Thanks to T-Boo, NY)
For Basic Diet #1

Mix:

3 packages frozen spinach (2 c. steamed fresh)

1 c. yogurt   3 c. flaked coconut

Blend:

4 eggs   1 c. yogurt cheese
1/3 c. tamari   1 1/2 c. kefir cheese
salt to taste   1/3 c. quinoa flour

Fold into spinach/coconut mix. Spoon into ungreased 2 1/2 qt casserole dish. Refrigerate for 1-2 days. Bake uncovered at 350° for 40-45 minutes. Allow to stand before serving.

VEGGIE ENCHILADAS
For Basic Diet #1

Chop into small bite-size pieces any of the following:

carrots   onions
green beans   bell peppers
corn off the cob   summer squashes
celery   mushrooms
parsnips   peas
radishes

Saute until tender. Remove from heat. Add:

2 tbsp. tamari   1/4-1/2 tsp. cayenne

Steam or lightly fry 12 tortillas. Fold tortillas in half and fill with a large spoonful of veggie mix. Top with fresh tomatoes and yogurt cheese or sour cream.

ENTREES WITH CHICKEN OR FISH

CHICKEN CACCIATORI
(Thanks to Corinne Smith, NY)
For Basic Diet #1

1 chicken, cut up   3 c. chopped tomatoes or tomato sauce
1 cup sliced onions   1/2 cup sliced green onions
1 cup diced celery   3 cloves garlic, chopped
3 tblsp. olive oil or butter   1/2 tsp. fennel seed
1 tblsp. parsley   1/2 tblsp. oregano
1/2 or 1 c. chicken stock as needed

Put oil or butter in large fry pan and saute garlic until tender. Add chicken pieces, a few at a time, until lightly browned. Remove to oven pan. Any time the pan gets dry add a little chicken stock and scrape around. Add onions, celery, and parsley to pan with scrapings and sute until slightly tender. Add to chicken in oven pan. Add tomato sauce or tomatoes, stir and place in 350 oven for up to an hour or until chicken is tender.

'CRABMEAT' DIP
For Basic Diet #1

Blend:

    1 qt. plain yogurt   1 package fake crabmeat (pollack)
    1/2 Tbsp. Worcestershire sauce   salt to taste

Serve with baked corn chips or cold, cooked or raw veggies.

CYNTH'S SHISH-KA-BOB
(Thanks to Cynthia Scott, NY)
For Basic Diet #1

Marinate cooked, cubed chicken breast in Tandoori spices and yogurt for 5-10 hours. (Tandoori spices -- 1/8 tsp. each ground: allspice, cardamom, cinnamon, cloves, tumeric.) Alternate with chicken on the skewers any of the following:

    tomato cubes   onion cubes
    mushrooms   chunks of green or red peppers
    zucchini cubes

Broil till done, turning once.

CYNTH'S SMOKED TUNA PASTA 'ALFREDO'
(Thanks to Cynthia Scott, NY)
For All Basic Diets

Saute in butter lots of:

    sliced mushrooms   chopped cilantro
    salt and pepper to taste   sliced Spanish onions (Chives for Diet #3)

Mix in food processor or blend:

    plain yogurt   1 tbsp cornstarch
    smoked tuna fillet   some of the onion mix

Stir fish mix into sauteed veggies. Gently heat (over cooking will separate yogurt.) Serve immediately over quinoa/corn pasta or sprouted sourdough toast.
Variations: Try different veggies with onion mix.

DELICATE SLEEPING FISH
(Thanks to Ruty Magidish)
For Basic Diets #1 and #2

Slice as thinly as you can:

      2 potatoes

Coat them with 3 tbsp. melted butter. With 1/2 potatoes, line a pie pan, over-lapping them on bottom and sides. Slice thinly 1/3 lb. fish (salmon, tuna, snapper.) Layer them over the potatoes.

Mix together:

1 clove garlic, minced	fresh tarragon, dill or dried thyme
1 egg	dash of white pepper

Drizzle egg mix over fish. Layer the rest of the potatoes, working in a circular motion from the center out. Bake at 350° for 35 minutes, covered. Uncover and bake for 10 minutes.

DIANE'S OVEN 'FRIED' CHICKEN
(Thanks to Diane McNulty)
For Basic Diet #1

Slice cooked chicken breasts into 1 1/2" strips. Dip strips into yogurt.
Toss into a strong plastic bag:

1 c. ground corn flakes	1 Tbsp. Herb de Provence
1/2 c. quinoa flour	1 tsp. paprika
1 Tbsp. garlic powder	1 tsp. pepper
1 Tbsp. onion powder	1 tsp. salt

Toss chicken strips in dry ingredients. Place on greased cookie sheet. Bake at 375° for 10-15 minutes or until brown.

DIANE'S SUSHI
(Thanks to Diane McNulty)
For All Basic Diets

Simmer until done:

1 c. quinoa	2 c. boiling water
1 tsp. butter	

Add:

      washabi and tamari to taste

Set aside to cool.
Cut into thin strips any of the following:

fresh, raw salmon or tuna	zucchini
cucumber	avocado
celery	green onion
let your imagination go wild	

Make the nori rolls: Dampen sheets of nori. Lay a small mound of quinoa length-wise down the center. Lay strips of fish or veggies down center. Start to roll the nori sheet using wax paper to control. Wet outside seam of roll when complete. Slice roll into 1" pieces using a VERY sharp, smooth knife.

    FOR DIETS 1 and 2: Serve with tamari, pickled ginger or mustards.

FISH STEW
(Thanks to Ruty Magidish)
For Basic Diet #1

Saute:

1 onion. minced	1/2 bunch fresh basil
2 tbsp. butter	7 cloves garlic, minced

Add and fry for a few minutes:

1/2 c. water	1 hot pepper, cut in half

1 stalk lemon grass (cut into large pieces to remove)
4 ripe tomatoes, chopped

Add and fry for several minutes:

1/2 lb. fish, cut in large chunks (try 2 different kinds)

Add:

4 c. water	1 can coconut milk (or 1 2/3 c.)
2 tbsp. fish sauce.	

Bring to a boil, then simmer for 15 minutes, covered. This dish is very satisfying and tastes even better the next day, if it lasts that long!

GOURMET BROILED FISH
(Thanks to Ruty Magidish)
For All Basic Diets

Mix together:

1/2 hot pepper, minced	2 tbsp. melted butter
2 cloves garlic, minced	1 tbsp. maple syrup

Coat all sides and soak for 5 minutes:

1/2 lb. fish, sliced

Broil for 5 minutes on each side. Serve on a bed of plain quinoa or Springtime Quinoa.

LOX AND EGGS
For All Basic Diets

Saute:

      1 med. onion, sliced   1/2 lb. mushrooms, chopped
      2 Tbsp. butter

Beat:

      4 eggs   1/2 c. yogurt or kefir

Pour into onions and cook. Just before the eggs are done, add cut up pieces of lox.

MARSHA'S COCONUT DIPPED CHICKEN
(Thanks to Marsha Porcell, NY)
For Basic Diet #1

Wash and dry 1/2 lb. skinless chicken breasts, cut into strips. Beat 1 egg.
Mix well together:

      1/2 c. corn flour   1/2 c. unsweetened flaked coconut
      salt, pepper, 1 tsp. garlic powder and curry powder to taste

Dip chicken strips into the egg and then into the dry ingredients to create a thick coating. Sautee chicken over medium heat in a pan with butter until done.

POACHED SALMON WITH DILL
For All Basic Diets

Boil:

      water   1 tsp. peppercorns
      1 bunch fresh chopped dill

Poach thick salmon fillets in water. Serve with yogurt and dill sprigs or make a White Sauce with yogurt and dill.

POTATO SALMON PANCAKES
For All Basic Diets

Steam unpeeled potato cubes till soft. Saute 1 large Spanish onion in butter.
Mix or blend both with added:

      butter   parsley
      yogurt   salt and pepper to taste
      1 can salmon, drained

Fry in patty form until golden.

TIDEWATER CRABCAKES
For All Basic Diets

Beat together in a large mixing bowl:

> 1 large egg
> 2 Tbsp. yogurt cheese
> dash Tobasco
>
> 2 Tbsp. melted butter
> 2 tsp. Worcestershire sauce(omit in Diet#3)
> 1 1/2 tsp. horseradish (without vinegar)

Add:

> 1/4 c. ground corn flakes (for Diet #3, use quinoa flour)
> 1 tsp. dried mustard
> 1/2 tsp. pepper
>
> 1 tsp. Old Bay seasoning
> salt to taste

Add and toss:

> 1 packet fake crab meat (pollack,) in small flakes

Form into patties. Cook in ghee or butter until golden.

YOGURT BAKED SWORDFISH STEAK
For All Basic Diets

Mix together:

> 1 c. yogurt
> sliced fresh ginger
>
> 1/4-1/2 c. chopped scallions (or chives)
> salt and pepper

Spread one half the yogurt mix in the bottom a baking dish. Place thick swordfish steaks in dish. Top with rest of yogurt. Bake at 325° for 20 minutes or until fish is tender.

YOGURT SALMON MOUSSE
For All Basic Diets

Chop in blender:

> 1 bunch fresh dill

Mix until dissolved:

> 1 1/4 pkg. gelatin
>
> 1/2 c. boiling water

Add gelatin and blend till smooth with:

> 1 c. yogurt or kefir cheese
> 1 lb. can salmon with juice
> 3 anchovies
> fresh pepper
>
> 1/2 tsp. lemony salt
> 2 dashes Tobasco
> 1/2 tsp. paprika

Pour into greased mold. Chill till set. Garnish with dill and yogurt.

COLD QUINOA SALAD
For All Basic Diets

Combine in a bowl:

2-3 c. Cooked Quinoa   1/2-1 c. sour cream or thinned yogurt cheese

2 c. chopped raw or cooked veggies (I love tomatoes, cucumbers, chiles
    and onions, but any veggies will work)

Add any of the following herbs to taste:

Chives   Basil

Onion powder   Marjoram

Garlic powder

Store in the fridge, this will keep for 1 1/2 to two weeks.

YOGURT CHEESE SPREAD
For All Basic Diets

Into a cup of yogurt cheese, add any of the following:

cayenne   basil

parsley   thyme

sage   pepper

garlic   onion powder

salsa   curry powder

marjoram   savory

OR:

dates, chopped   apricots, ground

maple syrup   cinnamon

nutmeg   cloves

allspice   ginger

APRICOT BUTTER PRESERVES
(Thanks to Ruty Magidish)
For All Basic Diets

Saute for 3 minutes:

5 ripe apricots, sliced   2 tbsp. butter

Add:

3 tbsp. maple syrup   1/2 c. water

Over med. heat, stirring constantly, cook until water is almost evaporated. Add 6 tbsp. butter and stir until melted. Pour into a jar. Cool. Serve on crackers, toast, breads and cakes.

Variation: Use a handful of dried apricots rehydrated in 1 cup of boiling water. When the water is cool, drain it off and save. Use as all or part of water needed in step two.

APRICOT FOOL
For All Basic Diets

Cook until soft:

     1 lb dried apricots and water

Blend 1/2 apricots and water with:

     1/2 maple syrup   2 Tbsp. brandy extract

Fold into 1 c. yogurt. Add rest of apricots. Serve straight or over brownies or pumpkin pie.

APRICOT PRESERVES
For All Basic Diets

Bring to a boil:

     1 lb. dried apricots, unsulphered, organic

     water to cover

Cook until soft. Drain off excess liquid. Puree. Maple syrup can be added, though it's rarely needed. Refrigerate.

    Variations:

     Use any other dried fruit.

     Add spices like nutmeg or extracts like lemon extract.

FIG PRESERVES
(Thanks to Ruty Magidish)
For Basic Diets #1 and #2

This one is best done with a food processor. You can do it by hand, but the texture won't be as smooth. If you are lucky enough to get fresh figs, skip the rehydrating process. Place in a bowl and cover with boiling water:

     1 pkg. dried figs (1 lb.,) stems trimmed off

When cool, puree or chop fine. In a heavy skillet melt:

     2 tbsp. butter

Add the fig puree and whole figs. Stir for 5 minutes over med. heat. Add and bring to boil for another 5 minutes;

     1/2 tsp. ground cloves   4 tbsp. maple syrup

Add 2 more tbsp. butter and pour into clean jars. Refrigerate.

    Variation: Withhold pureeing a few whole figs, cooking them along with the rest of the puree. Separate before pouring preserves into the jars and use them to top dessert or as a special treat.

MOLE SAUCE
For Basic Diets #1 and #2

Saute:

3 Tbsp. ghee	1 c. chopped green pepper
1 c. sliced onion	2 cloves crushed garlic

Blend:

1/4 c. chopped dried apricots	4 Tbsp. toasted sesame seeds

Mix in bowl with:

2 Tbsp. maple syrup	1/2 tsp. cinnamon
1 Tbsp. quinoa flour	1/2 tsp. cumin
1 1/2 tsp. salt	1/8 tsp. cloves
1 tsp. chili powder	1/8 tsp. pepper

Stir into sauteed veggies along with:

1/3 c. carob powder	3 c. veggie or chicken broth
1 c. tomatoes or paste	

Bring to a boil. Reduce heat and simmer for 15 minutes. Serving: Bake chicken in the oven with sauce poured over it.

SPINACH & POTATO CHUTNEY
For Basic Diets #1 and #2

Steam:

1 lb. spinach, chopped

Peel and cut into 1" cubes:

1 lb. waxy potatoes

Mix the spinach and potatoes in a pan and simmer in a small amount of water for 10-15 minutes. Drain and set aside.

Saute:

1 large onion, chopped	2 tsp cardamom
1 clove garlic, minced	1/2 tsp. coriander
2 oz. ghee or butter	1 tsp. each: paprika, ginger, and pepper

Add spinach/potato mix. Simmer 10 more minutes or until dry. Season to taste.

WHITE SAUCE
For All Basic Diets

Over medium heat, melt 2 tbsp. butter. Add, stir and bring to a bubbling state:

2 tbsp. quinoa flour

Stirring constantly, add in gradual amounts:

1-2 c. liquid (diluted sour cream, yogurt, diluted kefir)

When mixture is thick, add whatever else you desire.

Variations: Add tamari instead of dairy products. Or, add herbs for flavoring.

BASIC BORSCHT
For All Basic Diets

Clean, cook, cool and peel 4-5 med. beets.

Blend: cooked beets
1 c. water
1/4-/1/2 c. kefir or yogurt cheese
herbs to taste: garlic powder, onion powder, pepper.

Serve cold or heat, stirring constantly.

BORSCHT
For Basic Diets #1 and #2

In a large saucepan saute:

1 lg. red onion, chopped   3 tbsp. butter

Separately, steam until tender:

1 lb. beets

Grate cooked beets coarsely, add to onions and add:

1 lbs. tomatoes, chopped   1 sweet red pepper, chopped
2 cloves garlic

Make a paste of the following and add to veggies:

3 tbsp. barley miso   1/4 c. water

Simmer soup for 30 minutes. Season with:

1 tbsp. sweetener   tamari to taste

Let stand, then reheat or serve cold. Top with sour cream or yogurt.

CURRIED ZUCCHINI SOUP
For All Basic Diets

In a cover sauce pan, cook until soft:

2 lbs. chopped zucchini   1 c. minced scallions, onions or chives
3/4 stick of butter

Add:

2 c. chicken or veggie broth   1 Tbsp. curry powder
1 Tbsp. cumin

Cook and stir for 2 minutes. Blend in batches with an additional 1 1/2 c. broth.
Transfer to large bowl and add:

1 1/2 c. yogurt

Chill.

PUMPKIN SOUP
For All Basic Diets

Saute:

2 oz. butter   1 1/2 c. chopped onions or chives
1 1/4 c. diced celery   2/3 c. chopped leeks (omit for diet #3)
2 Tbsp. diced garlic

Add and simmer:

1 1/2 c. pumpkin puree

Add and bring to a boil:

2 gallons veggie broth   1/2 c. maple syrup
2 tsp. nutmeg   2 tsp. ginger

Simmer for 45 minutes.

Add:

2 c. yogurt

Serve.

TORTILLA SOUP
(Thanks to Trudy Baker)
For Basic Diet #1

Fry until crispy:

1/4 c. olive oil or butter   1-2 roasted jalapenos
5 cloves garlic   4 corn tortillas, cut in 1/2" strips

Add and boil for 10 minutes:

1 onions, sliced   4 oz. tomato juice
4 cups chicken broth

Add:

1 Tbsp. cumin   2 tsp. coriander
1 avocados, diced   1 bunches (1 cups.) chopped cilantro
1/2-1 c. grilled or smoked chicken breast strips

Simmer on lowest heat for 1 hour. Garnish with bits of kefir cheese, cilantro and
tortilla strips.

VEGETABLE CHOWDER
For Basic Diet #1

Saute:

1 1/2 c. chopped carrots   1 lg. onion, chopped
1 c. celery, chopped   1/2 c. butter

Add and cook until tender:

5-6 med. potatoes, cubed   3 ears corn, cut off cob
1/3 c. parsley, chopped

Mix together and add to the above:

5 c. diluted sour cream or yogurt	1/4 tsp. nutmeg
8 tbsp. tamari	1/4 tsp. thyme
2 tsp. paprika	pepper to taste

Simmer for 10 minutes. Stir in one bunch chopped spinach. Serve.

SPROUTED BEANS AND LEGUMES

FRIJOLES

Simmer together for 30 minutes:

5 c. sprouted kidney beans	1 clove garlic, chopped
1 1/2 c. water	1/4 tsp cayenne
1 lg onion, chopped	1/4 tsp. Cumin seeds
1/4 c. chili peppers, chopped	

In the blender mix together:

1 c. yogurt, kefir or sour cream   the above cooked and cooled bean mix
**Blended beans may need to be somewhat runny to get them to blend.
Don't worry, the extra liquid will cook out.

Pour them into a frying pan and cook at low heat for 5 minutes or more, scraping the bottom of the pan constantly. Remove from heat and let stand for 30 minutes. Repeat the 'refrying' process until the bean mix is at the desired consistency.

KIDNEY BEAN SALAD
For Basic Diets #1 and #2

Mix together:

1/4 c. mayo substitute (see dressing recipes)   1-2 tbsp. minced onion
1 tbsp minced parsley

Mix in:

2 c. sprouted, cook and cold kidney beans	
1/2 c. chopped celery	2 hard-boiled eggs, chopped

Season with any of the following:

pepper	sweet basil
oregano	cayenne
marjoram	ginger

Chill well.

Variations:

Use pintos, anasazi beans, or pink beans as a substitute.
Mix a variety of any of these beans.
Mix in finely chopped carrots, green peppers and/or cucumbers.

LENTIL KEDGEREE
For Basic Diets #1 and #2

Saute:

    1 onion, sliced   2 tbsp. butter

Add and simmer for 30 minutes:

    3 c. sprouted lentils   6 whole cloves

    4-5 c. water   1/2 tsp. cinnamon

    1/4 c. maple syrup   1/4 tsp. mace

    2 bay leaves   2 cloves garlic, minced

    6 whole small pod cardamom

Add and simmer for 1/2-1 hour or until moisture is absorbed:

    2 c. quinoa   2 tbsp. tamari

SHELLEY'S CHILI
For Basic Diets #1 and #2

Simmer for 3 hours:

    3 c. sprouted pintos beans   2 15 oz. cans tomato sauce

    1 c. celery, chopped   3 c. sprouted kidney beans

    1 c. green peppers, chopped   4 c. whole tomatoes or bits

    2 cloves garlic, chopped   2 c. tomato juice

    1 or more tbsp chili powder   1/2 tsp. cumin seeds

    2 onions, chopped   1/4 tsp cayenne

Enjoy!

SPROUTED BEAN CHILE
(Thanks to Toby Tarnow)
For Basic Diet #1

In a large, heavy saucepan, brown:

    2 lg. onions   3 tbsp. butter or oil

Add and brown well:

    sliced fresh garlic (to taste)

Add and mix well:

    2 lg. cans tomatoes   3 lg. gr. peppers, in strips

    4-5 c. water   1 lg. can tomato paste

    1 pkg. frozen corn niblets   1 qt. sprouted kidney beans

    2 tsp. cumin seeds, crushed   1 qt. sprouted anasazi beans

    3 bay leaves   1 qt. sprouted adzuki

    4 tbsp. chili powder   1/2 tsp cayenne

Bring to a boil. Reduce heat and simmer for 3 hours or until beans are soft and sauce is thickened.

SPROUTED BEAN SOUP
(Thanks to Toby Tarnow)
For Basic Diet #1

In a large pot of water add:

2 lg. onions, chopped	1 parsnip, sliced
3 c. sprouted beans	2 celery sticks, diced
2 lg. carrots, 1/4 " slices	1 lg. jar marinara pasta sauce
2 tbsp powdered kelp	dried dill weed, to taste
1 potato, diced	Sea salt and organic ground
2 c. corn pasta, elbow type	pepper, to taste

Bring to a boil. Stir occasionally as pasta has a tendency to stick to the pot. Cook over low-medium heat until beans are soft.

SPROUTED SOYBURGERS
For Basic Diet #1

Mash, run through a juicer or grind in a veggie grinder:

     5 c. sprouted, cooked soybeans

Add and mix well:

3/4 c. corn flour	2 tsp. oregano
1 onion, minced	1 tsp. basil
2 tbsp. tamari	2 tsp. garlic powder
1/8 tsp. cayenne (or to taste)	

Form stiff batter into thin patties and fry or barbecue. These patties freeze well.

SPROUTED PEA SOUP
For Basic Diets #1 and #2

Bring to a boil and simmer for 2-3 hours:

1 qt. water	1/2 tsp. marjoram
3 c. sprouted peas	1/2 tsp. oregano
1 onion, chopped	1/4 tsp. sweet basil
1 bay leaf	1 stalk celery, chopped
2 tbsp. butter	a pinch of sage

Blend soup until smooth, adding 1 c. water.
Saute:

2 c. mushrooms, sliced	4 tbsp. butter

Add to the soup:

sauteed mushrooms	1/2 tsp. tamari
1 tbsp. honey (or sweetener)	pepper to taste
1/4 tsp. garlic powder	

Heat and serve.

SPROUTED PEA STEW
For Basic Diets #1 and #2

Simmer for 3 hours, adding water as needed:

5-6 c. water	2 c. sprouted peas
4 veggie cubes	1/2-1 hot chili pepper, minced

Blend this mix until smooth. Return to pan. Saute:

3 onions, chopped	3 lg. carrots
1 small rutabaga, chopped	3 small sweet potatoes or yams, chopped
2 stalks celery, chopped	

Stir veggies into pea mix and add:

1/2 c. parsley, chopped	1 1/2 tsp sweetener, to taste
cayenne, to taste	tamari, to taste

Pour over pieces of sprouted wheat toast. Put dollop of yogurt or sour cream on top.

VEGGIES AND VEGGIE DISHES

CYTHN'S FENNEL SAUTE WITH TOASTED CARAWAY SEEDS
(Thanks to Cynthia Scott, NY)
For Basic Diets #1 and #2

Wash a bunch of fresh leeks and julienne the bottom half, lengthwise. Saute leeks in ghee till browning and caramelizing. Cut fennel bulb in half and slice thin. Add to leeks later, so then don't over cook. Brown fennel seeds in ghee with salt. Sprinkle on veggie mixture and serve immediately.

MARSHA'S GNOCCHI
(Thanks to Marsha Porcell)
For Basic Diets #1 and #2

Mix in a bowl:

1 c. potato flour	1 1/2 c. water
2 tbsp. melted butter	

Beat in 2 eggs. Dough will be very sticky. Grease hands well and roll the dough into little balls. Drop into boiling water; they will float. Cook for additional 2-3 minutes after they float. Remove from water with slotted spoon. Serve with: butter and pepper, pesto, Italian tomato sauce.

T-BOO'S TURNIPS
(Thanks to T-Boo, NY)
For Basic Diets #1 and #2

Bring cubed turnips to boil and discard 1st water. Steam cubes till soft. Blend with:
      salt and pepper, garlic powder, ginger, nutmeg, cumin
Add a little maple syrup to sweeten.

Bibliography

Ageless Body, Timeless Mind, by Deepak Chopra (Crown Publishers)

Creating Heaven Through Your Plate, (see recipe section) by Shelley Summers (Warm Snow Publishers, (800)235-6570)

Creating Heaven ON Your Plate, Volume II, (more recipes for diet programs outlined in above book) by Shelley Summers (Warm Snow Publishers, (800)235-6570)

Fit for Life, by Harvey Diamond (Warner Books)

The Human Body, by Iaasc Asimov (New American Library)

Let's Eat Right to Keep Fit, by Adelle Davis (Harcourt Brace Janovitz)

Magical Mind, Magical Body by Deepak Chopra (Nightingale Conant)

Nutrition Almanac, by Nutrition Search, Inc., John D. Kirschmann (McGraw-Hill)

Sugarfree Cooking, by Nicole Walker, 3116 W Nebraska St, Tucson, AZ 85746. (send $4.50)

The 12 Stages of Healing, by Donald M. Epstein (Amber-Allen Publishing)

For a free catalog of books at discount prices on alternative health and wellness, write to: Warm Snow Publishers, P.O. Box 75, Torreon, NM 87061 or call 800-235-6570 and request "The Whole Health Book Catalog."

Index

D

E

eating disorders 126
  anorexia 126
  bulimia 126
Epstein-Barr Virus (EBV) 10, 12, 18, 20, 30, 44, 57, 101, 112, 113, 114
eczema *See* skin problems: eczema
edema 20
eggs 23, 25, 36, 41, 54, 56, 57, 72, 92, 122, 137, 145, 167, 189, 193
enzymes 10, 11, 24, 25, 27, 28, 29, 30, 33, 36, 38, 39, 40, 41, 42, 43, 46, 47, 53, 54, 55, 56, 57,
    58, 66, 68, 72, 77, 86, 140, 153, 157, 161, 163, 167, 168, 169, 170, 176, 177, 181, 182, 185
epilepsy 20
eyesight 128
  eyestrain 128

F

fainting 20
female hormones 135, 137, 139, 140
fingernail ridges 19
fish 17, 22, 26, 33, 36, 37, 40, 46, 51, 52, 56, 61, 65, 69, 70, 91, 94, 96, 97, 114, 118,
    134, 153, 159, 160, 165, 166, 167, 169, 171, 173, 174, 175, 176, 177, 181
flus *See* colds and flus
food reaction 62, 66, 67, 156, 159
formula 95
fruits 22, 24, 34, 36, 38, 46, 47, 48, 51, 52, 61, 62, 87, 93, 98, 99, 100, 123, 160, 161, 165, 166,
    169, 203

G

gallbladder 10, 14, 26, 40, 55, 129, 130, 151, 162
gallstones 10, 20, 130
goiters 20
grains
  natural grain products 215
  regular 36, 56, 168, 173, 177, 181
  sprouted 23, 27, 36, 40, 56, 57, 58, 94, 99, 166, 168, 173, 175, 177, 181, 207 - 210
    spelt pasta 248
    sprouted breads 210, 211

H

hair loss 20, 130, 165
hangnails 19
hay fever 20, 101, 106, 107

To purchase an additional copy of *"Creating Heaven Through Your Plate,"* see your local bookstore or health food store. If unavailable, send $24.00 (includes shipping) to: Warm Snow Publishers, Box 75, Torreon, NM 87061. For credit card orders, call **800-235-6570**.

A companion book of recipes, *"Creating Heaven ON Your Plate, Volume II"* includes scores of additional recipes organized by diet programs outlined in this book. To be published Spring, 1996. To order, write or call Warm Snow Publishers.

For a resource catalog of health foods, grains, flours, and additional products which meet the diet needs mentioned in *"Creating Heaven Through Your Plate,"* call **800-235-6570** and request a free copy of *"The Summers' Approach Products Catalog."*

To receive a complete catalog of books at discount prices on wellness, holistic health and alternative medicine, call **800-235-6570** and request a free copy of *"The Whole Health Book Catalog."*